The Company Doctor

The Company Doctor

Risk, Responsibility, and Corporate Professionalism

Elaine Draper

Russell Sage Foundation • New York

The Russell Sage Foundation

The Russell Sage Foundation, one of the oldest of America's general purpose foundations, was established in 1907 by Mrs. Margaret Olivia Sage for "the improvement of social and living conditions in the United States." The Foundation seeks to fulfill this mandate by fostering the development and dissemination of knowledge about the country's political, social, and economic problems. While the Foundation endeavors to assure the accuracy and objectivity of each book it publishes, the conclusions and interpretations in Russell Sage Foundation publications are those of the authors and not of the Foundation, its Trustees, or its staff. Publication by Russell Sage, therefore, does not imply Foundation endorsement.

Library of Congress Cataloging-in-Publication Data

Draper, Elaine.
    The company doctor : risk, responsibility, and corporate professionalism / Elaine Draper.
        p.   cm.
    Includes bibliographical references and index.
    ISBN 0-87154-249-8
    1. Medicine, Industrial.   2. Occupational physicians.   I. Title.

RC963 .D73 2002
616.9'803—dc21   2002026992

Text design by Suzanne Nichols

RUSSELL SAGE FOUNDATION
112 East 64th Street, New York, New York 10021
10 9 8 7 6 5 4 3 2 1

—— Contents ——

—— Preface ——

MEDICAL PROFESSIONALS increasingly find themselves working in the corporate environment. Medicine has been undergoing dramatic changes as more and more physicians have gone to work for large organizations run by nonphysicians; these now include HMOs as well as corporations like Dow, Chevron, and IBM. They have joined the other professionals—such as engineers and lawyers—who have long worked for organizations run by people not from their own profession.

Professionalism in corporations is changing along with patterns of loyalty and independence at work. Although professional journals, speeches, and ethical codes still proclaim the independent professional judgment of corporate professionals, company doctors themselves in interviews often express deep conflict and anguish over the difficult decisions they must make. They describe falling expectations about what they can accomplish and wonder whether they should have taken another job instead. The tightrope they walk becomes shakier when they must give records to the corporate legal department and managers. I had expected that most would have inured themselves to such problems, reduced their previous status aspirations, and accepted the fact that their choice to do company medicine has advantages, such as regular hours and the chance to do some interesting work with large populations. Instead, I found many who were disgruntled about their working conditions and status, and many who reflected eloquently on their work and values.

The research I draw upon includes fieldwork, documents, historical and statistical materials, legal sources, medical and trade association data, and one hundred confidential interviews with company physicians, scientists, and government and labor officials across the United States. Data from professional journals, private surveys, and other sources give additional insight into corporate professionals. To illuminate the social context and meaning of corporate professional work, I have used quotations from the interviews (respecting the privacy of those who wished to remain anonymous) throughout my sociological analysis. I have included an appendix on research methods, which explains the interviews and other research I conducted.

I wrote *The Company Doctor* with several types of readers in mind. First are scholars—particularly those in the social sciences who are concerned with work and organizations, science and medicine, technology, and social stratification; those in medical ethics and philosophy who are interested in issues of choice, autonomy, and justice; those who study law and society; and those in professional schools of medicine, business, law, and public health who wish to examine the changing environment of professional work in corporations. Second, I hope this book will be read by non-academics who seek to influence public policy, including health professionals, corporate managers, labor officials, politicians, and government officials. Third, I hope to reach general readers interested in environmental health and in various social and ethical issues in the world of work.

Over the course of writing this book, I was fortunate to have the support and assistance of many colleagues, friends, and family members. For their contributions to this work, and for their valuable comments on earlier versions and parts of it, I wish to thank Dick Scott, Troy Duster, Kenneth Karst, Diane Beeson, Bill Domhoff, Ida Simpson, Frances Olsen, Laura Gómez, Rick Abel, Bill Freudenburg, Joyce Rothschild, Paul Adler, Dorothy Nelkin, Howard Aldrich, Gillian Lester, Eugene Volokh, John Bird, Jody Freeman, John Peters, Ruth Roemer, David Matza, Lloyd Tepper, Laura Nader, Ross Koppel, Robert Schaeffer, Anne Lawrence, Fred Bird, Angela Bean, Dean Belk, Richard Lippin, Tony Mazzocchi, Terry Lunsford, Nicholas Ashford, Sheldon Kamieniecki, Eric Frumin, Paul Billings, Sheldon Samuels, April Wayland, and the anonymous readers. Through the generosity of these incisive critics, I received invaluable intellectual guidance and encouragement.

The Stanford postdoctoral program in organizations research and the Institute for the Study of Social Change at Berkeley offered me the time and a vital intellectual community for launching the project. I especially wish to thank Dick Scott and Jim March at Stanford and Troy Duster and Diane Beeson at Berkeley for our spirited discussions and joint projects, which greatly enriched this study. Talks at organizations colloquia at Stanford and research conferences at Asilomar were engaging forums in which to refine ideas. A study of community perceptions of environmental hazards that I conducted with the National Jury Project gave me insight into competing conceptions of risks and responsibility for environmental hazards that proved useful for this book.

The Pacific Center for Health Policy and Ethics in Los Angeles provided a welcoming and collegial environment for sharing research. I am especially grateful to Alex Capron, Michael Shapiro, and Vicki Michel for many stimulating discussions. The Organizations Research Colloquium at the University of Southern California, directed by Paul Adler, offered opportunities to exchange ideas and related research with thoughtful analysts of organizational change. The Occupational and Environmental Medicine Program, with its residency training program in occupational medicine, provided a lively forum for presenting my research before an especially alert group of critics: those who plan to enter the field of occupational medicine. John Peters and his group of residents offered insight into occupational medicine in universities, corporations, and private consulting. Kenneth Karst, Robert Goldstein, Rick Abel, and Gillian Lester at the UCLA School of Law helped make a year there as a visiting scholar a stimulating time to complete the manuscript. Scholars affiliated with numerous programs and research projects gave me many opportunities to try out ideas and to discuss related research. In particular, I would like to thank Sylvia Spangler of the Human Genome Center at Lawrence Berkeley Laboratory; Bill Roy, who organized the UCLA Macro Sociology Colloquium; Kevin Starr of Embassy Residential College, where I presented this research; and Loïc Wacquant, coordinator of UC Berkeley's Sociology Colloquium Series. In addition, students in my graduate seminars on work and occupations and on field research—as well as my law and society students at UC Santa Barbara—offered valuable insights that contributed to this work as it progressed.

The professional staffs of several libraries and research organizations were helpful in tracking down elusive sources, including staff members of the Government Documents Library and the Institute of Industrial Relations at Berkeley, the UCLA and USC libraries, the Library of Congress and the National Institutes of Health, the House Science and Technology Committee, and the former Office of Technology Assessment. Jeffrey Colen contributed exceptionally capable research assistance, and David Fogarty gave me excellent documentary advice. Janice Tanigawa, Tuesday Poliak, and Judy Corbett offered expert coordination of grant support and secretarial assistance at stages of this project where it was most valuable.

Some of the central ideas of this study appeared first in articles and essays I wrote for the *International Journal of Sociology and Social Policy,* the *Berkeley Journal of Employment and Labor Law, Risk,* and *Contemporary Sociology* and in papers I delivered at meetings of the American Sociological Association, the International Sociological Association, the American Association for the Advancement of Science, the Law and Society Association, and the Society for the Study of Social Problems. The Russell Sage Foundation awarded me grant support, which I greatly appreciate. Early conversations with Eric Wanner and Jim March were especially helpful in launching the book project in a promising direction. The National Institutes of Health funded the crucial early stages of this research. A National Institute of Mental Health fellowship contributed to the study by supporting intensive three-year research training in field research methods. Several other research grants and fellowships provided valuable support, including awards by the Haynes Foundation, the Zumberge Faculty Research and Innovation Fund, and the University of California.

In preparing this book for publication, I have had the good fortune of working with excellent editors and reviewers whose careful reading and brilliant criticism of the manuscript challenged me to extend my analysis. I am grateful to Suzanne Nichols, director of publications at the Russell Sage Foundation, for her outstanding editorial judgment and support. Anonymous reviewers and other scholars at the Russell Sage Foundation offered cogent recommendations that helped me in revising the manuscript. I also appreciate the extraordinarily helpful editorial advice of Gene Tanke, Emily Chang, and Cindy Buck. Finally, my deepest appreciation goes to the men and women I interviewed, who generously shared their time and experience with me. I am indebted to these physicians, corporate managers, government officials, labor officials, and scientists, who spent many hours discussing their experiences and social issues with me. For their candid and informative responses, I am most grateful. I hope that this study contributes to a greater understanding of the dilemmas of corporate professional work, and thus to their more effective resolution.

Introduction

For a doctor to be successful in a corporation, you have to grow new wings, and the old ones atrophy.

—Major oil company physician

PROFESSIONALS INCREASINGLY WORK in corporations, where they are subject to the decisions of company managers and to economic and legal imperatives stemming from their status as corporate employees. Ironically, as their numbers have grown, their autonomy has diminished. This trend is particularly stark in the case of company physicians, who share neither the independence nor the high status of the solo practitioner (see Sullivan 1995; Freidson 1986, 1994; Hafferty and McKinlay 1993; Sassower 1993).[1] Many processes that transform corporate professional work generally—such as corporate restructuring, the ascendance of legal departments, changing labor-management relations, and management by nonprofessionals—profoundly affect company physicians.

Employers say they have lost a sizable part of their profitability to health-care costs in the last ten years. Companies become concerned about employees whose medical expenses are steep and have chosen to screen employees as a solution. Thus, companies have increasingly hired company doctors—physicians who receive a salary from the corporation to provide medical services to its employees. It is a company doctor's job to conduct medical tests, diagnose illness, and develop wellness programs.

1

Some also treat workers, try to control workers' compensation costs, and help set corporate policy regarding toxic chemicals, health, and employment. Company doctors, who are found disproportionately in large manufacturing and service corporations, help employers contend with health risks and costs—as is clear, for example, from their role in the Manville Corporation and other firms that have used large amounts of asbestos.[2] Their work is intrinsically conflicted, particularly for those in profit-oriented corporations that are not in the business of providing medical services. Nonphysician managers, who are increasingly attuned to the financial and legal dimensions of physicians' decisions, often limit physicians' discretion in testing and treating employees and in conveying information to them (see Hafferty and McKinlay 1993; Starr 1982). They also review the medical information that physicians collect on individuals in deciding who can be fired and who will continue to work for the company. The formal corporate structure, legal pressures, and career concerns lead company doctors to serve managerial goals by burnishing employers' public image, managing disability cases, reducing the threat of lawsuits, and setting corporate policy regarding employment and chemical hazards.

Company doctors, like many other corporate professionals, attempt to gain the trust of their corporate employers and, usually, the employees in their company. They describe obtaining the trust of others as crucial to their ability to do their work. As we shall see, however, being compelled to work in an environment of lost credibility and mistrust is a common predicament of company doctors. The skepticism or mistrust that employees often have toward company doctors is part of a broader social trend of eroding trust in physicians and, more generally, in the professional experts who are responsible for protecting health and the environment along with the public welfare. (On the erosion of trust, see, for example, Cook 2001; Garrett 2000.) A closer look at the shifting patterns of trust and credibility in the case of company doctors sheds light on these broader trends regarding trust in medical experts and other professionals.

In the mid-1950s William H. Whyte, in *The Organization Man,* analyzed the changes in values and work that accompanied expanding bureaucratization, and in *White Collar,* C. Wright Mills examined the new orientations to work among middle-level corporate employees (Whyte 1957; Mills 1956; see also Bendix 1956). "The organization man" was an apt description of that era's corporate professional employees, but times have changed. People increasingly are not organizational soldiers who avidly perform as they are told in return for corporate beneficence. Although professionals are still expected to do what their organization demands, they also read professional journals, belong to professional organizations, and have certain professional standards and concerns. The legal, political, and economic environments shape their work. Moreover, they no longer expect lifetime employment in exchange for loyal service to a corporation. For the early twenty-first century, "the company doctor" is a more appropriate metaphor for understanding professional and managerial work in large corporations, for the role embodies the conflicting demands that professionals experience in the globalizing corporate economy.

THE EMERGENCE OF CORPORATE PROFESSIONAL NORMS OF INDIVIDUALISM AND CONFORMITY

A growing percentage of the corporate workforce is made up of employees whose education and specialized knowledge lead them to consider themselves professionals. Their swelling ranks now include not only doctors, lawyers, and engineers but also newer professionals such as systems analysts and health technologists. Corporate professionals gain influence from their technical knowledge and strategic importance in the corporation. They increasingly have control functions and the formal obligation to speak up for employees, but they are not always permitted to do so. Corporate pressures influence the ethical framework and conduct of the people who work in corporate organizations.[3]

Professionals have never made entirely autonomous choices. But as large organizations invade more and more parts of our lives, these organizations and their social structures shape the social and ethical perspectives of professionals and constrict their options. Professionals have often been under pressure to serve as corporate functionaries when their own values or those of their profession clash with company demands.

In medicine the number of solo practitioners has declined steadily in the past several decades, so that employment has become the typical case for physicians. Working for a nonmedical corporation is no longer the stigmatized exception it once was. Conditions obviously have shifted in private practice and managed care, with greater oversight by corporate managers and regulators (see Robinson 1999; Scott et al. 2000). Professionals, of course, operate under monetary and regulatory constraints wherever they practice, but the constraints of working in a corporation are different from those of working alone or in a group practice. Corporate medicine differs in its control structures, its doctor-patient relationships, and its interpretation of confidentiality. However, with rapid change in the medical field and physicians increasingly working for HMOs and managed care systems, physicians in general have become more like company doctors. Those who work for managed care companies face ambiguities in their role similar to those that confront the standard company doctor. More specifically, they face the problems of maintaining privacy and dealing with conflicting allegiances between the patient and the employer.

Those are two of the problems that this book explores in providing a way to think about the changes in contemporary health care. Managed care organizations have brought to health care ascendant cost-cutting managers and limits on services along the lines that have characterized company medicine for years. Following the pattern well established in company medical programs, patients in the broader health-care system increasingly worry about whether their welfare is undermined by the impact of economic incentives and conflicts of interest on doctors.[4] Company doctors are worth close examination in part for what they reveal as harbingers of developments in our health-care system of managed care.

Physicians are the prototypical professional case owing to their traditional independence, extensive training, power, and high status. Yet the small-town physician in private practice, governed only by his or her professional code and unencumbered by organizational pressures, is an idealized model of the past. Professionals typically have not been so independent. Social workers, nurses, and professors have always worked as salaried employees, often for large organizations; engineers have traditionally been employed in corporations, where they have encountered dilemmas in the aerospace and nuclear industries. The fact of salaried employment does not itself say much about prestige and power. Professionals ascend or decline over time and in relation to other groups under specific conditions of employment, professional socialization, and organizational pressures.[5] Even many of those who have been self-employed have been autonomous only in a trivial sense, since they have depended on powerful, wealthy clients in limited markets (see Starr 1982). Self-employment does not necessarily signify real autonomy, success, or power. As we shall see, physicians working as independent contractors can experience many of the same pressures as salaried in-house professionals; indeed, they often become even more compliant with corporate managers' demands.

Research on the rise of professionals has emphasized their autonomy, specialized education, and privileged status. But early organizational analysis and research on professions showed little concern with corporate employment.[6] Since the 1950s, however, more research has been done on corporate professionals. Some of it is case study literature on particular professional groups, such as engineers, lawyers, and scientists.[7] Several major theories about professionals have addressed issues of professional norms and autonomy, casting these issues in terms of the extent to which professionals have the power and ability to direct their own work.[8] These theories have produced bold assertions about professionals' gain or loss of autonomy and control over their work, but usually without considering the ways in which corporate structures, internalized professional socialization, informal cultural dimensions of work, and the law have transformed professional work. In examining these processes, this book offers a critical analysis not just of the doctors themselves and of the corporations that employ them, but also of the broad social context that has created some of the need for company doctors' services and resulted in the corporatization of professional life.

THE PLAN OF THE BOOK

In chapter 1, I examine the prevailing images of corporate employment, the important effects that corporate downsizing has had on company doctors, and the reasons doctors give for going into occupational medicine. I show how a military background gives physicians a different orientation to their work than does a public health background.

Chapter 2 explores the loyalty and independence of corporate professionals such as company doctors by considering the demise of lifetime employment in companies, the rise of professional workers, and shifting patterns of individualism and conformity in relation to traditional values. I analyze the tension between ideal types of doctors in corporations—the white coat versus the team player—and the professional perils of team play. I show how company doctors respond to conflicting pressures on them by blaming themselves for failing to persuade managers of their value. They only occasionally report problems to internal ombudspersons, professional organizations, or outside agencies and have conflicted responses to employees' efforts to defend their interests. Chapter 3 then examines how company doctors' conception of themselves as team players affects the ways in which they define deviance and conformity within the corporation. They help managers remove workers considered troublesome or costly while, in dramatic contrast, zealously protecting managers at risk.

The next three chapters analyze specific aspects of the work of company doctors as a way of exploring the broad themes that are of major concern throughout the book—trust; loyalty to corporate employers, employee-patients, and the public; privacy; responsibility for health risks; and the direction of medicine. Chapter 4 examines critical issues concerning toxics. I consider the ways in which doctors use information about hazards to respond to publicity over working conditions and to persuade managers to act. I analyze the selective concern with toxics that physicians and employers show in their daily work and in their professional organizations. Chapter 5 examines the important role that company doctors play in drug screening. They have conducted tests while acknowledging that testing is ineffective or harmful—in part because other companies do it. Chapter 6 then discusses the pitfalls of screening for susceptibility as opposed to monitoring for environmental hazards and gives particular attention to questions about the limitations of using screening to identify "problem" employees. I consider three major examples of ways in which company physicians identify workers they perceive to be high-risk: their responses to genetic information, reproductive hazards, and stress claims. I analyze the social framework for screening that often results in the ineffective or inequitable treatment of employees.

The next two chapters turn to the changing social definition of the doctor-patient relationship in the corporate context, especially to the key issues of doctors' responsibility to inform patients, protect them from harm, and safeguard the privacy of their health information. Chapter 7 considers how company physicians use medical information in the workplace and examines the issues of privacy that arise in employees' medical treatment. I give particular attention to the large data banks and search companies that raise important questions about the control of information. Chapter 8 considers the powerful and growing impact of the legal environment on corporate professional work; legal pressures help to explain company doctors' and lawyers' ambivalence about providing information and taking preventive health measures. Changing liability trends and regulatory pressures concerning medical malpractice, chemical labeling, willful negligence, and discrimination leave corporate professionals feeling vulnerable and eager to shield themselves against legal sanctions. I analyze the relationship of law and medicine in corporations along with some surprising findings about the response of lawyers to workplace hazards. Lawyers have sometimes pressed for fuller disclosure of hazards and for preventive health practices while also working to control damaging information and undermine the credibility of critics who point to health risks.

Finally, chapter 9 recasts corporate professionalism in light of the fact that intensified professionalism coexists with intensified corporate control. I also suggest some directions for policy and some implications of this research for a sociological understanding of corporate professional work. Workplace medicine could be managed more rationally and fairly, with greater attention to health goals, confidentiality, and equity issues.

Chapter 1

Corporate Professionals
in Transition

*This is a very difficult profession, and people who enter it be-
cause it looks easy—regular hours, a lot of do-gooder preventive things that some company is willing to pay for that you
can't do out in private practice—probably aren't good students of this profession.*

—Physician in a major oil company

I N THE FILM *Outland,* the company doctor for a remote mining
operation heroically aligns herself with the forces of justice
(and the federal district marshal, played by Sean Connery), risking
her life and livelihood to combat a lethal drug scourge that the
company's general manager has knowingly helped create. Referring to herself, this self-described alcoholic "wreck" of a company
doctor (played by Frances Sternhagen) says: "You know, you
haven't your medical all-star here. Company doctors are like
ships' doctors. Most are one shuttle flight ahead of a malpractice
suit."[1] In the classic movie *Brief Encounter,* a general practitioner
going off to work in a hospital in Africa explains his special interest in preventive medicine and his passion for his work:

All good doctors must primarily be enthusiasts. They must, like writers and
painters and priests, have a sense of vocation—a deep-rooted, unsenti-
mental desire to do good. Obviously, one way of preventing disease is
worth fifty ways of curing it. That's where my ideal comes in. Preventive

8

medicine isn't anything to do with medicine at all really. It is concerned with conditions: living conditions and hygiene and common sense.[2]

The employees in the film *Salt of the Earth* live in company housing on company property, buy from the company store, and must pay twenty dollars to see the company doctor. A woman in labor needs to see a doctor, but because she is married to a striking mineworker, the sheriff refuses to search for him, saying, "The company doctor won't come to no picket line."[3] Ibsen's play *Enemy of the People* (1997 [1882]) portrays an environmental physician working for a municipality that is trying to promote tourism by advertising its medicinal baths. When he proclaims his opposition to their use after discovering that the baths are contaminated, he incurs the wrath of the bath owners, the mayor and other town leaders, and even his daughter. He fails to understand the insecurities of the citizens who might lose their livelihoods if the baths were to close.[4] In the famous British novel *The Citadel* by A. J. Cronin (1937), a physician who attends to miners suspects mine conditions as the cause of their diseases and publishes his findings on coal dust inhalation and silicosis. He is shocked to learn that workers receive no compensation if they fall ill. After his lab experiments are destroyed and his investigations sabotaged, the doctor leaves for a lucrative society practice. But later he defends a maverick practitioner successfully treating tuberculosis against the charges of threatened physicians. He rails against the inadequate training of doctors, their insufficient participation in research, and their intolerance of pioneers outside the medical mainstream.

These literary and cinematic works suggest some of the significant history of occupational and environmental medicine, as well as some of the dilemmas that company doctors can encounter. They also describe the conditions that pervade corporate employment for professionals. And in real life as well as in literature and film, physicians do not always side with their employers when conflict over employee health arises, despite the risk to their careers.

The terrain of corporate professional work is shifting as major social changes affect professionals' power relative to that of workers, managers, and other social groups. The profession of occupational medicine is changing, just as health care is being corporatized and managed care organizations are on the rise. The important processes affecting company physicians are similar to those affecting other corporate professionals (such as lawyers and engineers) and physicians in other corporate structures, such as hospitals. In many ways the story of company doctors fore-shadows the story of medicine and of corporate professional work.

A BRIEF HISTORY OF OCCUPATIONAL PHYSICIANS

The field of occupational medicine evolved as the new railroads pushed west from St. Louis in the 1860s and 1870s. In the 1880s the isolated mining, railroad, and lumbering companies hired doc-tors to treat the huge number of injuries and accident victims and, less often, to provide routine health care. Major corporations in the coal, steel, and automobile industries hired physicians to pro-vide emergency care and then opened their own hospitals and clinics to cut costs.[5] By the early twentieth century company phy-sicians were firmly established in the United States.

The railroad doctors were general practitioners and the pi-oneers of modern occupational medicine. They treated trauma and became known as "industrial physicians." Because the care of injuries was implicit in the term "industrial medicine," its practice was primarily the purview of surgeons. The negative reputation of occupational physicians before the 1950s was largely deserved, because the field was neither highly professionalized nor full of highly competent people. These physicians were in disrepute be-cause of the quality of care they provided to employees at a time when work injuries were common. Some of them had never gone to a formal medical school and had read only some medical litera-ture, so they could not get licenses in states like New York and Massachusetts when medicine upgraded itself. Most lacked spe-cialized training in occupational medicine, which was then rudi-mentary. Well-trained physicians in family or internal medicine had little interest in moving west to serve railroad workers. Many of those who did go west may have been trained in medicine but were maladjusted people—alcoholic, mentally ill, drug-addicted, social outcasts, or felons—who could not make it in other fields and had been rejected by their medical community.

Beginning in the 1910s, as states adopted workers' compensation laws, employers were required to report and pay for occupational injuries and illness.[6] These laws thus motivated employers to hire doctors. Large corporations hired physicians directly to see their employees, rather than pay for doctors through a state fund, so that they could contain medical costs and compensation awards. Manufacturing companies in chemicals, auto, and steel had medical departments because they had workers' compensation injury cases. In addition, workers in industries such as aluminum and steel negotiated early on to have companies put in on-site clinics. The doctors received wages and often coped with limited supplies, few colleagues, and nonexistent hospital support.

The mineworkers played a pathbreaking role in health care reform by creating the United Mine Workers of America (UMWA) Welfare and Retirement Fund in 1946. They set up clinics in isolated areas, such as southern Appalachia, and reviewed and certified doctors. The innovative way in which the UMWA delivered health care to miners and their families made joining the union especially attractive because members could get good-quality health care at a reasonable cost. With the development of health-care delivery infrastructure even in rural areas, the use of company doctors to provide health care in remote locations declined.[7]

The American Medical Association (AMA) was generally hostile toward companies providing treatment for their own employees (or selling services to the public) and lacked a serious program of overseeing occupational medicine as a specialty.[8] The medical profession and the AMA segregated plant doctors, and the best doctors typically did not enter that field. Company physicians were looked down on as professional outcasts, as practitioners who were not socially, economically, or academically in the same league as other doctors. An electronics company physician said:

I detest the term "industrial doc," but it fit the original concept of simply doing pre-employment physical examinations. The major reason companies had the "industrial doc" around was simply to have a cheap way to get their pre-employment physicals done on-site the way they wanted them, which was the way it was for a long time. Corporate America basically didn't want to be involved in the medical care of employees if they could help it.[9]

Henry J. Kaiser greatly influenced company medicine during World War II when his Kaiser Steel Corporation and its foundation formed a group practice called Kaiser Permanente. Using hospitals on company property near the shipyards, Kaiser operated a full-service medical program to treat employees and their dependents during wartime, before allowing people from outside the company to join.[10] Its group medicine concept—the forerunner of the health maintenance organization (HMO)—lowered insurance rates and enabled doctors to use expensive equipment. Kaiser retained local physicians, and the company medical director supervised plants from the home office.

Kaiser was certainly not typical; its resources were much greater than those of small companies, and health care was part of its organizational philosophy. More extensive in-house clinics such as in the Kaiser health plan gained a reputation for being "socialized medicine," partly because their comprehensive health-care services used panel doctors (which limited patient choice of physicians) and corporate and government administrators were major decisionmakers. A physician who worked for Kaiser Industries from the 1950s until the late 1970s said:

> We at Kaiser Industries and Kaiser Steel were always looked upon as a bunch of mavericks and socialists in the area of health care and labor relations. But the people who had some idea what direction medical care was taking, even back then, were studying this as the first prepaid health plan in the world, as it grew and prospered.[11]

Many companies hired doctors and developed a scaled-down version of the Kaiser model for company medicine, in the belief that having a full-time staff of doctors benefited the company. Companies like New York Bell ran clinics to deliver primary care to employees and their family members—an early use of managed health care as a cost-containment mechanism. To reduce health-care costs, many others, such as Tenneco and Uniroyal, established wellness programs that usually were not run by physicians trained in occupational medicine. Some companies, like the electricity producer Southern California Edison, developed an enormous health-care structure; others tried hiring an in-house staff and failed.[12]

Most company clinics were oriented to trauma and first aid and therefore held little interest for doctors trained in toxicology and epidemiology. But as occupational medicine evolved and information about health hazards from work accumulated, large corporations increasingly began to think of exposure issues as company problems. In the 1940s and 1950s major companies such as AT&T, DuPont, Dow Chemical, and Kodak developed substantial medical departments to study the health and safety effects of chemicals. Their practice of occupational medicine helped change the earlier image of the isolated company doctor.[13] The Occupational Safety and Health Act and Toxic Substances Control Act laws in the 1970s then increased the need for company doctors to test workers and made workers and their representatives better able to understand chemical hazards.[14] Still, companies generally did not manage their clinics aggressively to reduce exposure hazards, and employees routinely viewed the company doctor as an advocate for the employer instead of the worker.

THE JOB OF COMPANY PHYSICIAN

Today companies with a medical department typically have clinics that perform surveillance exams, including tests for hearing, lung function, and drug use. Companies hire doctors to evaluate suitability for certain jobs in view of medical conditions that could put a worker at risk for further injury or illness. Some physicians supervise fitness centers, health education, and wellness programs, while others travel worldwide to find doctors for employees and arrange for evacuations of workers in other countries.

Companies vary in the extent to which their in-house doctors become involved with the company's environmental staff. Some doctors are segregated into clinical aspects of occupational health, whereas others substantially influence industrial hygiene and safety or even conduct studies in toxicology or epidemiology. Company doctors also have been active in regulatory matters and lawsuits. They testify as to the company's liability for occupational disease awards and at OSHA rule-making hearings, and they make disability determinations for company compliance with the Americans with Disabilities Act (ADA).

Most companies deal with only a specific range of familiar health issues, such as the exposures to solvents and cumulative trauma disorders faced by employees of computer manufacturers. Company doctors may be allowed to provide only brief primary care or first-aid treatment during working hours because the company health insurance plan is supposed to cover most treatment: they must usually refer chronic or severe problems to outside specialists. Doctors who want follow-through control over patient care are thus likely to be frustrated in company jobs. Some complain of feeling like a second-class citizen because they must call somebody in the company's network of outside doctors to take care of individuals who need to be hospitalized. An automobile company physician said:

> Here you are almost like an urgent-care clinic or emergency room, where you take care of them for that episode and they're gone. You're certainly not the person who hospitalizes them. I miss closure, where you get to follow them all the way through and see what's going on. Coming from an internal medicine background, it was nice to take care of your regular patient's congestive heart failure and see him come around.

The job of a company physician providing clinical services is different from that of a medical director at company headquarters, who is responsible for managing programs nationally or regionally. They are in a sense two different breeds. Medical directors generally focus on the administrative aspect of occupational medicine: regulations, disability benefits, and union contracts. They advise management on issues such as workers' compensation and drug testing. Many of them seldom see patients, except occasionally to resolve a case.[15] In contrast, clinic doctors do primary-care medicine for people with cuts and fractures, minor illnesses, and occasionally more serious injuries. Some of them spend virtually all their time doing routine back-to-work physicals, examinations for new hires and for people exposed to various chemicals, and certification to perform certain tasks or to wear respirators. Lower-level plant physicians may have some latitude in determining what tests to order, but they may know little about occupational medicine beyond conceiving of it as primary-care practice in the workplace. Company doctors describe some medical positions as tedious, such as those involving repetitive cases of tendonitis and lower back pain. This publishing company physician, for instance, said: "Doctors practice medicine, and they are happier treating disease. I was disappointed because the job was dull—just physical exams. There was no challenge, really no medicine involved." Other doctors acknowledge the cursory or substandard medical procedures they have performed in corporations. A physician for a food services company said: "The city required that all food handlers have an annual physical, so I learned to do physicals at the rate of about fifty an hour. I also took care of workers' compensation accidents—cuts and burns mostly, broken bones."

Large Companies and Dangerous Jobs

Full-time in-house physicians are a large-company phenomenon. One oil company I researched had close to one hundred full-time doctors, a few part-time, and over two hundred doctors who contracted with the company to provide services. At its peak in 1983 another oil company had a $12 million budget with nearly two hundred people in its medical division: about fifteen doctors, plus nurses, epidemiologists, industrial hygienists, a biostatistician, chemical engineers working in a lab, a health and safety trainee, and a lawyer in the medical department who handled regulations and precautionary labeling of products.[16] The small number of doctors listed by some major corporations often gives an understated impression of their medical programs. For example, one company I researched had fifty doctors but also hundreds of contract physicians, over two hundred nurses, and a strong environmental department in addition to its medical department.

Even large corporations do not have full-time physicians in all their facilities. Physicians from headquarters travel to other facilities, sometimes worldwide. But these large corporations have the money, staff, and research capabilities to do things that small companies cannot do. They generally are more aware of their criminal, tort, and workers' compensation liability and more concerned with developing programs that could reduce costs and prevent adverse publicity. Large companies with in-house doctors and sizable medical programs generally invest more in occupational health than smaller companies, which often lack the resources to keep up with regulations and information about hazards.

Most U.S. workplaces do not have full-time physicians. Companies with two hundred to one thousand employees more often contract out medical services to clinics and hospital group practices. Small companies usually do not have even part-time in-house doctors—and an untold number of those who do fill such positions for small companies lack the training and competence to respond to dangerous exposures. Many companies—especially small ones—make the minimal effort to comply with regulations and do not even offer medical insurance.[17]

Corporations that face significant health hazards in their line of work hire physicians on staff or under contract to conduct tests and evaluate workers exposed to certain toxic substances. Oil and chemical companies and highly regulated industries like the steel industry, which historically have been criticized for the risks of their operations, are more heavily involved in occupational medicine than other types of companies. They are also more likely to have industrial hygienists and epidemiologists studying disease and toxicologists in the lab testing chemicals, and they are more likely to see efforts at controlling health hazards as a matter of corporate self-interest.[18]

Medical programs differ partly according to the type of company in which the physician works.[19] The job of occupational physician in a chemical or other manufacturing company may entail responding to hazardous exposures like solvents and heavy metals, whereas doctors in white-collar settings more often function as internists, evaluating clerical and managerial workers. Doctors in service industries such as phone companies and railroads have concerns about electromagnetic radiation and repetitive motion disorders, but many of their programs focus on fitness centers, smoking cessation programs, and related wellness issues. There are fewer corporate medical directors in the West than in the East, where more major companies have their corporate headquarters and where in-house medical departments first appeared in the older heavy industries.

Occupational physicians are distributed according to where the money is even more than according to where the hazard is.[20] The need to have occupational physicians monitor and control hazards is not closely correlated with where they are.[21] Large manufacturing companies are disproportionately willing to employ doctors, even though smaller companies have major health hazards. For instance, many shops that spray-paint cars have great hazards and high levels of toxicity, but only companies like Du-Pont and Dow that manufacture the paints are likely to employ a cadre of doctors, industrial hygienists, and toxicologists. Few health professionals watch over the paint shop, and inspectors monitor them less often. Yet people get sick in these smaller firms.

Training and Career Path

Company physicians were classified as general practitioners, not in a separate specialty, until the American Board of Preventive Medicine established an occupational medicine section and began certifying residents in the field in 1955.[22] In the late 1950s the field generally became known as "occupational medicine," and use of the term "industrial physician" declined. Occupational medicine is now established within departments of preventive, family, and community medicine in universities, primarily to train resident medical students and conduct research. These residency training programs have grown since the Atomic Energy Commission, the U.S. Air Force, and certain corporations began sponsoring fellowships in occupational medicine in the mid-1950s. But until the 1970s funding for resident training was minimal, and medical schools typically offered only an hour in occupational medicine in a four-year course of training. Even now students learn about toxicology and epidemiology but often are essentially unaware of occupational medicine because of their negligible exposure to it— typically only a few hours of training or less.[23]

Training programs expanded after 1970, in part because federal funding expanded and demand increased for trained physicians with the passage of the OSHA Act and the Toxic Substances Control Act, which created a market for trained specialists. More and more graduates of training programs at schools such as Mount Sinai and New York University were finding company jobs. Today demand has outstripped the availability of trained people in preventive medical specialties like occupational medicine, leading to a shortage of occupational and environmental physicians.[24] Beginning in the 1970s universities set up training programs funded by the National Institute for Occupational Safety and Health (NIOSH) to increase the supply of occupational physicians and nurses. However, government or foundation money remains insufficient to train an adequate number of people in the field.[25]

The American College of Occupational and Environmental Medicine (ACOEM) is the main professional organization for occupational medicine physicians, with about seven thousand members in the specialty, mostly employed in-house in corporations or in private clinics under contract to companies to provide medical services; few work in universities or government.[26] Corporate medical directors also belong to medical groups within trade associations such as the American Petroleum Institute. Full-time corporate doctors, a powerful minority of occupational physicians, still dominate ACOEM. Occupational medicine is primarily practiced by private physicians working in clinics, simply as part of their practice; these practitioners generally do not belong to ACOEM. Those who do typically also belong to their own medical specialty organizations, such as internal medicine and family practice, and associate themselves with occupational medicine to earn money.[27] The proportion of physicians in private practice–based occupational medicine in free-standing or hospital-based clinics, universities, or consulting firms is rising relative to the number of physicians employed by corporations.[28] In their interviews, two physicians, one from a retail sales company and the other from a financial services corporation, noted the change in company doctors' professional organizations brought about by the influx of contract physicians:

> The professional organization used to reflect this high-minded fraternity of people who were both employees and providing medicine inside a company, not for fees. Suddenly the professional society is split now, with profit-making consultants who are trying to drum up business. There has been a tremendous sea change in the commitment of the profession and the professional organization ACOEM, because most of our members now are outside consultants. That has deep implications. I feel disaffected from the society because the deep ethical center has changed from commitment to employees to profit-making.

> A professional society is responsible for maintaining standards, and medical directors are the role models who set the pace for the organization, as the well-established fraternity among occupational physicians. Now we're losing some of that collegiality with the reduction of corporate

medical directors and corporate programs. I am concerned about occupational health services provided by entrepreneurs who hire doctors, because they're less concerned about the quality and integrity of those doctors than with putting bodies in a contract.

Most occupational physicians were never trained and board-certified in the specialty. Only about 20 percent received formal residency training in occupational medicine, during which physicians learn industrial hygiene, epidemiology, toxicology, and administrative skills. The rest have taken a few courses or learned whatever they know on their own. This background is unlike most other specialties—such as surgery or internal medicine—in which members have had formal training in their field. As of February 2001, according to a spokesperson for the American Board of Preventive Medicine, the board had certified 3,026 physicians since it began certifying residents in 1955. A spokesperson for the American Board of Medical Specialties noted that about 2,500 of those board-certified physicians currently practice medicine.[29] Many work in universities or in government, so not many well-trained specialists with an extensive background in occupational health are available for companies to hire.

Corporate physicians dominate the residency review committee for occupational medicine residencies under the Accreditation Council for Graduate Medical Education (ACGME), partly because of the way residency review committee members are chosen.[30] Their dominance of the occupational medicine specialty differs from most other medical specialties, in which academic physicians typically provide the training, control the certification process, and run the professional organization. A physician from a major hospital and another from a university occupational medicine training program commented on the dominance of corporate physicians in occupational medicine:

Those corporate guys are managers who are on the road half the time; they don't have the peace of mind to write anything more than a letter or memo. They're not intellectually interested, and they have no incentive to publish—it's simply not their game. It's a shame! But they still control the American Board of Preventive Medicine, which certifies occupational medicine training programs. That's unique to occupational medicine. You can't find another branch of medicine where the academics don't control the body that determines training requirements.

Those of us in academic occupational medicine, primarily occupational medicine residency directors, have been trying to change things so that we have more of a voice in the profession and training. Our corporate medical brothers and sisters should have a strong voice, but not the only voice.

Many physicians already practicing would like to see the field grow, but they do not want to compete with more colleagues, who would exert downward pressure on their own income—an old story in medicine. Numerous medical board specialties limit the numbers in their field—for instance, through high failure rates on entrance exams—in part to avoid competition and the resulting reduction of their income (see Starr 1982; Freidson 1973).

Most board-certified occupational physicians who were trained in occupational medicine beginning in the 1960s graduated and went to work for corporations or government. The proportion of doctors who went into private practice specializing in occupational medicine grew in the 1970s and 1980s, so that by the early 2000s most graduates of university-based occupational medicine residency training programs—such as in the Harvard School of Public Health—were going into private practice and fewer were working for corporations, the government, or universities.[31] Many have established their own occupational health services and started contracting with employers in hospital-based or group practice–based companies. Graduates who want to practice clinical medicine have limited options.[32]

Occupational medical training programs generally follow the philosophy of the faculty members who organized them. Some residency training programs in occupational medicine are reputed to be pro-management, and others pro-worker or public health. The training, field placements, and anticipatory socialization for corporate employment depends in part on the program the person attends.[33] A university occupational physician who directs a training program said: "All graduates from our program for the past two years went into industry. Maybe it's because of the way we train them: they see a lot of companies when they're training, so they usually end up there."

Certification and residency training requirements for occupational medicine are changing. The requirement that four months of the two-year residency program be devoted to practical training on-site at a workplace traditionally had trainees placed in the classic corporate medical settings of the smokestack industries, even though U.S. workers also encounter hazards in services and government jobs. Since the directors of occupational medicine residencies have begun to lobby for change, placements for hands-on practical experience now may occur in settings outside heavy industry.

A barrier to attracting young, well-trained physicians to the field is that many see it as administrative work. As an oil company physician explained:

> We're trained in the field to develop programs to protect people from getting sick from hazards in the first place, not to care for people in hospitals. Most young people find that totally unappealing. The psyche of medical students is that they want to treat people; they're very clinically oriented. They want to go out and inject people, give them pills and examine them, cut them open and do all kinds of tests on them. This field of medicine is appalling to somebody like that; it's dull because they don't want to deal with paper.

Occupational medical training programs are not necessarily directly pertinent to what company doctors actually do. Companies usually do not hire physicians trained in occupational medicine at the entry level because their training, which is basically nonclinical and administrative, does not fit the entry-level job of seeing patients. Because of the way employers generally define the job, those hiring new doctors do not necessarily value board certification, and many of the physicians they do hire have boards in internal medicine instead of occupational medicine. A utility company physician said:

> Doctors who've come in with occupational medicine training aren't as good at taking care of patients. We do internal medicine 70 percent of the time, so I'd rather hire somebody as an internist first and then teach them what they need to know about occupational medicine than have them trained as an occupational medicine physician and have to learn internal medicine.

A doctor who can only make medical decisions, however, may also be more vulnerable in a corporation than a doctor trained in industrial hygiene and safety; the latter knows about the environmental impact of the company's toxic materials and how the company operates. Moreover, that person may be laid off less readily.[34]

Some large employers now demand advanced qualifications, as this chemical company physician explained:

> We've not seen board certification to be that important in the past, because our occupational medical program is a traditional program, but it will become much more important that people are certified, trained, and at least board-eligible as we go forward. We try to encourage all our physicians to get board certification.[35]

Because of the more demanding requirements that large corporate employers have established, physicians who want to work for them are thus increasingly motivated to become board-certified.

WHY DOCTORS GO INTO OCCUPATIONAL MEDICINE

Occupational physicians come from a variety of backgrounds: typically they are internists, family practitioners, and emergency room physicians from private practice and the military. In the past many chose to work for a corporation after burning out, having a midlife crisis, or failing to get work somewhere else, as with prison doctors; they came in with no special training or affinity for the field. The growth of occupational and environmental medicine, however, has brought doctors into corporate employment for more diverse reasons.

Business or Labor Background

Many company doctors said that they had been especially interested in working for a corporation because their father had been a businessman. For example: "My father was an engineer who always worked for large companies in some kind of major industry. I'm sure that influenced me." A few said that their father had been a factory worker or a "union man"—an unusual background for a physician. A physician from a mining corporation said:

> My father was an underground miner and a union man all his life. He also was a black lung recipient. We had two pictures on the living room wall: one was the good Lord, and the other was John L. Lewis, and you never knew who took precedence. I chose to come here because of my family and my cultural background in coal. I was raised in a mining town, and I know the culture, which has helped me very much; as I speak the language, I have no problems communicating with the underground miner and the hourly individual, where a lot of other people do.

Others, like these physicians from an auto company and a metals company, said they had been employed as industrial workers themselves:

> I'm the son of a machinist, so I'm used to working around heavy industry. I've worked in the shops with my dad and some other shops as well to support myself through college and medical school, so I knew the tooling and what went on and enjoyed that kind of thing.

> I was a steelworker and worked myself through school working in a steel mill. I never flaunted that, but I could identify with them. Following military experience and a short period of private practice, I realized that occupational medicine was very appealing to me.[36]

The mining company doctor had a different position in the company than his miner father, so I asked what he thought his father would say about that if he were still alive. He said:

> Before he passed away, he said he never thought that any son of his would become a company man, and he said that mostly in jest but with a little hostility. He had fifty years of being union and was what we call a shit stirrer. I said, "I can do more good in this position for the miners than I can loading coal."

Short Hours, Avoidance of Private Practice Hassles, and Money

Many people go into corporate occupational medicine because it is potentially an easier type of medical practice than others. Doctors from a primary-care background are drawn to the hours and steady income of company employment. Surgeons who deal with trauma on nights and weekends can find the hours devastating to their lives. Extra hours are not the rule for company physicians, and by five o'clock most can go home without being on call, so their sleep and normal life are not disrupted. An airline company physician said:

> I came from a private practice where I had my own patients and worked in surgery, the emergency room, and the intensive-care unit. I took care of critically ill patients that were immediately post-op—in circumstances when it was impossible to put down the responsibility except when I left town for two weeks and specifically arranged with somebody to cover me. I'm glad I'm out of that level of interminable responsibility.

Many people enter occupational medicine in their late forties or early fifties, like this aerospace physician:

> This is simply a transition between the much more stressful emergency medicine I was doing at the hospital and full retirement, and I wanted to taper off rather than retire completely. The work here is so much less stressful in terms of hours and patient load, which makes it much more pleasant.[37]

Some disliked certain medical trends and wanted to avoid the strain of private practice, including malpractice issues and third-party payer problems. As an oil company physician said: "I would never want to be in private practice now; too much garbage is involved in billing and fighting with the government, and it's just not pleasant anymore. All the fun has been taken out of it." Ironically, one aerospace doctor went into corporate employment because he did not like the business aspect of private practice. He said: "I went into solo private practice, but I didn't like being a businessman. And if I didn't like it then, I'd sure hate it now because it's an awful lot worse."[38]

Occupational medicine is not as lucrative as most medical specialties, but physicians are at the top of corporate salary structures, on a par with vice presidents and in some cases CEOs. Corporate physicians are usually paid more than physicians in universities and government practice but less than successful contract physicians—such as those doing physical exams at urgent-care centers—or consultants, who can make twice the income of a corporate physician.[39]

Contract physicians lack the prestige of cardiologists at the local hospital, but their work as consultants or vendors to many companies is generally lucrative. Physicians in corporate medicine may complain about limited staff or authority, or about how much more money successful contract physicians can make, but few seriously consider leaving; most quickly become accustomed to the secure income, short hours, and other benefits of corporate employment.

Military Background

The military is a common background for people in occupational medicine. Physicians who leave the military at age forty or fifty are unprepared to start a practice, and corporate employment offers work that is similar to what they had become accustomed to in the military. A chemical company physician said:

> Some doctors who come from the military into a corporation, unfortunately, can best be described as retired. They retired from the army, they're still retired, but they're working for somebody else. Some folks want a cushy nine-to-five job. They didn't work too hard in the military, and they don't work too hard for Acme Widget Company.[40]

Military physicians were among the first occupational health specialists in the United States. Physicians who went into occupational medicine beginning in the 1940s and 1950s typically were trained and practiced medicine in the armed services. The management style and core values of the military are different from those of corporations; nevertheless, military medicine makes a natural transition to corporations and an easier one than the transition from private practice. An airline physician said:

> Practicing occupational medicine in a corporation and in the military are almost identical, except we don't wear uniforms and address each other by rank. We report to a chain of command, either in an advisory capacity or a direct link, with line and staff functions. Many of our flight officers and mechanics are from the military and have been regimented to that way of thinking. A military physician has a lot more latitude and power than a corporate physician and doesn't face the cumbersome union organizations and federal laws applying to corporations. Otherwise, everything else is just as it was in the military.

Military physicians treating individual soldiers and corporate physicians treating employees face similar issues of authority in a chain of command. Both contexts certainly differ from the relative independence of private practice. However, the military's authority structure clearly differs from that in a corporation. Military physicians wear their authority on their uniforms and can write orders that will be followed worldwide, whereas in corporations doctors must be more willing to develop consensus among other parties, to compromise, and to incrementalize change. A publishing company physician with a military background had this to say:

> The military empowers people when they're given certain responsibilities, so that everything in the military is set down with clear lines of authority and responsibility. Most corporations want the leadership qualities you develop in the military, but they don't invest people with the authority commensurate to the responsibility load. So you wind up with a lot of responsibility but sometimes no power to change the process that would benefit the employees' health. So one has to learn different corporate political skills than one needs in the military.

A high-level physician for a conglomerate explained:

> People with a military background in the company are less open-minded, less ready for change, less likely to have a broad understanding of medicine, because from day one they have worked in such a structured, precise way. It's a different managerial style. They consider themselves elite and have dominated the field until recently. The military guys do well with the top of the corporations—CEOs, etc., but the new breed of physicians in their mid to late thirties are more professional and better physicians and easier to work with as colleagues than the physicians from the military.

Medical care is not the primary goal of either type of organization, but corporate physicians with a military background say that doctors have more influence in the military than in corporations because in a military division their job is to practice medicine. Although doctors in corporations as well as in the military serve to get workers or soldiers back to the workplace or battlefield, keeping the soldiers well is a higher priority in the military, so that doctors find it easier to make a case for health programs there. And unlike physicians in corporations, who must defend their activities within the overriding business concern of making money, military physicians do not have to justify their role to management in terms of profit and loss. The military is much more aware of the role that medicine plays in its success than is corporate management. Whenever the military goes to war, its leaders realize that the medical function is essential to success, whereas relatively few corporate managers appreciate the role of occupational medicine.[41] A major auto company doctor with a military background said:

> Medical priorities in the navy weigh heavily, because people are going off on a ship to a remote island somewhere or deploying to a carrier, so they are obsessed with making sure they are ready. They give all these shots and want Joe's bad knee looked at. It's more of a laissez-faire thing here in the corporation, where there's less concern about employee health because you go home at the end of the day.

Military doctors need not justify their importance in terms of profit and loss, but cost-effectiveness principles become important once they reach a leadership level in the military, as this publishing company physician with a military background explained:

> Maybe cost isn't reckoned in dollars in the military, but it's an efficiency issue: How best to utilize twenty people to serve forty thousand? Will you make them work sixteen hours a day in order to serve forty thousand people? You can say, "Get six hours' sleep. Here's your cot." It may not last long, but you can do that; you're in the military.

Physicians still operate largely within a medical subculture in the military. For instance, the basic ambience and subculture in a military hospital or medical research unit is medical, and physicians generally work among other doctors and report to doctors. In contrast, a corporate medical department is seldom large enough to create its own personal and organizational protection day to day, so the doctors spend more of their nonclinical time with engineers, lawyers, controllers, and human resources people than with other doctors. They are absorbed into the corporate world more thoroughly than doctors are absorbed into the military world, and more estranged from their base business and background than military doctors are.

In emergencies, naval doctors in particular can insist that medical considerations be given top priority, and their authority to do so gives them more independence than is available to company doctors.[42] An auto company physician with experience as a military doctor said:

> Decisions about medivac-ing somebody by helicopter or aircraft must be made sometimes. If somebody has an appendicitis on a small ship without a surgeon, you can definitely make things happen: they will send a helicopter and get the person evacuated off the ship. It's the same thing if somebody stationed on an island or a remote site falls ill or gets pregnant; you have the authority to say, "This person will be shipped back to the States."

Military medical budgets can be overhauled immediately in acute situations, so that some plans will be abandoned while everyone responds to the crisis. There are parallels in corporations. Exxon's budget changed considerably after the 1989 oil spill in Alaska disrupted everything the corporation was doing. Health expenditures are likely to be cut in financial emergencies because they do not generate revenue. A publishing company physician said:

> In the military you know when you're sent someplace you have an interval of time to achieve your agenda. Then, at the end of your three years, you walk away and leave it alone; it's gone. That military experience is an advantage. In the corporate setting you can have a goal that's approved this year; next year the company's in financial trouble and your pet may go. You learn the discipline of acceptance. I have around here somewhere the Serenity Prayer: to change the things you can, to accept the things you can't, and the wisdom to know the difference. That's a lesson learned quickly in the military.

Overall, however, a military background is not necessarily an advantage in ferreting out health hazards or in practicing occupational medicine. A physician who has provided medical services to companies and now trains occupational physicians explained:

> Retired military physicians were popular for corporate positions because employers knew they wouldn't talk back to them; they were team players who didn't know a lot about what they were in the middle of, and they weren't particularly well versed in occupational medicine, sometimes not even trained in it. A company would be relatively assured that they could

get away with an awful lot of disease creation without having to pay the bill.

The New Breed with a Public Health Interest

The field of occupational medicine changed in the 1980s and 1990s with an influx of public health–oriented physicians who were formally trained in occupational medicine in residency programs that attracted young professionals. This new breed is unlike many of their "old breed" predecessors trained in the military or Public Health Service, who were more likely to become company doctors as a last resort after becoming exhausted or failing in practice.[43] Few doctors in the 1950s came to the field by way of the residency-trained pathway because few institutions existed. That started to change in the 1970s, when many physicians with public health and environmental interests entered the field. They had a variety of motivations: growing environmental awareness; the Occupational Safety and Health Act, which required companies to have medical surveillance programs; NIOSH residency training money; and greater union interest. The trained occupational physicians among this new breed are more likely to have the skills to detect disease patterns when studying health records, so they are more likely to detect hazards in companies and to work with managers to design processes to reduce exposures. They are increasingly likely to go into management and direct health programs rather than work in medical clinics. The commitment with which they come into the field has rejuvenated it.

Although the public health fervor declined in the late 1990s, young residents still come through training programs with a strong preventive orientation. Occupational medicine preselects people who tend to have a broader perspective and to be more interested in social issues, in preventive medicine among basically healthy populations, and in health hazards in the workplace, such as asbestos or lead toxicity.[44] Training in occupational medicine reinforces that approach. Formal training and board certification permit occupational physicians to collect different information and interpret it differently than would be the case with the many company doctors who lack the knowledge, experience, and inclination to provide preventive services.[45]

Occupational medicine also attracts physicians who begin to see the value of prevention after years in practice treating the end-stage diseases of people in their sixties and seventies who have been, for instance, long-term smokers or alcoholics. They then see the need to get into the workforce when people are young to develop educational programs and protect workers from hazardous exposures. They become more concerned with environmental effects on large groups than narrow medical treatment of individual patients, as these physicians, from a utility and a conglomerate, respectively, explained:

> I thought of doing occupational medicine basically because I got burned out on seeing people die of end-stage kidney and lung and heart disease, and I liked the opportunity to do some preventive medicine. It seemed that all I was doing was prolonging the dying process, and that was not my idea of what I wanted to do as a physician.

> It sure beat the hell out of looking after people with sore throats and colds, and it was wonderful to have a global picture and to try to impact diseases administratively, rather than going out there in the trenches and putting a Band-Aid on everybody. Here you could mandate something that would benefit an entire population of people.

The new breed with a public health background, trained to go into preventive medicine, tends to have contempt for what they perceive to be the old breed's lack of training and interest in prevention, and that attitude affects the general environment of practicing occupational medicine. Two physicians, from a chemical company and a utility company, said:

> I started out in occupational medicine and was residency-trained. I am not a retread, I did not come to this field after I left the army or got fed up with family practice or some such thing.

> By the time I entered it, occupational medicine had made its most significant change: it wasn't just the company doctor there to make sure the laggards and sluggards got back to work and no one was gaming the system. Historically that's been a concern: Whose doctor are you, anyway?

Unlike most company physicians, university physicians have considerable freedom to pursue preventive strategies and conduct research into occupational disease and environmental health.[46] As academics, they typically have more extensive research capabilities and tools than those available to doctors in corporations. They also train medical students to be occupational medicine practitioners in corporations, government, and universities. They can consult with employers to suggest preventive measures after they evaluate workers, and they can advise unions on projects. An occupational physician who does consulting and finds corporate positions for occupational medicine residents said:

> There is an old, historical split between corporate-based medicine, which was the dominant form of occupational medicine for decades, and the academic side, in part because we operate in mutually exclusive worlds: our training, our concerns, our daily jobs, and the pressures on us are different. Corporate doctors depend on lawyers and various other people before they hand over documents and submit evidence on hazards. I don't envy the limitations they operate under or sympathize with what they have to do, but that's the life they chose.

Nonetheless, although corporate physicians have less freedom to pursue preventive measures than academic physicians, corporate physicians who have the public health goal of prevention in occupational medicine try to take positive measures against occupational illness, despite the fact that concerns such as cost containment have become so important to their employers.

IMAGES OF CORPORATE EMPLOYMENT

Trained occupational physicians are at pains to distance themselves from the image of the company doctor before the days of public health training and occupational medicine certification. As these physicians in publishing, telecommunications, and chemicals stated:

> When you're a company doc, you have to realize that employees don't think you can make it in private practice or anywhere else, so you have to live that down. That's why I have all these diplomas and plaques on the wall.

> Even ten years ago a lot of leftovers were in occupational medicine— people who strayed from medical practice or were gearing down their medical careers. I won't call them "rejects," but they certainly weren't the

pick of the litter. Doctors in occupational medicine now are generally more skilled and have greater managerial potential.

Occupational physicians in the earlier era were the orphans of medicine, having no respect for ourselves or no respect within the broad profession of medicine—not fitting in, not being taken seriously by mainstream medical people. We were embarrassed for good reason. The field was viewed as a rubber stamp of big business, where corporate paychecks completely controlled doctors. Even worse, it was simply a field that attracted doctors who couldn't get a job in a hospital or practice because of alcoholism or emotional disorders, so they got a job in a company doing physicals or what have you.

The perception that company doctors have an unfavorable reputation continues to this day, as these two observers noted:

The image of occupational medicine within medicine in general is that it is a place for somebody to retire, prop their feet up on the desk, and read the *Wall Street Journal* and goof off. I was not impressed with the docs in the company I met over the years before I came here. That was not too comforting.

Status is important to physicians, and the status of the occupational physician is about the same as the status of the military physician. Being a military doctor is just very secure, but you don't go to a cocktail party and say, "I'm a major in the army," and have anyone tell you their health complaints.

Some doctors' images of corporate work were fairly accurate before they went into it because they had been placed in corporations as part of their occupational medicine training fellowships. They were thus less likely to be disillusioned about their role in the company or their low status in the medical hierarchy.

With pervasive changes in doctors' working conditions and improved training through residency programs, the reputation of doctors in corporate or large group practice is better than it was thirty years ago, when the vast majority of physicians were in private practice.[47] A generation ago the best physicians worked in solo offices, but medicine has changed dramatically since then.

Physicians now have different aspirations and take jobs in corporations less reluctantly; a growing number of them see this field as intellectually respectable. A bank physician, a utility physician, and a physician who has provided medical services to companies had these comments:

> When we were in medical school, they introduced us to what used to be called "industrial physicians," and of course we thought they were hacks: people who couldn't make it in practice anywhere else went into industrial medicine. But as time went by, better physicians have come into occupational medicine, and now people are saying to me, "Do you have any jobs down there?"

> There was definitely a derogatory thought about company docs in the old days—that they just took care of injuries for the company and made sure that patients got back to work as soon as possible, possibly to the detriment of the patient. I was concerned about the company doc stereotype, and I know all my friends thought I was crazy coming here. Now they are coming to work for me. Things got switched around in five years.

> My generation of graduates of medical school all expected to go out into private practice, and the best of us would become well known in the medical community, and that was a goal; obviously you'd make a lot of money if you did. Now the best graduates from medical school *hope* to be on the staff of Kaiser because it's the only job security left. Private physicians are dying. *Everybody* anticipates working for an entity; it's no longer a failure like it would have been for my generation.

Physicians are increasingly less embarrassed about being called company physicians. The stigma of corporate employment has diminished. But even with the influx of public health–trained physicians, the reputation of occupational physicians as poorly qualified and in the back pocket of management remains.

DOWNSIZING AND THE OUTSOURCING PENDULUM

As old corporate jobs disappear with shifts in the U.S. economy and global competition, many companies have cut the size of their in-house medical staff. Occupational medicine has changed dramatically as corporations contract out their services to hospital-based programs and free-standing clinics. Contract doctors do physical exams and provide services to companies a few hours a day or by being on call. Corporate employers decide which in-house services they need to retain and make strategic decisions to cut human resources, shifting costs by using vendors rather than in-house employees. Many companies that once had full-time doctors have replaced their medical director with a nurse-run first-aid unit; some have replaced their entire medical department with twenty-four-hour or late-hour walk-in urgent-care clinics for minor emergency services, where individuals can go without an appointment.[48] Small companies hire hospitals and clinics essentially to serve as their medical departments. Large corporations that pare back clinical services may still retain in-house medical directors to supervise programs and provide medical advice related to lawsuits, government-mandated programs, and disability management; then they bring health professionals in only for specific tasks, such as dealing with environmental hazards and crises. Companies that hire contract physicians have in-house doctors design the program, choose the people to fulfill the contract, and monitor their performance.

Especially in times of budget cutbacks and reorganization in corporations, medical considerations are not foremost in managers' minds. Also, fewer doctors are required to run in-house programs after general company layoffs. Doctors have tended to be concentrated in older manufacturing companies rather than in the service corporations that have grown so rapidly in recent years. Much of the need for physicians in manufacturing operations disappears with the loss of manufacturing jobs.[49] Moreover, the belief that an annual physical exam is necessary has declined, necessitating a smaller medical staff. A chemical company medical director said:

> When I came into the company in 1970, we had 144 physicians; we are now down to thirty-nine, and I'm still reducing. When I first came into the company, physicians did hands-on physical exams on everybody, and we still do, but we're changing that traditional, physician-oriented physical exam to more of a wellness evaluation that will be less physician-intensive. We'll use nurses more than physicians and eventually wind up with fifteen to twenty physicians instead of the 144 we had. We think we're doing a better job now and not sacrificing anything. Other companies preceded us.[50]

Most major manufacturing corporations have downsized in some way, partly because of the restructuring and leveraged buyout furor that swept across corporate America in the 1980s and 1990s.[51] Laying off employees and hiring people under contract is a pattern that extends far beyond the medical department. Health services seem no different from anything else that distracts from the company's main business, whether it is manufacturing chemical products or providing telecommunication services. Companies whose business is doing medical exams take over occupational medicine from the corporation's internal resources, just as a contractor may handle food services, media relations, research and development, legal functions, and pension administration better or cheaper than employees can. Companies make extensive use of contractors as a buffer so that they can lay off contract employees rather than regular employees when demand declines. Externalizing programs to contractors who require no commitment gives management flexibility. Employers that contract out medical services can change vendors more easily, decide to eliminate the whole service, move it off-site, or choose from a menu what they want for their employees. And they do not have to pay health or retirement benefits to contract employees.

An important factor that leads to outsourcing company medicine is the explosion of entrepreneurial companies designed to exploit the trend within major corporations to concentrate on their major product or service and eliminate whatever else they can. Companies could not buy outside expertise as easily twenty years ago because fewer vendors were in business. Classified ads in journals and the ACOEM employment referral service reflect this change in the complexion of occupational medicine practice. Physicians in free-standing occupational health services do exams for companies as a way for hospitals to gain patients and expand their business. Beginning in the 1980s large group medical practices added occupational medicine specialists to treat employees for workplace injuries and disease along with personal illnesses, a service that became more lucrative as workers' compensation reimbursement increased.[52] Trends in medicine have encouraged people to become contractors in for-profit occupational medicine clinics. Vendors solicit potential corporate clients by aggressively marketing their cost-cutting packages of services as substitutes for in-house programs. They propose to do physical exams for less money and persuade managers that their services are necessary. A physician who has provided medical services to many companies and a consumer products company physician said:

Now all corporations get promotional material from consultants: "We come in from the outside; you don't have to worry about litigation and malpractice. We're generally smarter, younger, better-trained, and it'll cost you a lot less." Companies buy that.

Some vendors can make themselves sound like God's gift to humanity who will solve all your problems and your health-care bills never will go up. Well, they wouldn't be in business if it were all so wonderful—they would be retired by now after having made their fortune. It just doesn't work that way. There is no magic bullet. A large body of evidence on the opposite side says that you lose a great deal by contracting out, and obviously our management here still agrees with that.

Economies of scale make having in-house physicians more cost-effective than sending everything out, especially when employees and facilities are geographically concentrated. Outside contractors often provide medical services more efficiently than in-house doctors could for small companies and those spread out in many locations. It makes sense to dedicate equipment, facilities, and full-time in-house medical staff to service a company with a critical mass of five thousand people in one location, but not for a company of fifty employees. Whether companies provide health services in-house depends in part on the company's geographic layout and what the company does.

Company physicians argue that employers and workers lose quality by not having in-house medical services. In this view, having physicians in-house to interact with management, see people quickly, and provide the types of services to employees and managers that company doctors can provide is better than what employers receive from outsiders who do not understand the organization or managers' expectations. Corporations may save money by using outside contractors who say they can do the same job at lower cost but then in fact do not provide the same program. A computer company physician whose employer decided to outsource all the disability management that the company's internal staff had once done said this: "It's absolutely chaos. People came to expect a certain level of understanding and service in the company with a strong corporate culture and a lot of history behind it. Suddenly it all changed and isn't managed well."

Companies have gone back and forth, to some degree, on the business decision of whether it is profitable to keep physicians in-house. Company physicians, perhaps too optimistically, describe a pendulum. Some say they have seen medical departments come and go several times, with companies already having gone through several outsourcing cycles over thirty years. New management may suddenly end company medical programs and do only what they absolutely must by law, then the pendulum will swing back toward in-house corporate services because of an expanding economy, or because employers recognize that such services enhance employee productivity and decrease company costs and human suffering. Employers may also realize that they are not getting the level of performance their outside contractors had promised them. In this view, corporate medicine follows the business cycle in regard to decentralizing or centralizing.[53] These oil company physicians said:

> Contractors say they'll do everything for ten dollars, then the light goes on later. Companies realize they paid more money than they thought, they lost control of what happens to the employees, they lost all preventive health care. Managers say, "Gee, if we pay a lab over here and the doc over there, and we pay because our environmental waste-treatment guy got into trouble, then why don't we get our own doctors?"

> I've seen companies grind all the way down to a bare-bones staff that burns out struggling to keep doing everything, and finally get a contractor to do it all. Eventually workers' comp costs get worse. Employees who could have been effectively helped now cost the company money because committed people who understand the company are not doing that work. They boot out the unsatisfactory contractor and come full circle, hiring their medical staff again.

American business and social trends are not now moving in the direction of bringing services in-house, but circumstances could once again lead corporations to hire more physicians. Interest in worker protection erodes as employers lose their economic competitiveness, whereas after conditions improve the field tends to expand and attention to health issues increases. Businesses that have outsourced many functions generally build back up again when prospects for the company revive. Managers could learn that abolishing corporate medical departments is not working. They may see that contractors who lack expertise or knowledge about workplace conditions are unable to offer good advice.

Companies contract out in part because it looks cheaper, then become dissatisfied once they see high turnover in the canned programs offered by outside vendors, who seem oblivious to company operations whenever managers try to discuss their services with them. Occupational medicine is also likely to return as an in-house function if a disaster occurs. For instance, workers at Allied Corporation who manufactured Kepone (chlordecone) began showing severe neurological symptoms. Kepone is an organochlorine insecticide that causes reproductive effects (specifically altered sperm transfer), pleuritic and joint pains, liver disease, tremor, and other chronic and acute effects (Lemasters 1998, 227; McConnell 1994, 853–54). One university occupational physician recalled:

> There was an economic downturn when I came into the field in medical school in the mid-1970s, and a lot of industries were outsourcing, cutting back. Then people began to realize the value of what they had lost. Allied was a good example. They felt one reason their Kepone disaster caught them by surprise was that they didn't have any in-house health specialists. So they swung the other way and started to build up a big program and now are starting to shed some and go the other way. It swings back and forth, just as business goes through cycles.

An additional reason companies may rebuild their in-house medical departments has to do with OSHA requirements. Although responding to OSHA rules has become part of company operating procedures, new OSHA laws could spur the growth of corporate medical departments if employers perceive a greater need for physicians to respond to the new rules.

Medical practice in general and the occupational medicine field in particular are undergoing an enormous transition. Physicians who work in corporations are becoming more professionally oriented and better trained. They have better qualifications and a stronger public health background. Paradoxically, many corporations are laying off in-house professionals just as these professionals are becoming better trained—and therefore in some ways more valuable to the corporation. In transitional periods like the present time, seemingly contradictory things happen simultaneously. More physicians now come into occupational medicine with a public health background and advanced training, even though economic pressures on employers to cut back on preventive measures also are greater. Even the exceptionally well-trained, more public health–oriented "new breed" of occupational physicians can be laid off. It is not only cost, however, that leads corporations to lay them off. As we shall see in the next chapter, in-house doctors may cause other problems for employers, such as those related to loyalty and credibility.

Chapter 2

Loyalty and Professional Perils for Corporate Team Players

If you go into occupational medicine in a corporation, you'd better understand you're working in a business, with business-men in charge. If you choose to move to Alaska, you'd be a fool to complain about the weather.

—Oil company physician

When you deviate from team spirit, you have to make sure you explain clearly to the management team that you're pur-suing a greater good. If you can't do that persuasively, you've lost it in a corporation.

—Physician who has provided medical
services to companies

THE DOCTOR-PATIENT relationship of hallowed tradition is trans-formed in corporations. Employers, nonphysician managers, insurers, and other third parties now play a role along with doc-tors and patients, even more than in private practice. Doctors worry about company costs and liability, and they often have con-siderable direct contact with other corporate sectors—such as le-gal, personnel, and environmental departments—that influence medical decisions.[1] Management may even try to tell doctors how they should differentiate between one diagnosis and another. The increasing pressure on professionals to serve as "team players" who serve the ends of employers and insurers affects not only company doctors but also physicians working for managed care firms and other types of corporate professionals as well. However, in the transformation of physician loyalty, company doctors are further along on the general trajectory on which doctors in a wide range of organizations are moving.

THE LOYALTY IDEAL AND THE REALITIES
OF COMPANY MEDICINE

The ethical code of the American Occupational and Environmental Medical Association proclaims that "physicians should accord the highest priority to the health and safety of individuals" in the workplace and environment.[2] It advises physicians to communicate to workers "any significant observations and recommendations concerning their health" and to keep medical information about individuals confidential.[3] Doctors can use the national organization's ethics code to justify their actions when they are caught in conflicts with management, as when managers demand to see employees' confidential medical reports. Doctors can use the code as a weapon to support their right to take specific actions.[4] A physician who served on the ACOEM ethics committee said:

> The code is our protection. You can always point to that and say, "I can't do this because of the ethics code," if you have some external body to lend validity to your claims. We asked members in a questionnaire study what they use to help them decide what to do when ethical conflicts arise in their practice. I was totally surprised that the most frequent answer was "the code of ethics." The lesson I learned was, we'd better take a good look at the code and make sure it says what we hope it says, because people actually use it.

When asked about loyalty and possible conflicts such as those that the *Journal of Occupational and Environmental Medicine* discusses between serving patients and other goals, company physicians say that in general they do not face such conflicts and personally have not felt torn.[5] For example, a railroad company physician said:

There is no conflict between serving the corporation and serving the patient in occupational medicine. The function of the corporate physician is to serve the corporation, and part of doing that is to try to keep the workers healthy.

Others described labor-management conflict or legal constraints as surmountable with appropriate interpersonal skills of tact, mediation, or even psychotherapy. They said such skills were needed to perform the sometimes delicate balancing act that corporate employment requires. As a chemical company physician said:

Understanding how you deliver health care under conflicting pressures is a non-issue. It's an issue only for people who lack maturity and a clear understanding of the values of delivering health care in a way that meets society's other needs. I've never really come into conflict with management or been faced with unresolvable win-lose circumstances.

A close examination of professionals' own conceptions of loyalty and their work orientation can deepen an analysis of divided loyalties and work satisfaction. Physicians who generally assert that they experience no conflicting loyalties give many examples of just such conflicts when they discuss their own work. A long-time physician from a major airline described the challenge of adapting to the competing pressures of corporate employment as akin to that in a dysfunctional family:

I grew up thinking that fair was fair, and it's hard for me to give that up in this corporate context, but it's not compatible with working for a large company, which is almost a perfect analog to living in an alcoholic, dysfunctional family: the parents fight all the time, and you can never predict what will result. You do the same thing twice and get yelled at once and approved of the second time. Each parent tries to seduce you to support them against the other. The CEO is like the paternal figure, and the people who work at his level are deceitful and misrepresent the company's actual resources according to whatever they need at the moment, and they are greedy. My raises over the past ten years were less than 1 percent per year; our CEO went home with over $30 million last year.

Although doctors are raised to observe the ethical command that the patient comes first, some have modified its traditional meaning. A computer company physician said:

I view the company as my patient. I get involved in-depth in the medical policies and the whole culture around the company. I enjoy working closely with ten or twelve people in the human resources team: personnel professionals, EAP [employee assistance program] managers, labor lawyers, so I feel like part of a family and part of that team.

Employees are skeptical about company doctors' loyalty to them and the strength of a doctor-patient relationship, as this union official argued:

I've dealt with company doctors on committees and panels debating the issues. I've rarely met a company doctor who didn't go through a little ritual of proclaiming his independence, professional integrity, and commitment to workers' health and well-being. But I've never met a worker who has anything good to say about a company doctor, over my twenty years in occupational health, working with local and international unions and workers' groups. It's not even a topic of debate: company doctors are not trusted. People go to them out of necessity, as the stop they have to make on the way to a real doctor if they get injured or sick on the job. But they don't expect medicine from them. Coal miners talk about company doctors with a sneer and use colorful language to describe them—such as Babette, the whore. They have almost a mythic status among coal miners because of the history of doctors who worked for the company. Miners resented the fact that part of their pay was deducted to pay for a doctor they didn't respect or have control over, who was just an instrument of management to screen people out of jobs or deny the existence of occupational disease.[6]

A doctor for a telecommunications company acknowledged this negative view:

You're perceived as not being a "real" doctor; you're management no matter what. Unions think that you're an enemy if you belong to the company; they discredit the company doctor as biased on the side of management and send people to their own doctors.

Doctors often blame workers for not trusting them. They are more likely to do so in companies with a highly adversarial management-labor posture or a strong union. Rather than acknowledge the real conflicting interests and power dynamics, doctors and managers often simply condemn employees' mistrust as irrational. For example, a metals company physician said: "People have their own personality problems that interfere with accepting any positive concern about their well-being."

Sometimes doctors admit that employees may mistrust doctors for good reason. Metals company physicians said:

The workers have a strain of paranoia, but there's certainly a basis for it. People have been dealt with arbitrarily. Situations of true conflict between the individual's perceived needs and the needs of the corporation are inevitable.[7]

Even in this day and age a doctor is thought of as working for the company. It's a hangover from the old days of just out-and-out exploitation of good, hardworking generations of people. It has to do with the environmental and familial and work aspects of the mining culture, and the geographical areas of the country we're involved in, such as the bowels of Kentucky and West Virginia, where you still don't dare walk down the street as a company man after dark. It's almost a hatred. I'd have a problem if they didn't know who I was and I had a company hat or jacket on.

It is reasonable of patients to see that even if a doctor-patient relationship exists, the doctor works for the company and must attempt to serve the employer's interest in order to survive on the job. A telecommunications company physician said:

The major loyalties are with the employer who provides your paycheck and a company that you want to see successful. People are kidding themselves with the idea that physicians are able to separate themselves as physicians—to isolate medical issues and not see the needs of the employee or the company. It's a nice objectivity that doesn't exist in real life.

A textile workers' union official agreed, saying, "You can count the cases where doctors take workers' side on the fingers of a long-term meat cutter."[8] However, some corporate physicians take bold chances, such as engaging in national legislative battles over workplace health or health-care reform. Those who are not fired typically work for companies with either an unusual tolerance for professional dissent or employee organizations that strongly support them. Professionals in that rare and relatively protected position may have conflicting motivations, unlike those who are interested only in their careers and therefore remain essentially unconflicted about anything their employer wants them to do.

Doctors tend to have strong beliefs about whether unions help the medical department or impede what doctors say should be done. Doctors at some corporations say unions overall have been a positive influence and an ally of company physicians in working for employees' health. At times unions have commissioned studies, pressured negligent companies, and supported medical programs that doctors believed companies needed. A utility company physician said:

> Here the union is strong and into employee rights. Some doctors may view that as a pain in the butt, and it is at times. But it's not necessarily bad, because it keeps things honest and it keeps you as an occupational physician thinking. Individuals will be put upon and not given their rights unless they have a strong constitution and are willing to fight for their rights. That's the fact of the matter.

In contrast, doctors at many corporations perceive that unions have been adversaries standing in the way of what company physicians want to do. They believe that union fears are overstated and that unions have been a hindrance by advising employees not to cooperate with the medical department, so that nobody then participates in their programs. They say unions exacerbate health problems and adversarial relations with management when they seize upon a health hazard and publicize it. Unions may invite NIOSH in to do a study or use health issues to foment agitation. Unions have opposed in-house occupational physicians and argued that third-party physicians be used instead. An airline physician said:

> We have disagreed on various issues, such as medical arbitration and the weight program for flight attendants, which the union has fought for years and even tried class-action discrimination suits over it. Often decisions as to whether employees can go to work are at odds with what employees want. A lot of them feel we're only interested in serving the company's need to get them back to work at all costs, regardless of how they feel or what their needs are in getting well or being productive. They fear that the corporate physician is management's puppet.

Many doctors say that government regulations have made unions unnecessary. For example, they argue that OSHA and the Environmental Protection Agency (EPA) now address safety issues that unions addressed in the 1930s and 1940s. The Consolidated Omnibus Budget Reconciliation Act (COBRA) and the Employee Retirement Income Security Act (ERISA) dissuade companies from denying people their benefits, and government regulatory bodies like the Equal Employment Opportunity Commission (EEOC) and rules such as those of the Americans with Disabilities Act (ADA) protect employees.[9] Despite the fact that the percentage of people in unions has been small and declining for many years, some doctors refer to unions as "big labor," as if they were a mighty counterweight to managerial prerogative. A chemical company physician said: "Big labor and big management have a lot more in common with each other than they have differences. Big labor, big management, and big government become involved in causes, and the worker gets lost."

Company doctors sometimes say that they can gain a reputation for making impartial judgments based only on facts, and that their loyalty to the medical profession makes them nonthreatening to managers and workers. However, doctors inevitably become involved in individual cases involving issues such as workers' compensation, layoffs, disability, and health benefits, and when labor and management run into conflict, it is virtually impossible for the doctor to be accepted as a friend of both sides equally.

TEAM PLAYERS VERSUS WHITE COATS

Company doctors describe the ideal professional as a "team player," but this does not simply mean someone who works well with other people in a complex organization. The corporate model of loyalty and service to the employer is in tension with the medical profession's model of loyalty to the patient and advocacy for health. In the corporate culture it is understood that team players have access to resources and power, whereas "white coats"—with perspectives typical of the solo private practitioner—are ignored, held in contempt, or terminated. A textile company doctor said:

> Being a good occupational physician in a corporation requires a person who has the ability to be patient, to shift with the paradigms within the business, and to sense what the people you work for value and try to see if you can bring your values into alignment and get them incorporated into their values.

Corporate managers often consider professionals outsiders who are not businesspeople and must earn their spurs through years of trying to be a team member. Those who cannot make themselves seem to be team players either leave or remain at a low level. But team players and white coats are "ideal types"; most people and most careers are a blend of both. Team players appear to be loyal, in that they follow corporate directives and pursue their employers' goals. But their preferred approach is not solely to serve the company. Rather, they are team players who bring professional and career interests to their corporate roles. *Being a team player is the new kind of professionalism*. Professionals define it in terms of individual career, self-protection, and survival in corporate employment. When professionals operate as team players, they usually are not sacrificing for the good of society or even for the good of the corporation. Their apparent loyalty to the corporation often stems from a fear of losing their own job or concern about their career opportunities.

Company doctors are under constant pressure to cast their medical judgments in profit terms and show the business value of medicine, but they cannot do that when their services are simply good for the employees' health. The doctor's opinion and medical priorities often prevail in a clinical setting, but implementing an idea or policy within a corporation requires building consensus among people with diverse perspectives and recognizing that the good health of employees is only one need of the corporation. A physician for an oil company said: "You need to be aware of the priorities of the large organization that surrounds you to find successful ways of getting your programs to move forward while at the same time supporting the business objectives."

Many corporate doctors who favor the white-coat approach actually wear a white coat or have one hanging prominently in their office, whereas those who favor the team player approach often wear a white shirt with a tie at work.[10] White coats are more likely than team players immediately to mention professional competence and board certification in occupational medicine as important for company doctors. The very characteristics that team players say are so detrimental for company doctors are ones from private practice that white coats advocate, as this banking industry doctor did:

> The best corporate physician is one who makes the best private physician, caring for people and not letting anything from the business interfere with the relationship of taking care of people. What's good for the person is usually good for the corporation, and what's good for the corporation is good for the person. Good medicine is good medicine.

Someone who puts on a white coat and says, "I'm a doctor. Leave me alone," is often the person who fails in the business managers' terms. An oil company physician said:

> Occupational physicians must be opportunistic to be able to survive in the corporate arena. The standard medical education does not equip doctors to be relevant to what a corporation needs out of doctors, and old-style doctors sooner or later will be goners if they think their white coat and stethoscope and reputation and aura of respect alone will be sufficient in the corporate world.

Team players are more likely than white coats to have a background as a military physician, whereas white coats are more likely to be drawn to occupational medicine because of a public health interest. A military background shapes the corporate doctor's expectations about what he or she should do and makes screening employees more palatable. Unlike medical training, military experience also prepares doctors for simply carrying out orders, such as performing whatever tests management asks for.

Publishing and Speaking Constraints

Company professionals experience constraints on their ability to publish and speak, to conduct studies of suspected exposure hazards, and to draw attention to problematic working conditions. Managers and company lawyers set up screening procedures out of concern over the use by professional staff members of the company's name. Doctors may collect information on what seems to be a disease pattern among employees that they want to publish, give a paper on, alert employees about, or publicize, but few of them collect information that could demonstrate a health hazard, partly because of how employers have defined company doctors' jobs. The constraint may work more effectively in companies with a strong, more polished reputation. These physicians, with major computer, chemical, and pharmaceutical companies, said:

Publishing is a problem, no question about it. There's a tremendous filter, levels of approval; the image of the corporation is their life. And people have the job to jealously protect that image. Executives are assigned whose sole job is to promote and protect that name.

An executive officer of the company once told me, "I don't care where you are, whatever comes out of your mouth represents the Company, *period.* You always have to remember you are partially wearing that hat."

We would have liked to have published findings or conducted studies in many cases, but the legal department looks at anything we want to publish closely and vetoes half of it. It's fifty-fifty whether or not they permit it. They have a protocol, and you go through the system.

A physician who has provided health services to several companies said:

There are clearly examples of tangible impediments to research and publication. I have had that problem, where I've ended up with the result in research projects, and the employer says, "This is not the result we want to see." The company would object, and we'd write the paper to leave out some things and emphasize others. It was not cricket. In some instances it means either leaving the job or the company asking physicians to leave their job if they publish, particularly people who have done the work in-house. But they usually just let it slide and don't publish.

Employers who ask outside researchers to do studies for them typically ask for no publication of the findings, the right to review before publication, or advance notice that will give them time to prepare their response to the anticipated public or government reaction to the published findings. Many university-based physicians reject insistence on no publication or on prepublication review. Employers increasingly take an "advance notice" approach when working with them, in contrast to their more restrictive approach with in-house physicians.

The performance of professionals as team players is not necessarily by edict. They typically accommodate employers without necessarily being told to do so. The constraints typically operate as subtle injunctions that professionals tend to take for granted and cooperate with rather than as formal proscriptions. When professionals censor themselves, they may not perceive any prohibition at all.

The MBA and the MPH

Team players say they wish they knew more about the economics of running the business. They mention an MBA business degree as not only desirable for a company physician but perhaps more valuable than a master's in public health (MPH) or even board certification in occupational medicine. They say the MBA is the more pertinent degree in part because business courses cover the kinds of things they will decide in corporations and as consultants to companies, such as budgeting and determining whether the funds they allocate have a good return. Doctors argue that the occupational physician in today's environment must be a good businessperson to survive and a good manager to reach the upper levels.

Doctors also may wish they had an MBA because they lose too often when they advocate for the medical program. Having an MBA, they think, might improve their prospects. Management may see an MBA as a basic guarantee that a physician understands business management and administration. Feeling insecure after seeing many medical departments shrink, physicians may perceive a managerial aura around the degree and think that it could help them sell their programs to managers who may know nothing about medicine.

Doctors consider themselves socially isolated in the corporation, having been socialized as physicians and segregated as a result. People with MBAs learn a new language and way of thinking, and it is certainly not the way doctors are taught to think in medical school. Although almost no one in occupational medicine has an MBA, many company physicians nonetheless crave business training. A physician who has provided health services for companies and a publishing company physician explained:

> Doctors have a yen for an MBA degree because they want to be socialized the same way that MBA people are socialized so they'll hear people differently and respond to them differently. I'd like to be able to throw up the charts for business projections and costs and all those things. People feel like they are missing an important part they can't touch—they're socially isolated. I feel it so strongly I can taste it when I sit in meetings. I think, *I want to be in this group*. I want to be able to say something in these meetings and not have anybody say, "Pffft, he's a doctor." If you're a

physician at high levels in management, where you have nothing but MBAs with business training around you, you feel a gap, a lack, socially disadvantaged.

We got a master's in public health when I did my residency; for this kind of practice in occupational medicine we should have gotten an MBA and not an MPH, which we never use. What's it good for? Sure, the courses on occupational diseases are fine, but a master's of business and business courses—cost-benefit ratios—would be more practical than the public health stuff in a position like this. Physicians in most cases want to progress in the company, and the MBA will shine more than a guy with an MPH when it shows who understands where the business is going. The CEO will say: "This guy talks my language." If you're a physician, you'd like to be able to talk the language of the CEO.

In sharp contrast to the team players who covet MBA degrees, white coats generally see an MBA as less important for a company physician than an MPH degree or strong training in toxicology, epidemiology, industrial hygiene, and environmental health.[11] A chemical company physician who takes this approach said:

An MBA might be as important as an MPH if you define occupational medicine as managing health-care economics, if that's the way this field wants to go. But if it wants to be a scientific discipline and advocate for worker health, it has to stick to the notion that we're trying to understand the relationship of work to health, and let the benefits managers focus on bailing out their corporation's health-care cost problems. That's not occupational medicine, the way I understand it.

Company physicians cannot successfully sell themselves as a substitute for an MBA because they are too expensive. Physicians can never divorce themselves from their medical roots, because that is the unique skill for which they are being paid. Even without an MBA, company physicians can gain an understanding of business either through their occupational medicine residency training, when they rotate through corporations, or through their on-the-job experience. They can learn enough economics and business to be effective, but an MBA is unnecessary for the work they do and they need not try to compete with the MBAs.

Over time, corporate physicians generally identify less and less with the public health concerns that motivated them when they were younger to enter the field. Their work draws them away from the traditional public health search for links between work exposures and disease, and they do less and less preventive medicine, if they ever did. Many also associate public health with the political left and advocates in the American Public Health Association (APHA) rather than with the concerns of physicians in ACOEM. They are pulled toward the MBA and a business orientation, but also pushed away from public health medicine as their knowledge and interest in it fades. An occupational physician who has worked in corporations and government said:

> Once you get into corporate medicine and you get all the secondary gain with the money and security, then the socialization you desire in this milieu is business socialization. Sure, corporate work has a little bit of public health and preventive medicine, but that's what the advocates do, and you're not with those people anymore and that's not your job. You need some of it, but you spend less time in an eight-hour day doing that than doing business planning.

Routes to Success Within Corporations

Doctors who seek to thrive as company physicians must be able to adapt to the corporate culture, which doctors describe as contrasting sharply with hospital or medical school culture. Engineers tend to dominate in industrial corporations, as an oil company physician explained:

> You have to find out what their receptors are, basically what they want to hear, how they want to hear it. Company physicians are among engineers basically trying to render medical decisions comprehensible to people who think in right angles. Our corporate culture is dominated by an engineering mentality, and it's implicit in how day-to-day business is run, which is quantitative, precise, black and white, with minimum appreciation for probability, judgment, intuition, creativity. A lot of it is totally foreign to doctors by nature and by training.

Company doctors become more powerful within corporations and successful in the eyes of other corporate physicians when they function as benefits managers and cost-containment experts who help manage their corporation's enormous health costs, including group health and disability insurance. This role of the company doctor as benefits manager extends far beyond the traditional model of taking care of the sick and injured and thus has little to do with the typical education and training of clinical physicians.

Other company doctors become successful in corporations that perceive a need for them to attend to potentially costly occupational and environmental health hazards. These corporations are more likely to hire doctors and provide resources that can make the physicians more influential. When risk management within a company is a significant issue, company doctors also become important by helping employers interpret and respond to hazardous substance regulation. Despite these routes to success, powerful physicians in companies remain atypical.

Company physicians often refer to one particular doctor as the model of the successful occupational physician in a corporation. As a chemical company physician said: "Bruce Karrh at DuPont became a vice president able to integrate that with becoming a leader in occupational medicine. He took an interest in the business aspects of DuPont, which many doctors have either a hard time doing or choose not to do." Karrh was in a huge corporation where handling occupational and environmental medical issues could have major effects on the company. He became a powerful company doctor in part because addressing health and speaking publicly in ways that management favors has been of such strategic importance within DuPont. So Karrh traveled extensively with the CEO and held a prominent position in company decisionmaking, roles that go beyond being a team player.

After a corporate decree that costs would be reduced by $1 billion, DuPont cut its medical department, shifting to greater use of contract physicians. Karrh became responsible for health benefits as well as occupational health. When I interviewed him in the mid-1990s, Karrh said that in fundamental ways he no longer functioned as a physician:

> If I retired, the company wouldn't replace me with a physician most likely. They'd get a manager, because that's really what I am. We don't really need a doctor in my position. Health-care benefits is my primary job now. They don't need a doctor to do what I do.[12]

He said several times that he has had a strong relationship with management, and that is the reputation he has had with other occupational physicians:

> I have great respect for management, and management respects me. I respond to what they need. My number-one job is being responsive to what management and employees need, and walking that line between the two is what I'm here for. The biggest problem I have is making sure that management recognizes that what is good for the employees is good for them, and if I can stay in the discussion long enough, I've never had a manager that didn't come around to that way of thinking. I don't go to the mat on everything. I figure out those battles that are worth fighting all the way, and those that if I give them up we won't lose anything anyway and the employees won't lose anything.

In a second unusual case of a company doctor becoming highly influential in a corporation, Manville made Paul Kotin a vice president, not just director of medical affairs. Like Karrh, Kotin was a strategic person in a company with known major health hazards.

Learning to "Pick Your Battles"

One main way in which doctors become team players is by, as they say, learning to "pick your battles." Doctors sound the theme again and again that they must do this to avoid becoming isolated in the corporation. Two physicians who have provided medical services to many companies said:

> You have to choose your battles very carefully. You have to say to management, "Okay, I won't go to the mat over these fifty-fifty things," where it's not real clear. Management could be right, the worker could be right—who knows? I won't alienate the legal department or my co-employees over it. I want to go to the cafeteria and have somebody sit with me.

> Being a part of a corporation, making team decisions, a physician wears velvet handcuffs. You're quiet about it even if you don't like what's going on.

Physicians sometimes wish they could initiate and act on ideas without the many constraints of being a team player. But they speak of a balance, a maturity, and the need to pick their battles carefully and marshal evidence to go to bat for a few things. One chemical company physician said: "Picking your battles is part of being a good politician. You can't fight or win them all, because you're perceived as constantly tilting at windmills as soon as you try to do that."

Company physicians face loyalty dilemmas that are invisible to them because they take the form of pragmatic self-censorship. They do not always try to persuade managers every time they see that something would be good for health, because they know it will not always succeed. Instead, they may simply drop such proposals without putting them forward or giving them serious consideration.

Shooting the Messenger

Professionals do not always side with their employers, but they are under pressure because they may be fired or frozen in the corporate hierarchy if they bring problems that may require a costly solution to their employer's attention and advocate expensive remedies. Professionals have reason to be skeptical of management's willingness to back up those who speak out based on their professional standards, because employers may indeed shoot the messenger.

Some managers insist that they want to be the first to know about any problem; they reward doctors for informing them about problems and punish those who do not. However, physicians who have tried to get management to recognize health problems and take action to solve them are often punished for bringing bad news to managers who decide that knowing about hazards creates problems for them. Company doctors seek to protect themselves by not telling managers what they do not want to hear, but they feel obligated from time to time to do just that, as happened with this physician who has worked for several companies:

> I'm always free to run things that come up several levels up the flagpole. One way to silence people is to say, "That's fine. Write it up in a memo, and then we'll look at it." Then you never hear about it further. That's the most benign way of stymieing things. Sometimes things are just not politically acceptable. They just tore one up and threw it in my face because of the liability. They said, "I just don't want to talk about this. Just forget it." It

wasn't a smoking gun. I was speculating and could have been wrong. They didn't want to hear about it and didn't want me to pursue it. I got the message.

A physician with a major pharmaceutical company said:

> Most large medical departments report to human resources, which is not a good reporting relationship, because they don't know the ins and outs of your program. They say, "Give me no waves, keep everything calm." You can't always do that in a workplace setting.

Management may consider a message from company doctors especially odious if they believe it really comes from resented government regulation. An oil company physician said:

> Because you often do things that the government tells corporations they have to do, you can be tarred with the same brush. It makes us look like we're just one of those regulators every time the government passes another law that you have to comply with. We're a necessary evil: "If we had our choice, we wouldn't have you. But no, the government makes us do these things, so I guess we have to have you around."

A doctor for a major oil company knew about a physician colleague who was terminated because he brought bad news to the company executives in the interest of protecting the company. He said that at the annual meeting the CEO said, "We don't shoot the messenger." The physician said, "They do say they don't shoot the messenger. *Normally* they don't."

Doctors feel threats to their security, even though most could go out into private practice and survive. A publishing company physician said:

> I don't want to go into private practice because it's hard out there with managed care and doctors in private practice are hurting. It's not the time. You always pick your time and your place when you want to make some pointed remarks. There's no sense rocking the boat at this stage of the game.

Such team-playing company physicians subdue their concerns about preventive health largely out of personal concerns about job insecurity and the effects on their career.

THE DEMISE OF EMPLOYMENT FOR LIFE

The career concerns and team-playing strategies of corporate professionals such as company doctors exist within the broader social context of declining corporate loyalty to employees. In most American workplaces, the bargain of the 1950s—that if you were loyal to the organization, the organization would be loyal to you—is far weaker today, or altogether absent. Professionals have agreed to be corporate employees, but where are the secure employment and the paternalism that employers have traditionally held out as their end of the bargain in exchange for employee loyalty? The contract has been altered as employers have responded to intensified competitive pressure and globalization.

Corporate departments (such as medical and safety departments) are being constricted and defunded. Whereas experienced employees were once especially valued, many companies now view them as a costly burden, seeing advantages in hiring new people at bargain prices. Corporate professionals recognize this diminished commitment to long-term employees, despite their employer's rhetoric to the contrary. When employers can vend out or eliminate entire operations, employees appear to have become little more than costly factors of production in employers' calculus. Slogans to the effect that "people are our most important asset" seem unconvincing when a company is reducing benefits and laying off workers.

Loyalty to the company has declined along with the company's loyalty to its employees. In the Depression and shortly thereafter, employees felt they needed to show they were loyal to their company and would avoid missing work at all costs—partly out of loyalty but also partly because of higher unemployment, greater desperation, and less extensive compensation for work absences. The pervasive sentiment now is that individuals must look out for themselves and cannot assume that their job will exist tomorrow, even if they work hard and appear committed to their employer.

Cutbacks and diminished loyalty also affect the welfare and morale of professionals. Corporate professionals who see downsizing and layoffs all around them increasingly do not expect employers to be loyal to them—and they are less loyal to their employers in return.[13] One long-term doctor with a strong public health background in a major computer company referred to the "backhanded indifference" managers have shown toward employees:

> Longtime employees are viewed as a millstone. Our implied contract of full employment and loyalty has been broken; the company's undergone a major change. My feeling is that people are not loyal to you, and you don't owe any loyalty to them either. Along with that major change comes the feeling that people are less important. Teamwork is less effective; people aren't as willing to sacrifice and do things for the corporation as they might be, unless it's out of fear—they desperately need the job.

Social and economic forces extending beyond the corporation have largely driven the change in loyalty. When competition intensifies and profit margins decline, managers in struggling U.S. corporations become persuaded that their employees are not cost-effective. They have traditionally sought to regain momentum by relying on layoffs, short-term remedies, and unilateral managerial decisions. Loyalty will always be a casualty of that process, which appears likely to continue.

Clearly the percentage of the workforce that does temporary, part-time, or contract work is high and growing (see Barker and Christensen 1998; Lester 1998; Tilly 1996; Abraham and Taylor 1996; Callaghan and Hartmann 1991; Plovika 1996). At the same time managerial mobility has increased as professional managers move from company to company to advance their careers, bolstered by MBA training and executive headhunter services. Significantly, increased job mobility and the demise of secure employment have markedly different effects on these two groups: it benefits many upwardly mobile professionals and managers, but it hurts lower-level or older workers with fewer job options.

The perspective of the CEO certainly affects how doctors treat workers' health. Priorities are set differently in more autocratic, hierarchical, or centralized corporations than in less autocratic environments. Many companies are highly sensitive to their company image and how the public views them. Companies that serve the public more directly (like Arco and IBM) have public personas that they avidly protect. A CEO's sense of noblesse oblige and long-standing support of employee programs boost company medicine. CEOs who believe workers are to be valued and respected are more likely than others to provide good benefits, be more responsive to employee and public concerns, and preserve services to workers during intensive cost-cutting. Their companies are quite different from those that have a hard-nosed, don't-give-an-inch style and view employee services grudgingly as a necessary favor—like the lunch counters of the past. The overall corporate culture thus facilitates or impedes employee programs. In a company culture that puts a priority on employee services and preventive health, professionals tend to have more influence.

Although the overall corporate culture affects whether the occupational medical program is beneficial or not, the medical department may not benefit from a favorable corporate culture without the CEO's support. It does not matter who the medical director is, or even if there is one, if senior leadership is not already persuaded that in-house medicine is good for employees or the business. A corporate medical director might spend years building up a program only to see a new CEO dismantle the whole department because "we're in the business of producing oil, not health care."

Increasing globalization is another force that tends to erode management's loyalty to employees. Community and labor organizations find it overwhelmingly difficult to curtail managerial prerogatives and to create alternative employment and environmental policies. (On globalization, see Schaeffer 1997; Barnet and Cavanagh 1994; Greider 1997; Madrick 1995; Thurow 1996.) Declining loyalty to employees and communities does not result from impersonal economic imperatives alone, however, but rather from deliberate managerial choices about how to respond to competitive conditions. Employers have chosen layoffs over other available policies and dismissed social costs as mere externalities when evaluating alternative courses of action.

CAREER PERILS FOR CORPORATE TEAM PLAYERS AND LOCATING BLAME IN A GLOBALIZING CORPORATE ECONOMY

As corporatization and globalization advance, many company professionals are losing their jobs and showing considerable anxiety. Having become accustomed to the corporate culture over many years, they anticipated retirement as they reached age fifty-five but have found themselves being eliminated instead. Companies may sometimes hire them back part-time as contractors, expecting them to generate support for their remaining time on their own. These once-protected in-house professionals must then market themselves outside the company in order to pay their own office rent. They have by necessity become transformed into self-promoting entrepreneurs set loose to sell themselves in a competitive marketplace.

In-house doctors who adopt a team player strategy often let themselves become complacent and their medical skills erode, thus making themselves vulnerable to replacement by competitive private consulting firms. Few are highly qualified professionals who would thrive in private practice, even if they could have done so in the past. For example, company physicians generally do not conduct research and publish, circulate much with outside professionals, or develop their clinical skills after years of corporate employment. The flip side of successful cultural adaptation is that it then makes reentry into the world of outside corporate medicine difficult or impossible. Professionals in corporations develop skills and ways of working that are not as useful outside the corporation. For many, the bargain they made has obviously not worked out in the new milieu.

Professionals generally respond to intensified career perils by becoming more avid corporate team players. But company doctors' strategy of being a team player and serving the company with great loyalty has partially backfired in terms of their own careers. In addition, their loyal team play in some ways has undercut their usefulness to their employer—such as when they testify and conduct research on behalf of the company and try to persuade management of their usefulness.

Credibility in Testimony and Research

Corporate physicians who testify in a regulatory agency or court carry an enormous burden, because their employment status can be seen as diminishing their credibility. Their usefulness to their employer becomes limited when their testimony at hearings is increasingly discredited.[14] A chemical company physician said:

Anytime someone starts defending a company, they're suspect. I have more credibility as a company spokesperson because I am a physician, but still, being a company spokesperson means that I'm immediately looked upon as suspect until I establish my own integrity in the situation and work my way through it. People attack your integrity if they don't like the message you bring. I've had my integrity attacked many, many times.[15]

A government physician who has worked in corporations and has heard a great deal of testimony by company physicians said:

A corporation commits hara-kiri when they get one of their own to testify. If I was their legal counsel, I would say, "We don't want these inside people. Get the big name at the university, who will come in and say what we want him to say or agree with us, but who isn't *one of us.*" Then people will say, "Look, he's not on any payroll. Sure he gets an expert-witness fee, but what he says arises from his own understanding, sometimes even his own research."

The reputation that many outside expert witnesses develop for being consistently on the employers' side damages their credibility. Some companies therefore seek favorable testimony from physicians who have a good scientific reputation but have rarely if ever testified. They hope that this lack of previous exposure will make such experts more credible. A physician in a large transportation company who has been made responsible for finding consultants who will testify in litigation on behalf of his employer had this to say:

I try to get the best physicians I can with the greatest credibility possible. And the other side tries to get the best doctors they can. We all tend to use the same people over and over. The doctors for both sides get to know each other after a while. The best doctors don't always like to testify in court. They like to make their living practicing medicine.

Companies increasingly seek university researchers to do their corporate studies because the public generally regards the findings of academics as more credible than those of company researchers (see, for example, Dembe 1996; Sheehan and Wedeen 1993; Jasanoff 1995). Particularly on sensitive topics, even large corporations with research capabilities are now likely to conclude that they should not do research themselves, lest they invest a great deal of money and still not be believed. One company, for example, discovered a statistically significant excess of kidney cancer in a broad cross-section of its employees. To determine whether company exposures were the cause, it contracted for a study from university researchers. Acknowledging the reduced credibility of in-house work, a physician involved in planning the case-control study said: "We, of course, contract out for that kind of work." Corporations still fund the research and programs, but having researchers from outside the corporation helps distance the companies from the results. An airline physician pointed to credibility problems for in-house staff evaluating radiation hazards from counterweights on the airplanes:

> We had to calculate how much risk people working on these weights had and then offer them appropriate reassurances or test them if we thought they had been exposed. We wanted to reassure the workers that it didn't require emergency procedures, but we didn't have enough credibility in the company, so we hired an outside health specialist to come over and consult with us so that she could say the things we'd been saying that the workers didn't believe.

A large pharmaceutical company bought another company that had dumped dioxin on horse trails, thereby killing horses, damaging the environment, and creating serious health risks. Company practices resulted in a major lawsuit and huge compulsory cleanup efforts in conjunction with the government (through the Superfund).[16] It cost millions of dollars to clean up the polluted areas. NIOSH conducted studies of the effects of dioxin on employee health, and company management considered doing its own parallel study but decided it was not worth the trouble. As a physician in the company explained:

> NIOSH and some other pharmaceutical companies came in here to find out whether our people were being protected. We thought about doing a duplicate sampling, but even if the company study was different, could we defend our study as the correct one, more trustworthy than NIOSH? It might seem we were trying to cover up and distort the facts. Doing our own study could undermine people's trust in the findings, and maybe it would create more problems than it would solve. It would have been hard to evaluate our study and theirs, one against the other.[17]

In addition to the career perils that physicians face when their corporate employment impedes their ability to conduct research and to testify credibly, physicians can present problems for employers by being too pliable, too accommodating, and even too agreeable in doing what they are told. A metals company physician and an occupational physician who has provided services to companies said:

> People respect fairness and objectivity. The worst behavior that a physician could engage in is acting in such a way that he's perceived to be a tool of management of the company and as making decisions based upon expediency. Yet physicians can be under intense pressure to do just that.[18]

> People in corporations say, "I hired a doctor, not another goddamn MBA. Why can't they just be doctors and say what doctors are supposed to say?" Even upper management still wants corporate physicians to be doctors. They criticize doctors because they have gone too far in trying to get upper management to accept them. You were hired as a physician, you are called "Doctor," they expect responsibility. So you lose something if you go too far.[19]

A physician who acknowledged that he lacks credibility with employees and the public said he could still take comfort in the respect of his physician colleagues:

> The discouraging things are the attitudes of the public—lack of credibility, bought man, company agent. Everybody knows I'm the company doctor. Once when I went to a meeting with our citizens' advisory group in Florida, one member got up and said, "Well, you're the company doctor. You're paid to do this." And I said, "I hope that you'll look at the evidence and disregard who pays me." The reward of this kind of work comes from being trusted and of having something to contribute that people think has value. My peers in major corporations call me a lot; and it makes me feel good when peers want to know what I think about things. Fifty docs call me up to ask my advice, and I call them. Nothing is more rewarding than the respect of your peers. That's the reward of the job.[20]

Nonetheless, team-playing corporate professionals who avoid giving bad news to managers do not help employers stay out of trouble. Those who practice this sort of professional loyalty simply undercut themselves as well as their usefulness to their employers.

Self-Blame and Selling Oneself to Management

Company professionals maintain that they must be able to sell themselves and their programs to management, as part of being effective team players. Those who learn to communicate their needs in managerial language, proving to finance people the value of what they do, enjoy a favorable reputation within their company. In the military those who successfully justify a program almost always get the resources to carry it out; the sales job is usually done at a high level, and an order comes down to all military units (comparable to a large corporation's manufacturing units) to comply with a specified number of dollars and personnel. In contrast, corporations typically require internal competition for resources, which entails a sales effort at all levels.

Professionals say that their company will decide not to use their services if they are not smart enough to show the company where they have saved money. While the legal, financial, and operating departments are considered indispensable, medical departments may not be. Physicians say they fail by hiding behind their professional expertise and feeling they deserve acceptance in the corporation without paying their dues as team members and learning enough about the corporate priorities and hierarchy to sell themselves successfully. Survival, from the professionals' perspective, thus hinges on how well they market their skills and their contribution to the company.[21] A metals company physician explained:

> I don't blame corporations for their decision to eliminate medical departments; I blame the medical people for not having shown management their value. I would blame myself if the medical department were eliminated tomorrow. Obviously I had not done a good enough job to be considered as valuable as some other function within the corporation.

Among company professionals, belief in the need to sell their own programs supports a belief that they themselves are responsible for their own limited power and resources in corporations. Like the automobile workers in Ely Chinoy's *Automobile Workers and the American Dream* (1992 [1955]), or the laid-off workers in Katharine Newman's *Falling from Grace* (1988), professionals tend to blame themselves for their plight. (On American values of loyalty, commitment, and the "American Dream," see Bellah et al. 1985; Sullivan 1995.) They believe their company has pared back in-house professionals because they themselves have not done a good enough job of selling management on the economic value of their services. By talking extensively about good communication and leadership skills, corporate professionals suggest that their programs were cut because they lacked those qualities; they may even suggest that certain organizational problems are the result of their own inadequate tactics or psychological deficiencies. Nevertheless, having grown up believing in the fairness of the system, they find it difficult to relinquish that faith. Thus, the American Dream survives even when it eludes them personally.

It is clear, however, that professional services are outsourced even when professionals communicate well. Downsizing has a force that overpowers personal characteristics. The current dynamics in American corporations are such that companies that are restructuring cut functions that appear peripheral to their business regardless of how compelling the professionals' personalities have been. Although many managers would say that they think the contributions of professionals are valuable, company decisions about cost-cutting tend to override such assessments.

Professionals cannot always find another job readily. Some who are fired set up consulting firms to try to do for other companies much of what they did for a single corporation, while others find jobs at least roughly comparable to their previous company job. For some, the opportunity to use their skills is difficult to come by.[22] Nevertheless, the impact of a layoff on a professional is seldom as serious as it is for a factory worker who is dismissed a few years before retirement age.

Many employers who praise professionals' performance in crises (such as handling a chemical leak or treating an executive suffering from a heart attack) still devalue routine programs in times of cutbacks. In addition, professionals who act skillfully may nevertheless find managers angry with them, not because they are poor salespeople but because they have failed to meet managers' expectations. Physicians, for example, can be criticized for not identifying company health hazards even though the corporate structure effectively discourages them from doing so. In such cases, despite the pattern of individual self-blame, it is the corporation and its management that create the conditions that cause the loyalty of team-playing professionals to backfire.

RESPONSES BY CORPORATE PROFESSIONALS AND EMPLOYEES

In general, professionals who want to do a good job, behave ethically, and protect employees and the public find themselves in an isolated and vulnerable position. Employees with a grievance against the company can turn to their union, but few corporate professionals belong to unions, and most of them have nowhere to turn for effective solutions to serious problems that the employer will not remedy. They are in a conflicted position, for example, if they know that company processes are dangerous but that management will not spend the money necessary to take effective preventive steps.

Some companies have established internal mechanisms—such as quality circles or ombudspersons—intended to allow individuals more freedom to express their views.[23] However, corporate professionals recognize that they risk offending management by providing information about work hazards to internal committees, unions, or the government, because it will usually be clear where the information comes from. They find it difficult to protest company policies even when the employer has procedures for reporting errors, illegal activity, and unethical conduct. A physician in a conglomerate described the ineffectiveness of reporting even major problems to people inside the company:

> It's common in large organizations to have an ombudsman people can call to report ethical violations, but reporting within the company to an ethics committee never gets anywhere. I used to get involved in those types of things. You get all these anonymous tips because people usually don't give their names out of fear. You have nothing to substantiate them, and you're still stymied: What will you do with this information? Will you prove it right?

Overall, empowerment and participative management programs have somewhat improved corporations as workplaces. But compared with the sectoral shifts in the U.S. economy that constrict employment options and the corporate structures that limit the power of professionals relative to employers, their impact is largely symbolic. In addition, recourse for those who wish to report ethics violations and protection for corporate whistleblowers are limited.

Corporate Whistleblowers

Although corporate professionals generally are not encouraged to bring costly problems to management's attention, when they do and are rebuffed, they can make an outside entity—such as their professional organization or state regulatory agencies—aware of them. Whistleblowers frequently are not disgruntled marginal employees but rather people in quality control, health and safety, and other parts of companies whose job is to identify problems and address them. They blow the whistle when they think the organization is responding inadequately to a problem that it has a responsibility to solve (see Rothschild and Miethe 1999; Glazer and Glazer 1989). But most corporate professionals do not blow the whistle when they find major hazards in corporations. They know that whistleblowers have suffered retribution in the past and that managers have kept them out of the informational loop after concluding that they are not reliable team players—that is, persons who solve business problems as managers define them.

Physicians rarely act like an organized rank-and-file employee when they protest company policies.[24] Instead, they may defend their position by saying, "As a physician, I find this policy unethical"—a means of protesting employer actions that is unavailable to regular employees. Physicians at university clinics who see employees become advocates who support union demands and provide technical expertise for unions more often than corporate doctors, largely because they are more detached from corporate control and generally freer. They more often report hazards to OSHA or state health departments on their own volition relative to company physicians, who are more constrained by their employment status. Adverse economic conditions for their employer exacerbate their lack of recourse.

Some physicians who believe that their past actions were ineffective in response to health or environmental hazards admit feeling guilty about their limited or failed efforts, as did one doctor who described blowing the whistle on a submarine hazard years ago. The doctor discovered the submarine risks because people confided in him when he was on-site. After his whistleblowing, operations shut down for a week, but management did not want to take further action. He said:

> When I was first with the company years ago, I truly was a whistleblower on an unsafe submarine program we had. I went to the division president, who acted as the judge and convened an investigation into unsafe procedures and shut down the operation for a week, then brought in all the people to give their versions. Everybody who needed to covered their butt, and finally everything was whitewashed. The decision was, "Operations start tomorrow morning at seven A.M. We'll ensure that checklists are always used." Nobody was shot at dawn, nobody was drummed out of the corps. They weren't demoted or fined, and the good guys didn't get any promotions out of it. It just sorted people out so everybody knew who was on what side, so to speak. The bad guys continued in their role. It went right to the top of the division. I lost a lot of respect for that individual [the division president] after it was over. But he must have had significant pressures on him to keep the program going and keep everybody happy.

People were angry at him for causing trouble, as they saw it, and he felt isolated. And though he remained confident that he "did the right thing," he assumed a quieter role after he saw that his whistleblowing had little effect on company practices. After he retired from the company, he learned that a citizens' medical organization was sponsoring a committee to investigate his former employer for creating environmental hazards. He called to volunteer for that committee but was rejected because of his possible bias. Though disappointed, he recognized his continuing loyalty to the company:

> I would have found that investigating committee intellectually stimulating and could have gotten a lot of guilt over my work in the company off my back. But then, since I still have stock in my retirement plan, my retirement income down the road will go down if their stock goes down. So that definitely is a conflict. You feel loyal once you've worked there. And of course, I still have a good close relationship with a lot of the executives and baseline workers there, so I do have emotional ties—can't get away from it.

Generally the higher their position in the corporate hierarchy the more corporate professionals believe they can influence company policies. Those who are vice presidents, for example, have a forum different from the one available to those who report to a second-level employee relations manager who reports to a vice president. When upper management tells them to go out and look for or resolve problems, professionals with entire units reporting to them have more flexibility and resources. But even some who have a high-level position in a large corporation are not consulted on important company matters.

Self-Policing and Ethics Violations

It's up to us in the profession to set standards and maintain quality.

—Oil company physician

If their employer refuses to take remedial measures, company physicians can report exposure hazards to their professional organization, ACOEM. Despite ACOEM's pronouncements of physician loyalty to patients and the fact that its members may confidentially counsel individual physicians, company doctors with complaints about improper practices have had little real help from this and other professional organizations. ACOEM's ethics board has not imposed sanctions on physicians for following their employer's directives or formally censured them for ethics violations, even when serious injury or breaches of confidentiality have been involved.[25] A physician who served on the ACOEM ethics committee said:

> Normally we use the code of ethics as our basis when somebody brings a particular problem to the ethics committee saying, "A member of your organization is doing this, and we think it's wrong, and we'd like your opinion." The ACOEM ethics committee uses the ethics code to make a decision, but I haven't been impressed with what happens after we make a decision. You have to wonder, what's the use of having a code as an organization if nothing happens to an individual who you think broke it? That's the point we're at now.

An ACOEM member physician who knew about a suspected ethical violation brought the matter before the organization's ethics committee. A committee member said:

This was a clear violation of something we found in the code, and the committee of about ten people unanimously agreed that something should be done about it, which is pretty rare. I assumed we would get rid of the person or at least punish him publicly for doing something so bad for so long. We recommended to the judiciary committee that they should look into it and do something about it, but because this person was a well-known old boy in the system, the board of directors decided to just do away with the judiciary committee. Now there is no punitive function left. We were overruled, and the person is still acting in violation of the code. We on the ethics committee were all stunned, as were some of the board of the directors, but clearly a deal had been cut somewhere. Everybody had known the person as a friend or socially for a long time. Nobody wanted to take it on. It is awkward in a situation like that. But to allow people to remain when they have clearly violated what everybody else expects members to live up to is a mistake. If no one will do anything, then you don't stand for anything, and being on the ethics committee is a farce because we waste our time spinning our wheels. And why do it if the code of ethics is a farce?[26]

Millman (1977, 97–119; 1981) analyzes a similar pattern with medical mortality review boards, describing the functioning of these boards as "a cordial affair" that shields fellow professionals from repercussions for their actions and seldom sanctions them. Company doctors rarely punish deviance among their own. Nevertheless, corporate physicians, like other professional groups, argue that they can best police themselves. (On the professional self-regulation of lawyers, for example, see Arnold and Kay 1995; Devlin 1994; Gallagher 1995.)

IN-HOUSE WORK AND THE PROBLEM OF "INDEPENDENT" CONTRACTORS

Much of the literature on professionals and general intuitions about direct employer control would lead us to expect that in-house doctors would be more malleable and compliant with employer demands than doctors who work for multiple employers but otherwise do much of the same work day to day as conventional company doctors. However, a closer look at in-house professionals and contractors results in some surprising findings regarding loyalty and independence.

Company doctors themselves maintain that employers who outsource their medical departments to cut costs face pitfalls because outside vendors are less loyal than in-house physicians, who know the company and can perform the services better. It may be false economy, they argue, for employers to focus on the money they save by paying contract physicians only for a limited number of hours. As an airline physician said:

> Supervisors know us and talk to us face to face daily and sometimes hourly, so they trust us more when talking about a particular patient's medical problem than they would when talking to some physician they may never see or hear from again. They are much more willing to believe us and accept our judgment that an employee cannot work than the judgment of a fee-for-service vendor who has fifteen contracts with other airlines and no particular interest in us.

Employees see benefits to having doctors from outside the company because they are treated by someone who may be more objective, freer to give an independent opinion, or less stigmatized in their eyes than the company doctor. That may be worth a great deal, but either way the company pays and typically retains control over services. A contracting doctor who has also worked as an in-house physician said:

> An outside contractor can be more independent. We are not employees of the companies, which gives us a lot more leeway. I still feel at times that employees see me as a company doc. When push comes to shove and I have to tell somebody that they can't go back to work when they want to, or if I won't put them off work when they want, then I get the distinct feeling that they think I do this as a company representative. I've never liked that, but it goes with the territory. When I say, "I'm not an employee of the company," they say, "Yeah, doc, but who pays you?" (*laughter*) The distinction *is* a fine one.

From the perspective of physicians, contractors may be able to arrange better job security for themselves than physicians working for one company. Two doctors who provide contract services to companies said:

> After I left the company because they were going down the tubes, I made up my mind that I would never tie myself to one industry or depend upon one source of revenue for the practice. So I set out with forethought to put

together a group of clients, and over the years we lost some and gained others, and it worked out. It's given us a wider base of support to fall back on.[27]

Financially I'm better off as a contract physician than with a company. I don't have to worry that they'll fire me; or if they do fire me, I only lose an account, not my total livelihood. In a corporation the stakes are different.

Although corporate professionals have lost autonomy, contractors who take on what in-house physicians had done are not truly independent. Many of them start out with small-to-medium-size company clients, and then their desire for better cash flow and greater security leads them to seek bigger companies that buy larger blocks of their time. They scramble for business and sometimes are less aware of their professional obligations than in-house doctors. Three physicians who have provided medical services for companies said:

As a consultant, you have a lot of leeway to say anything you want—especially if you don't want to be paid again.

Consultants get into the same routine as an in-plant doctor. They get sucked into cost containment, supervising nurses, attending safety committee meetings, doing some glad-handing and routine stuff rather than being given carte blanche to get involved in the company. Some are exceptions who gain rapport and start to do more. But by and large, corporate consultants have not done anything more than the older breed of corporate physicians thus far, and they don't have much more influence—they're just happier.

Most people in practice [as contractors] feel that to keep customers they must be more compliant, which means providing services they think are not medically indicated, or not providing services they think are medically indicated, because it's the client's wish. It's driven by competition.[28]

One contracting doctor lost his biggest corporate client, and considerable income, for not doing what the client demanded:

We've done this contracting work now for fifteen years and nobody ever fired our group, but we've had some companies go belly up and I've fired a company in effect. I removed my physicians from a situation in which a sizable client blatantly tried to get us to shade opinions and put people back to work before we felt they should go back. We didn't do it, and it took us about two years to make up for that major loss financially. But it made me feel good (*laughter*).

Another contractor lost half his business when he published an article about an electronics industry hazard, because employers saw him as no longer trustworthy. He stated:

> When I started talking about health issues in the semiconductor industry, I began losing clients in private practice, and I had to calculate how many other kinds of clients I'd have to get to keep the practice alive. That's the way they play hardball. I imagine a lot of things ran through their minds: "What does he know about us? He's been taking care of our patients. Has he compiled data?" Many of them asked me if I had files.

Both these professionals experienced great pressures as contractors to set aside professional standards. In some ways so-called independent contractors may be company doctors as well—in the sense that they may be at least as dependent on the companies that employ them as in-house professionals. Physicians in the private sector under contract to companies must earn their fees; their work will disappear if they cannot recognize and provide what corporate management wants. This fact of life is ignored in much of the literature on professionals, which sees in-house professionals as captive and contractors as largely independent of corporate influence. (For a discussion of occupational physicians inside and outside corporations, see Walsh 1987; Jacobs 1995.)

The Puzzle of Corporate Cutbacks

Many large corporations pare back or eliminate their medical departments even though doctors try to persuade management that having physicians in-house saves the company money in lawsuits, regulatory violations, workers' compensation claims, and lost productivity. The fact that some employers are shrinking their medical departments suggests that they are unconvinced that having physicians on staff cuts costs. In-house staff expenses are harder to control than contract services, which companies can easily cut. In addition, the medical department has always been considered a service unit rather than a line or operational unit that makes money; medical services tend to be targeted for outplacement when management perceives that they are too costly a burden. An oil company physician and a physician who directs an occupational medicine program said:

> Companies are not necessarily cutting down on the program, but this corporation, like many others, doesn't seem to care what you spend on contract services as long as company employees aren't doing the work and it doesn't cost people in the company.
>
> Medical services do not generate income. Although it may cost as much or slightly more to outplace, it comes out of a different pocket. They reduce a salary slot. That looks good and indicates tight management.[29]

However, the cost factor does not entirely explain the outsourcing of medical services, because some corporations know that contract services are not necessarily less expensive than having in-house physicians.[30] Among the other factors at work are a changing marketplace, corporate culture, the expanding supply of contractors, and employers' interest in spreading liability. Having contractors share liability with in-house professionals may insulate companies from their own employees' decisions. In this view, corporate professionals themselves are in a sense to blame for their own decline because they present too great a legal risk. Although employers may still be held liable for contractors' work, they are correct in believing that they are likely to reduce their overall legal liability by shifting to outside contractors.

Issues of control also affect corporate decisions about whether to retain or farm out medical functions. Employers who can afford it may believe that having in-house doctors enables them to control situations better. In contrast, managers who eliminate in-house medical departments often believe that outsourcing gives them more control. An oil company doctor said: "Some of our managers would like to outsource medical because they think it would give them more control and get around them dealing with us."

Another reason employers eliminate medical departments involves corporate turf. Other units, such as security or safety, may covet the medical department's resources for services like acute care or drug testing. In addition, corporate managers may see other difficulties with having a medical department. A doctor who worked in an oil company said:

> Medical departments are perceived as creating problems. If we didn't have doctors who treated people and listened to people's stories and said, "Oh, yeah, that's work-related," maybe no one would complain about it. One refinery manager here said to me in a meeting, "Most of us come from small refineries, and we notice that refineries that don't have clinics have fewer injuries."[31]

Fewer reported injuries does not necessarily mean fewer actual injuries, however. Smaller companies are less likely to have sophisticated health programs and reporting practices. In addition, employees in companies that use only contract physicians may decide not to report an injury, such as a strained back, because it would mean having to make a trip downtown to the clinic; they may choose simply to try to recover on their own instead.

Greater professionalization and higher aspirations for what they can accomplish in corporations also make company physicians less malleable. Medical departments have in some ways always been a thorn in the side of management. The new breed of company doctors may be especially threatening because of their expertise and concerns about confidentiality and ethical standards; they may appear less likely to be team players than the former family practitioners or military physicians. Problems of physician loyalty thus help explain the trend toward replacing in-house physicians with contract physicians.

CONCLUSION

It is important to recast the problem of professionals in corporations. As we have seen, professionalism and corporatization are not always opposing pressures. Professionals are in fact gaining and losing power in corporations at the same time.

To some extent, occupational medicine is becoming more professionalized and the quality is improving, even in smaller companies that hire part-time physicians instead of big in-house staffs. As corporate physicians become more professionally oriented and better trained, larger companies more often rely on their expertise—as is economically reasonable to do once employers spend the money to hire professionals. Employers who are aware of a higher level of specialization now sometimes seek out people with training in occupational medicine or even board certification in the field. The field of occupational medicine is growing in universities—more conference papers are being presented and the caliber of research has risen—and some physicians have been trying to upgrade the profession.[32] This professionalization also encourages doctors to advocate for worker health and do so more competently.

At the same time, however, current economic and social pressures in some respects work against the professionalization of physicians in corporations. Corporate and legal pressures wrest important professional decisions away from doctors and put them in the hands of corporate management and the courts. In-house doctors are under increasing pressure not to advocate for employee health but rather to serve the employer's needs by containing health costs, reducing employee benefits, reporting fewer illnesses, and avoiding liability for disease. Thus, even as occupational medicine is becoming more professionalized, there is rising pressure on corporate physicians, whether in-house or outside the company, to comply with managers' wishes, which are often in conflict with employees' interests and preventive health practices.

—— Chapter 3 ——

VIP Health Versus Eliminating the Thorn in the Side of Management

Any honest medical director in a Fortune 500 company will tell you that his or her capacity to survive or thrive is highly dependent on personal relationships with senior executives and their function as the executive's personal physician or advocate.

—Chemical company physician

Some corporate managers and supervisors . . . send trouble-makers to the medical department to see if they are psychiatrically or physically sick. They like it that way, because they don't want to fire somebody as a troublemaker, but they can get somebody out who has an illness.

—Chemical company physician

MANAGERS OFTEN SEND to company physicians those employees whom management otherwise considers a problem—the individuals who are, in one doctor's words, "a thorn in the side" of management. When physicians screen these individuals, they routinely turn information about their health over to management; in contrast, they generally guard information about *executives'* health carefully in what I call VIP health care in the workplace.

Physicians and managers have sought medical explanations for troublesome employee conduct as well as for accidents and absenteeism. In doing so, physicians have helped medicalize managerial problems. At the same time they have also cooperated with management in demedicalizing legitimate medical concerns by, for instance, focusing on psychological explanations for the health effects of chemical exposure.

REMOVING THE THORN IN MANAGEMENT'S SIDE

Managers will sometimes send people they view as troublemakers to the medical department for evaluation in the hope that doctors can discover some medical, drug, or psychological problem. These individuals include whistleblowers and union activists, people who attempt to uncover health hazards, individuals who miss work or who are involved in accidents, and people they simply do not like. They tell doctors they suspect a problem and want it diagnosed, sometimes with the implied request to recommend removal of the employee from the workplace. (Managers who have a role in determining the physician's pay raises and promotion can exert particularly heavy pressure of this sort.) A physician from a large metals corporation said:

> Everybody will go out of his or her way to accommodate an employee who's well liked who has an impairment, but plant managers look for an expeditious way to get rid of an individual who is a thorn in management's side. A time-honored way to do that is for the individual to be considered disabled and unable to return to work, and of course the physician is the mechanism by which that happens. That's probably the most common source of pressure from management for a plant physician. Management sends the person in for a consultation and an opinion from the physician as to whether that person is fit for work, with or without work restrictions. It's very evident that the person is a thorn in management's side by their reluctance to accommodate him.[1]

Employers use the doctor's evaluation to determine—or justify—whether employees should be prevented from returning to their normal duties. Permitting employees to remain at work with certain restrictions does not solve the supervisor's or employer's problem. If the medical department identifies a drug or psychological problem or disease, they may recommend that the person be sent out on disability. Their recommendations also may result in the worker's termination.

Employees are sometimes sent to a psychiatrist or psychologist because managers claim that they have problems with authority or cannot get along with fellow employees—behaviors that leave considerable room for interpretation. Managers' use of physicians to label and remove troublesome employees is similar to the treatment of people considered deviant or troublemaking as psychologically or medically sick in the former Soviet Union, where dissidents sometimes were imprisoned in mental hospitals. (On Soviet physicians, see Field 1957, 1966; on deviance and medicalization, see Simpson and Simpson 1999; Fox 1977; Conrad and Schneider 1992.) Assessing an employee's alleged psychological problem presents a particularly difficult case for a physician when people who have an interest in getting rid of the person present the evidence. As a physician with a major chemical corporation commented:

> People whom management doesn't like, whether they are troublemakers or have performance problems, are sometimes sent over to us to evaluate. That's called Russian psychiatry: you're sick if you're a troublemaker. That's the way psychiatry is used in some cultures: you're sick if you're a dissident or if you disagree with the party line.

Some company physicians conduct or supervise psychological testing designed to reduce theft, pilfering, absenteeism, and safety hazards. Employers often direct these tests at particular groups, such as security officers and employees with access to restricted areas. They also test those they consider "problem employees." A union health official said:

> One mine instituted a very sophisticated policy of screening applicants in an area of the country where the union historically is very strong. They screened people out using psychological testing and they brought in families for interviews. They wanted to make certain that people were not going to be voting for the union. It has been very successful. They have kept the union out.[2]

Management also uses doctors to try to find a psychological explanation for physical or behavioral symptoms that workplace chemical exposure may cause. These psychological analyses deflect attention from workplace exposure hazards. As a doctor who performs psychological assessments of many such workers from the chemical industry and other industries said:

> We see cases of people who fall under the rubric of multiple chemical sensitivities. They have seen many other doctors, and some doctors say, "This is an immunologic disorder." Others say, "This seems hysterical." Invariably they get to a psychiatrist to try to piece out what might be going on unconsciously to cause them to have these various sensitivities.

An example of the demedicalizing of health hazards is the dismissal of workers' complaints of medical symptoms from chemical exposures as merely "psychogenic illness."[3] Here is how an airline physician psychologized workers' medical complaints:

> Many times the employee and company disagree on whether the worker can go to work because of an issue that is not even related to their job that they are unable or unwilling to deal with. It may be a very significant personal thing in their lives or in their past history that may never have surfaced before. We're trying to make a better person. Then they will automatically become a better employee because they become more productive and dependable, whereas in the past they may have hidden behind a lot of medical disorders.

Employers also call in psychiatrists to evaluate whether a person's claim of repetitive motion injury is psychological or malingering. A psychiatrist who evaluates many workers for employers defended his practice of identifying employees who claim physical injuries from work as malingerers, an assessment that supports employers' interests:

> We see claims of repetitive motion injuries involving some question about whether this person is exaggerating their symptoms or trying to get out of a work situation for some other reason. The supervisor or the person's shift changed so that a working mother who comfortably arranged child care is now put on swing shift where she can't get a baby-sitter, and within a week ends up developing symptoms that allow her to leave that work setting for a time.[4]

Sometimes managers reprimand workers who go outside the company for medical care or advice about symptoms that may be work-related. By viewing such action as insubordination rather than as a legitimate physical complaint, management *demedicalizes* legitimate medical concerns.

Employees can go to the medical department voluntarily, but supervisors have the right to order employees to go there to determine whether a medical issue has contributed to performance problems. Physicians know that when an employee arrives by supervisory referral, he or she is considered a "thorn in the side" of management. As a physician for a chemical company said: "Some corporate managers and supervisors unfortunately like to use the medical department as the way to get people out of the company instead of dealing with performance."

Of course, employers do not need to go through doctors in order to fire an employee. As a textile union official said: "They have plenty of other ways to finger people and blacklist them, get rid of them, harass them. Employers don't have to question supervisors' loyalty, whereas with doctors they do."[5]

Nevertheless, managers often ask company doctors to examine employees for behavior problems that may in fact reflect managerial inadequacy. A physician for a major chemical company said:

> It's not always crystal clear whether the manager or the subordinate is the problem. There might be a psychoemotional component, but it's unusual to have a prominent medical component—the guy doesn't need pills or anything like that. Managers refer people to medical after their failure to confront and deal with a bad practice that gets totally out of control. It's a management issue, and it happens all the time. It's like attendance, which is a management issue and not a health issue.[6]

Company doctors sometimes help employers remove employees whose union activities prove troublesome. A union official who assisted with one case said:

> The company wanted to get rid of [the employee] because he was head of the health and safety committee and caused the company a problem as a union activist. Somebody who's entirely healthy could also suddenly get sent to the company doctor, who pulls something out of thin air. That's clearly unethical and a reach, but some companies might go that far with doctors willing to put their basic practice on the line by playing that game. The usual scenario is that the company just decides the worker's condition

is serious enough that he shouldn't go back to work at all, whereas other people with similar injuries are doing the job quite well.[7]

Employees have better protection in unionized workplaces, especially when the company tries to get rid of a worker through a psychological determination. An official with the United Steelworkers of America said:

> The removal of somebody based on a psychological evaluation as opposed to their behavior is a pretty easy grievance to win. If somebody hits somebody in the workplace or goes after somebody with a club or takes off all their clothes and pretends they want to do a high dive into a ladle of hot metal, then that's behavior. But if there's nothing like that in the background and no infraction of the rules, and somebody is just sent for an evaluation and the doctor says the person is schizophrenic or delusional or paranoid, then we won't lose that case.[8]

Nonetheless, whether or not employees are represented by unions, managers and doctors often cooperate in removing employees from the workplace. This is part of a more general process by which doctors help solve managerial problems and limit their health and employment costs.

DISABILITY COPS

Employers expect company physicians to testify, advise them, and submit evidence on the causes of occupational illnesses in order to determine the health care and benefits that sick employees are entitled to receive under workers' compensation. Company physicians' decisions about assigning risk help determine who must pay the costs of occupational disease, including medical bills, lost work time, unemployment, and custodial care.

Physicians frequently testify as to whether an employee's illness is due to work or to non-work-related causes. For example, a person may have lung scarring either from on-the-job asbestos exposure or from smoking. Whether the disease is due to workplace hazards and therefore compensable by the company is important to the employer. Those who testify for the employer on workers' compensation claims generally know that their job is to try to find a non-occupational cause for a worker's ailment and to provide a judgment that would serve the company's interest. Although it can be difficult to determine medically what exactly caused an employee's disease, employers in many cases rely on physicians to defend their corporation by testifying that the workplace could not possibly have caused a disease. Corporate physicians rarely take the plaintiff's side or argue that specific chemicals are so hazardous that they require stricter regulation. In the absence of firm evidence, pressure from employers and company attorneys inclines them to downplay the effect of occupational exposure in causing disease. Company physicians identify workers they perceive to be high-risk or deviant; they refer to themselves and other company doctors as "rub-out artists" who help managers get rid of employees by showing that their health problems are not due to the workplace. Many in-house physicians who testify in workers' compensation cases say they feel strong pressure from their employer to prove that the illnesses of workers are not work-related. Some physicians say that their predecessors in the company job were fired or had left because they did not adapt well to that pressure.

Managers expect company physicians to police illness and disability claims and to try to bring individuals back to work. They expect physicians to identify which workers are "gaming the system," manipulating disability claims in order to stay off work. Company doctors claim to use objective criteria in deciding whether to send people back to work. They often say that reassigning injured workers to lighter duties rather than sending them home is in the best interest of both the employee and the company. Nonetheless, the dependence of doctors on their employers for their salaries can limit their ability to diagnose people and advise on disability claims objectively.

Filing a claim against a company can be expensive for a worker, who may also risk being barred from employment elsewhere. Two physicians, with a chemical and a utility company, respectively, described their attempts to persuade employees not to file workers' compensation claims:

> I tell people, "There are better ways to go through life than lining yourselves up with lawyers and having negative opinions about the company that you work for. Get on with your life and do something positive." I see

these people who are completely consumed by getting back at the company, and they are miserable. I feel sorry for anybody who gets mired in this whole workers' compensation mess. The lawyers end up getting most of the money anyway. And they are not giant sums of money, especially considering the amount of energy it takes to go after it.

I try to talk patients out of filing workers' comp cases, because I know the dynamic, what the payoff and time commitment will be and what it will do to them. They may have trouble getting another job. I try to make it clear to them that workers' compensation is the last-ditch desperation protection. There are a lot of other answers. I say, "I don't think you want to do this. Let's see if we can work somehow within the bureaucracy." I still have to sign off on a lot of them. It's not a good system.

Company doctors complain about workers taking advantage of time off and disability benefits. Here are three representative comments from airline, aerospace, and telecommunications company doctors, respectively:

Employees tend to take advantage of the system as much as they possibly can. Sending someone home rather than keeping them at the work site is definitely in the interest of the patient, but it may not be in the interest of the company. We sometimes find ourselves between a rock and a hard place. Our hope and goal is that whatever is in the employee's best interest is also in the company's best interest. We do everything we can in our power to minimize the number of lost workdays.

You don't have the same degree of satisfying patient-doctor relationship as in private practice. It tends to be an inherent adversarial relationship, and you have to constantly be on the alert for people just trying to get out of work or establishing phony claims.[9]

I don't like trying to be a policeman; that's not why I got into medicine. People have very generous sick time and workers' comp time in our company. Some people are legitimately sick for a long time, but some stay out for as long as they can get away with it.

Company physicians either initiate or go along with their employer's policy of getting rid of or refusing to hire workers who have already filed claims. That hurts employees' ability to work and leads to long-term disability. An occupational physician who works with company doctors on evaluating employees' disabilities said:

An injured worker who gets involved in a workers' compensation battle is labeled a troublemaker, and the company would rather get rid of that person than find him a new job. Instead, the employer puts him on disability and then terminates him after the disability benefits run out. Even if I clear him medically to return to some form of work, management makes no attempt to find another job for him.

Employers sometimes have doctors outside the company serve much the same function as in-house doctors: evaluating an employee's fitness for work, reviewing qualifications for long-term disability or workers' compensation benefits, and assessing drug abuse or behavioral problems. Companies can choose which doctor they want to rely on for opinions about health effects, especially when the evidence is ambiguous. Their economic interest is to avoid using a doctor with a reputation for giving high estimates of occupational health hazards. The need for physician testimony has spurred the growth of an entire industry of medical-legal physicians. In litigated disability cases, the plaintiff and the defendant company typically line up medical experts to testify before workers' compensation judges. These experts are usually pitted against each other in testifying about return-to-work issues, vocational rehabilitation benefits, need for modified duty, or the work-relatedness of the injury or disease. In third-party liability cases, the two sides hire their doctors to prove their case; lawyers clearly do not pick these doctors randomly. The doctors are largely predictable. One set of doctor says, "Exposure and the onset of disease have a reasonable association," and the doctors opposed to them say, "It hasn't been proven yet." An auto company doctor said:

It's generally known within the industry which doctor is known as a rub-out artist. It's someone who is hired to kill the case and get the claim denied. They will say that this person's ailment is the result of something other than the workplace, or say there are no physical findings for it.

A railroad physician who gives about twenty-five depositions a year said:

In most of our cases that go to court, the men could work if they were motivated to work, and I'll testify to that fact: "Based on the medical information I have, this man could do this job if he wanted to. I will let him come back to work if his doctor releases him." So I put it back on his doctor. If his doctor releases him with restrictions, I'll have a work-capacity evaluation done on him and still let him come back to work with specific restrictions. Every city we operate in has doctors and attorneys for the plaintiff who will say and do anything. When I get a report from particular doctors, I don't believe a word they say because they just say what the lawyer wants him to say.

Company physicians testify at congressional and regulatory hearings as well as in lawsuits regarding corporate medical liability. They have testified on exposure standards for benzene, vinyl chloride, sulfur dioxide, cotton dust, and on basic OSHA risk evaluations. With few exceptions, they defend their corporations or advocate government standards that require personal protective devices instead of more costly engineering controls. The Labor Department hearing transcripts include examples of doctors testifying for companies at public evidentiary hearings on setting standards. An OSHA official said:

> Doctors argue the case of whoever employed them. Companies that employ physicians employ them to say that a substance is not as dangerous as OSHA thinks it is. A lot of physicians who testify for companies think that the rules and regulations that we promulgate are totally unnecessary. I think the doctors believe what they say, but sometimes companies pay them very well to do that.

Company doctors and employers rely on outside doctors to make fitness determinations. If an outside physician says that an employee can work, the company doctor may then allow that person to work, even if his clinical judgment suggests that the employee is at increased risk and should not go back to work. Outside doctors are sometimes unwilling to sign documents supporting their decisions about an employee's fitness, however, because they then may be liable for that employee's actions. A publishing company physician said:

> Some decisions are hard to make, such as when people take legal medications that may impair their attentiveness and reaction time. For example, drivers for our circulation trucks who take medication for a legitimate physical condition have to deliver a truckload of newspapers to various stops in the early morning hours when it's dark and rainy. The question arises: Are they safe to drive, or do they endanger themselves or anybody else? Typically under those circumstances we request the treating physi-

cians to make that statement in writing: "Do you think that this man can drive this truck doing these kinds of duties at this hour of the day, taking this medicine with his condition? Doctor, sign the piece of paper." If the doctor signs, we accept the doctor's opinion because he sees the patient. If the individual has an accident and it becomes a matter of record through subpoena, that doctor will have to defend his decision. If the doctor's unwilling to sign it, then we may well limit the duties of the individual based on safety.[10]

Company physicians frequently say that private physicians have an economic bias to do whatever the patient wants, or whatever will make the most money, such as treating a continuing disability. Private physicians therefore are willing to exaggerate workplace hazards to accommodate their patients' desire for disability leave or other company benefits. Company doctors challenge private doctors who support workers' claims and say they misread test results and facilitate employees' illegitimate absences from work. A doctor with a large metals and mining company that uses 1,500 local doctors around the country to evaluate employees said:

How do you deal with chronic absenteeism and a fellow who keeps coming in with excuse slips from local doctors? We periodically run across physicians who have become an excuse-slip factory. We simply approach them professionally, which works for a little bit, and then they are back into the same thing again.

An electronics company physician said:

We have doctors in the community who are a real black eye to medicine. I call them "medical prostitutes." They are very biased in how they approach the patient and always blame the employer and make it look like the employer has purposefully done something negative to the patient. They may perceive us as just the hired gun of the company, but it's not true. I always make the best decision for the patient, and I don't consider expense. They think they do the patients a favor by giving them a month off for a hangnail. Time and time again they just give people an inordinately long time off that costs society a lot of money and costs patients a lot too, because most don't get their full salary during that nonproductive time, and eventually the employees get a reputation for needlessly missing a lot of time, and it hurts their career.

While criticizing private physicians, however, company doctors tend to minimize the effect of economic motivation on their own decisions, even as they proceed to demedicalize employees' medical complaints.

VIP HEALTH

Physicians are obligated to declare employees fit or unfit for work. This obligation, however, does not always extend to executives. Whereas physicians who screen workers routinely turn over the information to management, in general they carefully guard information about the health of executives, creating what could be called VIP health care in the workplace. Occupational physicians say they know of few examples in which company doctors have released adverse health information about an executive to management, even when it might be the right thing to do or the best way to protect the company. On the other hand, their evaluations routinely hamper the careers and employability of lower-level workers who may be at increased risk for future problems. A chemical company doctor said that in evaluating risk to employees, he considers whether they are higher or lower in the company hierarchy:

> Physical workers who lift, push, and pull aren't much of a problem. I would say, "Let's take him out of work exposure to hepatotoxic chemicals and put him in another kind of work." Somebody who is lower in the hierarchy *is* more readily exchangeable and the company hasn't made a huge commitment. But you expect senior officers who go to the Far East for three to five years to have a tremendous effect on the company. If I know that an executive who is being considered for a new assignment has a problem but is doing okay today, I do not recall my ever having interceded to disrupt that promotion.

A financial services company physician who routinely screened employees said he was known for keeping the health risks of executives absolutely confidential:

> When I know an executive has a cardiac or neurotic problem or whatever problem but is ready to move up into a job with more responsibility, travel, pressure, and tension, my job is to persuade him to allow me, as his

advocate, to go to the person he reports to and explain that he could do that work but that certain accommodations have to be made, and what the reason is for them. I'd keep my mouth shut if he said no, even if I knew that he was heading for serious trouble.

A conglomerate physician and a chemical company physician emphasized the importance of keeping executive health information absolutely confidential:

We deal with the CEO and the top three or four layers of the company. Men in corporate America do not have many places they can open up to talk, but people will come to talk if an in-house physician develops a relationship like a mother superior with them. We pick up an enormous amount of disease early by doing executive physicals here, so we have a chance to do something and modify behaviors. You lose everything if you lose confidentiality; that's the bottom line.

In my eighteen years with the company I have never been in a situation where a health issue has been a consideration in advancing an executive—let's say, a vice president advancing to a president—*never!* That's probably an unfounded fear on the part of the executives. I have never heard of a physician reporting on an executive's health to others in the company.

Much of the work of physicians even ten years ago involved periodic executive medical exams that had a business-related purpose but did not fall under the medical benefit plans. Corporations required their executives to have annual physicals, including a chest X-ray, EKG, barium enema, and sigmoidoscopy. The goal was to detect people with early signs of disease and save money by intervening early and keeping managers healthy. Many companies rejected these tests as not cost-effective; after billions had been spent testing CFOs and CEOs without symptoms, the evidence from actuarial tables indicated that they were not living longer because of it. Although companies increasingly rely on HMOs or company health-benefit plans to cover such exams, many doctors continue to do executive physicals of top managers who have little or no exposure to occupational risks. In addition, company doctors sometimes serve as the personal physicians to top executives. A physician with a financial services company said:

> One company I knew had a medical director who was a longtime personal friend of the CEO, who was worried about dropping dead from a heart attack and wanted a physician at his elbow, and decided the physician was a good gin rummy player, so that's that. Many medical directors got their jobs because they were physicians related to the CEO.

Company physicians also act as medical advisers to executives who have their own personal physicians. The medical department generally enjoys more power, status, and resources if it treats the CEO and top executives. The opportunity to advise high-level executives on health matters is especially important for medical directors and physicians who clinically evaluate executives. Physicians who treat executives for health problems, help them choose outside specialists, or otherwise advise them can ask for favors, such as support for an expansion of the company's medical program. Two physicians, with a chemical company and a power company, respectively, said:

> A large corporation is an extremely political environment. We all do personal favors for people; that's how we get things done to a degree. But physician colleagues in corporate medicine abuse that practice by having a paper occupational health program and for years only taking care of executives and totally ignoring the rest of the program. That happens all the time. If you helped an executive take care of a personal need in the past, you can always go in and say, "I want this program." The executive will often get it for you, aside from business merit, because they feel you've done something for them in the past, so it's a tit-for-tat arrangement.[11]

> My practice includes almost the whole legal department. I take care of all the lawyers, so I have a personal relationship with them. The fact that I see the lawyers in this setting as patients makes them more understanding. They would not dictate to me or interfere easily. If the lawyers were getting health care somewhere else, then they probably would be arbitrary and dictatorial, looking down at the health-care department. But since we take care of them, they want us to do what's best for patients, which is them. So it's more of a hands-off approach and more collegial. This closed system makes the dynamic a lot different. It's extremely significant.

As with other leaders, the health of corporate VIPs conceivably could affect their careers, but physicians tend to prop up their leaders and keep executives' secrets (see Post and Robins 1993). Some doctors, like this chemical company physician, have expressed ambivalence about the role of personal physician or medical adviser to executives:

> Seeing top executives as patients gives you power to "have something" on them, to know something about them, and knowledge is power. It's a double-edged sword to be viewed as the executive doctor. It works *for* us in that we have access to the most senior people in the corporation on a personal level, which is exciting and gives us enormous opportunities. The downside is that we can never be treated as equivalent on the same playing field as other business managers. It contaminates our capacity to be viewed as a member of a management team. Some senior executives always view us as the doctor, and it's a very tricky job to be in. You're playing with fire, because you're playing with the bodies, but more so, the psyches of the senior people in the corporation, and they know it and you know it. How you handle yourself in that role and manage the health information affects whether you succeed.

The special access that many corporate physicians have to executives strains their relationship to other managers. In addition, employers may fear physicians, as a chemical company physician explained:

> The reason medical departments have generally not thrived in corporations is that the current crop of leaders of Fortune 500 companies fears doctors. They are afraid of us. No one other than occupational physicians has the capacity to bear the burden of the secrets of the CEOs' bodies and minds. They are afraid of having the medical department become too powerful. Somehow they think that it doesn't fit with their power games and control over employees, and that we represent a force they can't quite understand or control as much as other forces within the corporation.

As this argument suggests, managers may fear doctors in part because they stand for employees' health. The role of doctors as advocates for workers' health is threatening to executives who view workers as their adversaries, as they usually do in companies that are highly adversarial in their management-labor relationships. The whole occupational medicine field is founded in part on a liberal concept of having workers who are healthy. A physician for a conglomerate referred to company doctors as a silent irritant that managers cannot fully trust:

> Management just doesn't trust anybody with an MD—somebody who isn't
> an engineer who has something to do with a product that makes money
> for you, or a lawyer that keeps you out of trouble, or somebody in finance
> that helps you keep your money. And we are a "burden" people—that's
> the term; indirect, a burden. Burden departments are departments that you
> must have to function but that don't make a damn thing for you. That's
> true of occupational medicine and any support function. Perhaps there is
> reason for their distrust, because, frankly, I still consider myself to have
> more loyalty to my profession than to the company, and I think that's why
> I'm paid. You don't want a hack; you want somebody who's a patient-
> advocate who can keep the corporation out of trouble.

In addition, a visit to the company physician can challenge an executive's self-image. As a chemical company physician said: "When the CEO and president walk into the occupational physician's office, they are in a dependent situation, which they loathe."

In an unusual but telling case, one prominent physician told top management about an executive's personal health problem that he thought threatened the business. For this he was fired, even though management agreed that the information he provided did in fact help the company. Management saw him as disloyal for betraying the confidence of an executive and wondered whether he would someday pass on information about their own health or personal problems.

Company physicians and top managers sometimes treat lower-level managers much like low-level employees, as when they use medical information to defend their actions in firing a manager for nonmedical reasons. A physician in an aerospace company discussed a case in which he defended the employer's interest by withholding important medical information from a lower-level manager (who had been fired) but continued to feel guilty for having done so. Another physician in the company had failed to identify the employee's cardiac problem in the company's annual physical examination. The cardiac problem was causing sleep apnea, and sleep deprivation was causing him to fall asleep in meetings, which was one reason he was fired. The employee had not gone to a private physician, who might have told him what was wrong. The medical director said:

> They brought me the record and asked me what I thought about it after he
> left the company and filed a wrongful termination lawsuit. So I looked at

the data and said, "Well, yeah, there *is* evidence that this difficulty was there." Then I asked the doctor involved, "Did you talk to him about this problem?" He said he didn't. I told the attorneys, "We didn't do a good job; we screwed up." During the trial the company lawyers called me as a witness regarding this medical information and said, "Just answer questions yes or no when you're on the stand." They didn't ask, "Would the very fact that we failed to give him some information have been important?" Then I waited for *his* attorneys to ask me questions, but they didn't. I wanted him to win his suit, but he ended up losing it.

Medical departments in many companies have remained small or shrunk as corporate legal departments, human relations, and public relations staffs have grown. Although management's primary motivation for cutting in-house doctors is to reduce costs by contracting out medical services, their fear of doctors contributes. The fear and mistrust of physicians may be largely unjustified, however, since doctors generally do not report on the health of executives; once they uncover a physical or psychological problem, they tend to protect the executive's confidences, in stark contrast to their treatment of most employee medical problems.

Despite the higher percentage of company doctors today who have specialized training compared with thirty years ago (or any other previous time) and the increasing professionalization of their field, the long-standing function of company doctors in identifying medical reasons that justify removal of employees, protecting the confidences of the executives they advise, and demedicalizing legitimate health concerns remains important to employers as a reason to have physicians in-house.

—— Chapter 4 ——

Toxics and Workplace Hazards

I doubt that there's a problem—but I also have to say that we never looked.

—Metals company physician on the issue of metals exposure and declining cognitive function

If you get a whiff of smoke in a corporate setting, you had better go look to see whether there really is a fire.

—Physician in a large medical center's occupational medicine clinic

WORKPLACE HEALTH HAZARDS produce an array of diseases in people who are exposed to them, ranging from skin damage to emphysema and brain tumors. Employers and the physicians who work for them have various motivations to reduce toxic exposures, including cultivating good relations with their employees, protecting a skilled workforce that is difficult to replace, and avoiding regulatory fines. They focus on chronic exposure hazards for several reasons: because prosperity allows them to hire in-house staff to address those risks, because management perceives that laws require them to do so, or because the company or industry recently has had an embarrassing or expensive chemical problem.[1] A major chemical company physician said:

We had a horrible catastrophe in the company recently when our plant blew up. That has set the tone for the way most health professionals have spent their time since that day—doing accident prevention and response, which is a much cruder level of activity that we should be able to avoid by now. As the economy improves, [we] physicians and industrial hygienists get involved in more sophisticated issues of occupational medicine like chronic effects of exposure on workers.

Employers hire doctors to deal with routine toxic hazards as well as accidents, as related by this airline doctor and a contracting occupational physician who formerly worked in-house:

We see virtually every kind of toxic exposure and environmental hazard that you could imagine here, and that's the part that makes this a medically exciting job. I went to lectures eight hours a day for two weeks when I took the occupational medicine mini-residency, and in every lecture I'd say, "Oh, yeah, we had one of those last week."

We tend to get companies with exposure problems, safety problems, labor problems, workers' comp problems, looking for help. Many of them are in the so-called smokestack industries, chemical industries, utilities that have never had much occupational and environmental and industrial hygiene expertise. Many are companies in trouble one way or another. They need our kind of services.[2]

In this chapter, I consider employers' and physicians' selective concern with toxics and their use of information about risks in responding to publicity over working conditions. I also consider ways in which doctors use hazards to persuade management to act and the approach that their professional organization takes toward toxics. An examination of high-profile cases that the media have covered or that professional organizations have reviewed brings to light some problems of professionals in corporations that are obscured by the daily routine in these workplaces.

TURNING AWAY FROM TOXICS

Whether to use medical technologies to diagnose occupational disease, whether to design studies to identify disease patterns, and whether to support engineering controls to reduce exposures are not entirely medical or scientific decisions. Identifying health hazards and linking them to working conditions raises the nonmedical concerns of the legal staff preoccupied with corporate liability, of the marketing staff worried about product sales, of the public relations staff concerned about adverse publicity, and of managers worried about medical costs. Employers conduct studies and medical surveillance programs because government mandates them, or because workers demand services through unions, or because employers favor reducing health risks in any case. However, employers often support expensive surveillance programs without putting the study findings to much use in protecting health. They could undertake studies based on epidemiology and animal data to identify new risks—which is how hazards from asbestos, lead, and coal dust have been established. More often, however, they have a journal of negative results—conditions they describe as not hazardous. Their desire to avoid discovering and dealing with new problems leads them not to look. Although employers sometimes inadvertently design studies and tests so as not to look at exposure, the outcome is the same as when the effort is deliberate.

Managers have a general understanding that they must comply with the law, but most tend to take little interest in health issues unless the law requires them to do so or the related costs appear large. Even then, management delegates these issues to the lawyers, doctors, other health professionals, and regulatory staff.

Identifying disease patterns is seldom defined as an organizational goal. Corporate physicians may conduct medical tests and work-site wellness studies, give executives inoculations, and provide medical care without focusing on hazardous conditions in the work environment or helping to control them. Others are more concerned about negotiating major medical policies, deductibles, and copayments than about toxins in the work environment. The diagnosis rate for occupational disease has improved over the past thirty years, partly because physicians' knowledge about occupational medicine has grown and government action (as from OSHA) has expanded concern with occupational disease.[3] Still, ignorance of health hazards or denial that they exist limits the money that employers spend on preventive medicine. A physician in a large metropolitan medical center's occupational medicine program said:

These company physicians aren't focused on occupational disease. A doctor could sit in the plant and not know what goes on there. But even doctors who do poke around don't do the right tests and find out much anyway, due to their own limitations and training and money and the context. Their big mistake is that they don't match exposure with health outcome. You can't say anything about occupational disease unless you know what the exposure is. Employers usually don't use their medical surveillance information well.

Employers are concerned about what they would do if they found a workplace hazard. Reasons for the employer not to want to know about it include production or economic pressures, fear of publicity, desire not to alarm workers, the cost of remedial measures, and concern that knowing about a risk may leave them more liable for resulting disease. Employers have strong incentives to downplay or understate workplace disease and not to present evidence of a possible new workplace hazard. They do not necessarily want to hear about health hazards that might require expensive engineering controls, especially when they confront budgetary constraints. As an oil company physician said, "They don't want somebody coming in and saying, 'Oh, my God! You have to change your procedures here—it's unsafe.' "

Although part of what drew public health–oriented doctors to the field in the first place was their interest in eliminating exposure hazards, employers typically do not encourage doctors to uncover new occupational health problems or reward them for doing so. When doctors do suspect that a workplace hazard exists and ask that resources be spent to address it, managers may treat them as whistleblowers or troublemakers. They may regard concern with mitigating health hazards as too tentative, troublesome, or expensive, given their different priorities. Doctors hear employers claim to be acutely concerned about environmental hazards, but they usually conclude that management does not really want to know about hazards, or that their job as a doctor is to allay people's fears and not create fears by pointing to possible risks. A pharmaceutical company doctor explained:

Managers say, "Let sleeping dogs lie," in a lot of instances, as in the asbestos litigation. Certain people above me have made comments like, "Don't make waves. Show me the dead bodies," which means: "Unless you have absolute proof that it's a problem, I don't want to hear about it."[4]

Physicians may still conduct surveillance, look for further evidence, and wish to intervene with a preventive approach. Doctors tend to do considerable data gathering to support their recommendations so that they do not approach management unprepared. They may recommend that the company change work practices, substitute certain materials, or install enclosures and other engineering controls, but the organizational imperatives militate against this. Doctors generally lack the authority to institute many health policies on their own, or to shut operations down if they feel a serious hazard exists. They can argue that hazards should be abated, and they may be able to persuade management that the company should be more proactive in the area of health, even though this is not what management wants to hear. Company physicians find themselves in a difficult position when their recommendations would cost a great deal of money.

Some physicians and managers pursue an alternative strategy: asserting that a health problem does not exist without having done research into it, in the belief that such an assertion protects them from liability, adverse publicity, and demands for costly remedies. Two physicians, one in a chemical company and the other in a large medical center's occupational medical program with extensive experience with company doctors, said:

> We think intelligent self-preservation is important. It wouldn't be our failure to warn if we never found out what this stuff does, so maybe we shouldn't look.

> Physicians who recommend new work practices don't always meet with favor because the changes are expensive. Therefore, some physicians elect not to look, because what you don't know needn't provoke reportage and insistence on some kind of preventive response. Some physicians choose not to say much about problems they see.

However, there are countervailing pressures that encourage research and remedial action. Some employers can see that it may be in their financial interest to look for and remedy problems, especially after the asbestos debacle and the publicized bankruptcies of many companies that had known hazards. A physician employed by a manufacturing company said:

Managers never want to know there might be a health problem, but they're in trouble if they don't know, if OSHA comes in inspecting and citing them. So they may not relish the information, but they need to know. That's one reason you have to have good rapport with the plant manager, so if you come with bad news, they say, "Damn it! I'm sorry you have to tell me that, but what can we do?"[5]

Having an inadequate physician or monitoring program creates trouble for companies when physicians fail to have appropriate medical surveillance in place, to record illnesses appropriately in the OSHA log, or to delegate that authority properly to someone else.[6]

The Failure of Doctors to Recognize Occupational Disease

To assess workplace hazards, occupational physicians would need a good knowledge of the toxicology of the various products and would have to examine the work environment to check for safety precautions. They also would need to review workers' compensation and other data, talk with industrial hygienists and safety officers, and be familiar with the techniques of controls, such as respiratory protection and ventilation.

A major reason occupational disease is underreported is that many doctors either do not know how to recognize it or design tests that bear no relevance to exposures. Most board-certified occupational physicians with skills in epidemiology and public health who work in large corporations hold administrative and policymaking positions, but the doctors who actually treat employees working under their direction are not certified themselves. Analyzing aggregate data, looking for disease patterns, and putting in place prevention programs requires a knowledge of clinical occupational medicine and epidemiology that these clinicians often lack. Family practitioners and internists may be good at doing routine physical exams and acute trauma care without understanding the nature of production processes or how to assess exposure. They generally look at individuals rather than at the patterns of illness, and they do not collect information in ways that would make them likely to notice a disease trend that warrants further study.[7] Doctors may lack access to broad health data across the company or information on health effects on the com-

munity and consumers. More often they focus on occasional clinical puzzles—such as an employee who appears to have an allergic
reaction to a company's gasoline additive—with little knowledge
about how to detect long-term chronic occupational diseases,
which are more insidious in development and have a less obvious
cause. A union official and a physician who has provided occupational medical services to corporations said:

> Occasionally physicians will render an opinion that's not in concert with
> the production or finance or legal people. Then they put their morals back
> in hibernation for the next six months and don't ask the questions they
> ought to ask about employee health or put into place the data systems that
> they would long ago have had on-line if it involved any of a zillion quan-
> titative measures of the company's performance. But they don't ask for
> information about employees whose health is seriously affected. It's hear
> no evil, see no evil, speak no evil. So they collect a wealth of data about
> employee health, but none of it for preventive purposes. The company
> needs somebody to process the health disputes that come up and write up
> all these nondisability determinations for workers' comp cases. If doctors
> render the occasional controversial opinion, great![8]

> Doctors are part of an employer public relations effort. It's like, "We buy
> health and dental insurance for you, we give you this or that, and people
> in white coats in the company make sure you're safe here." But most in-
> plant health departments are there as window dressing to provide execu-
> tive physicals and do minor injury visits. They're not there to develop a
> broad preventive medicine program.

Employers that choose inadequately qualified physicians to be
responsible for the company's medical programs seem uncon-
cerned with the quality of a doctor's training and experience. An
MD seems sufficient for them. A high-level oil company physician
stated:

> Managers take for granted that you are technically competent, that you
> know your field and know what you're doing—and that only gets you to
> zero. That gives you nothing beyond baseline, because management
> thinks that a doctor's a doctor. To them all doctors are worth one point.
> Just as they assume you can fix cars if you come in as a car mechanic, they
> assume you know everything there is to know about the human body and
> how to fix it if you come in as a doctor. Companies give a semi-articulate
> doctor of osteopathy from Iowa talking about cardiac surgery the same
> weight as a Mayo Clinic–trained cardiac surgeon.[9]

In addition, workers and the general public are unaware that occupational medicine is a specialty requiring special training, and that to get clinical treatment they may need to seek another specialist (a cardiologist for chest pain or an orthopedist for sciatic pain, for example). This contributes to the misdiagnosis and inadequate treatment of occupational disease.

If in-house doctors often fail to spot occupational disease, farming medical services out to practitioners who know little about the nature of the companies they serve simply exacerbates that problem. Contractors usually work for many companies and do not inspect workplaces or attend joint labor-management health committee meetings; nor do they know much about the typical exposures in a workplace, which in-house people are more likely to understand. They may be called in to handle embarrassing leaks, spills, or lawsuits, then told to leave once the crisis subsides. They may visit the work site one day each week or each month, depending on the company's size and the services they provide. But most contract physicians do not visit their patients' workplace.[10] Small companies generally do not pay physicians to come out and learn what workplace dangers exist if employees complain about them, whereas in-house doctors can walk over to look, for example, at possible respiratory hazards and arrange for samples to be taken. Employers and in-house physicians often fail to provide adequate job descriptions to the contract doctor or ask for physical exams directed at those job requirements.

A detached service that basically conducts exams may not provide good mechanisms for proactive occupational medicine used to prevent disease. Contracting clinics principally are interested in the walking wounded rather than extensive health surveillance of exposure to toxics like benzene or asbestos. Some in-house physicians derogatorily call a contractor a "doc-in-the-box"—someone who knows little about conditions at work and gives substandard care. Companies also lose continuity when physician turnover is rapid in clinics and when contract doctors are unavailable to follow up on risk factors after they perform exams. As an oil company physician and a conglomerate physician explained:

> Contractors get paid for piecework. You can buy from a contracting organization all kinds of piecework or rent a medical director to come in to do

some things, but you can't get from a contractor the kind of commitment and interest in seeing things through that you get from in-house doctors. They are not paid to evaluate someone with a seizure disorder and try to find the right work-restriction formula to get the man at work so he can support his family and help him out of his depression about his affliction. Contractors *never* want to spend a lot of time on something. They don't even know who's in the organization or who to call, they don't know much about the culture or hear other issues that are raised. They are asked to do one thing and just won't know to do anything more.

Outside consultants don't know the plant processes or employees like someone who is there day in and day out, and this is a tremendous disadvantage. The result is that the plant manager becomes the corporate physician and decides what program to have because no one else is around to advise him except the outside consultant, who's the wrong person to ask; that's like asking the barber if you need a haircut. The manager knows that, so he doesn't have anyone to turn to and just may do nothing.

The quality of contracting services varies widely. Some outside services provide only superficial health screening that costs hundreds of dollars per employee but remains irrelevant to workplace exposures. Others with a national reputation have highly qualified, seasoned physicians who understand epidemiology, toxicology, and industrial hygiene and provide a full menu of quality services.[11] However, few physicians trained in occupational medicine in the United States are not already working in corporations, government agencies, or research settings. Contractors who know little about occupational medicine nonetheless see it as an opportunity to expand their business and earn more consistent income. Contractors are not short for work because they are not in oversupply, but their work is competitive in part because only some groups are knowledgeable, while other operations that bring minimal expertise will underbid to do medical surveillance in companies. A physician in a large medical center's occupational medical program said:

I once consulted to a hospital where the director wanted to set up an occupational medical clinic as a way to bring patients into the hospital and make money as the outside consulting group marketing health services to local companies. We knew companies had terrible exposure problems just looking at the workers' comp records. I asked him, "What will happen if we find problems in some of these companies that result in workers' comp claims? What will bring those companies to us the next year to obtain our services? Why wouldn't they hire someone out there who will be more compliant with them?" The hospital director then asked me, "Couldn't we just get our foot in the door and avoid identifying some of these things and then do better later, but at least maybe the first year not find so much?"

That question gets to the heart of the matter. Physicians who do a good job in occupational medicine will find exposure hazards and do other things that stand in the way of a company pursuing its economic interest without regard to health considerations. Companies may wish to avoid buying the services of physicians who cause them trouble. Independent firms that now market their services to corporations are faced with that issue; they must persuade employers that they are more likely to be held financially liable if hazards are not identified and remedied. Corporations may choose instead to hire contract doctors who know little about occupational exposures in part precisely because they do not want to have illness traced to its workplace causes. When health services are removed from the workplace, doctors are less likely to understand what goes on there or to focus on work-based problems. However, an on-site internist or family practitioner hired without training in occupational medicine will cost more but give no better service than any local contract doctor. Thus, companies that contract out save money without losing expertise.

Nurses and the Search for Occupational Disease

An important reason company programs do not target occupational disease is that nurses with little knowledge of preventive medicine and toxic chemical exposures now run major parts of these programs in many companies (although a few physicians run clinics without nurses).[12] Employers often expect nurses to minimize lost work time and promptly refer out to a private physician anyone with what looks like a workplace-related illness. Then the illness is unlikely to be reported to workers' compensation or treated at the employer's expense. Nurses typically have less power than doctors and do not disobey the directives of physicians and managers, who expect nurses to do what they are told. Some companies use nurses for some of the same purposes they have used doctors, but they generally rely on nurses to do a narrower range of clinical functions. Medical programs suffer when nurses extend their reach beyond their level of competence. A physician who ran a medical clinic without nurses said:

> Having nurses run the program makes life easy: it's what the nurses want, and it's the community standard and the way things have always been. Nurses run the system in a company health department: the passage of paper, who does what when; that's how things get done. Doctors don't usually get involved in that. Corporate doctors will have World War III if they come in and say, "Oh, no, I'll diagnose all this occupational illness and practice a level of medicine that requires my background." Doctors either come into companies and nestle into the system and let the nurses continue to run it or they have problems. With rare exceptions, electronics companies use nurses as pawns to create the illusion that someone in white is making the workplace safe, without investing in more corporate physicians. That gets them in trouble, though, if their bad health statistics are uncovered, because that hurts the industry from a public relations standpoint and even financially.[13]

ACOEM encourages close involvement of nurses in occupational medicine.[14] As a physician who provided services to corporations said:

> The ACOEM tradition is to have an annual meeting, with the nurses meeting on one side of the convention center and the doctors meeting on the other. But it makes no sense; they don't share the same level of scientific presentation. It'd be better for the image of the science of occupational medicine to stop this. They say they can't because exhibitors won't cover the overhead convention cost without tens of thousands of people. What other medical specialty anywhere meets with nurses? It's those old, comfy relationships between doctors and nurses that you find all the way through the politics of the College [ACOEM].[15]

In other settings outside corporate medical programs, nurses at times have been outspoken advocates for alternative treatment policies and have been among the leading voices expressing concern about health risks.[16] However, in company medical programs, nurses generally lack the training to identify and prevent occupational disease. They are less likely than company physicians to be charged with conducting studies of potential workplace health risks, and they have less authority than doctors with which to pursue health hazards. Aside from whatever concern nurses may have for the health of employees and the public, the delegation of company medical programs to nurses tends to be associated with an even greater focus on the treatment of injuries, routine clinical care, and basic screening tests than when doctors have a stronger hand in running medical programs.

Condemning Animal Studies and Concern with Multiple Chemical Sensitivity

Many company physicians believe that toxic chemical issues are becoming an increasingly less pressing concern.[17] Along with corporate managers, they generally maintain that current work conditions are safe, or that occupational hazards account for a small proportion of chronic illness relative to other factors such as diet, smoking, stress, naturally occurring carcinogens, personal lifestyle, and genetic constitution. There is little need to search for toxic problems, they believe, since the problem of work-related disease has been largely solved. A chemical company physician who repeatedly refers to "so-called toxic chemicals" found workers' concern about chemical hazards at work to be misguided: "Chemical plants or oil refineries today are not very dirty places anymore. The job of cleaning up the work environment has been done. That's not a big scientific issue." An oil company physician said:

> Occupational disease now is virtually nonexistent. We have laws on the books controlling work exposures to infinitesimal levels. The fundamental hazards associated with work have changed. From major exposures such as miners' black lung and asbestosis and birth defects from lead toxicity, we've gone now to repetitive motion injuries and ergonomics of video display terminals and tight building illness giving people headaches, which may be psychogenic.

Company physicians sometimes dismiss research on toxics that is based on animal studies, despite the standard use of animal data in scientific research, or say that the reproductive hazards of workplace substances are of little importance. These two physicians, from a chemical company and a pharmaceutical company, said:

A lot of what has gone on in the area of reproductive hazards and cancer is based on animal data. That model of dosing rats and mice with chemicals just hasn't been effective. A great deal of data is missing because we've studied rats, not people, and the rats haven't given us the data.

In actual fact, we don't know what causes most birth defects. The causes we do understand generally have nothing to do with the workplace. They give very high doses of a chemical to a rat, thousands of times higher than the workplace level. About the level where you start killing pregnant rats, you start noticing some minor changes that probably just indicate severe maternal toxicity rather than teratogenicity. I wouldn't be particularly concerned about it.

Acute exposure to an organic solvent can cause headaches, nausea, and a generalized malaise for a day or two; some individuals claim that these symptoms return with subsequent exposure to materials other than those they were initially exposed to. Many doctors reject this claim of multiple chemical sensitivity and focus on psychological causes. As a physician who evaluates workers for chemical companies explained:

We're starting to see illnesses that are a variation on a theme of the hysterical presentations of the nineteenth century. It's like Pavlov's dog. This group of employees is very suggestible. They search out and ultimately find a clinician who will reinforce their beliefs that they have something seriously wrong. Then they know they are really sick. Usually they go through some unusual type of treatment protocol involving massage or sweat treatments. Clinical ecologists see these patients as similar to cancer or AIDS patients, and yet studies don't show the same type of demonstrable physiological or immunological evidence and no double-blind studies show that the treatment they advocate is any more effective than placebo treatments.[18]

An airline physician concurred:

We have employees who claim to be victims of multiple chemical sensitivity syndrome and tight building syndrome and bad air in the airplanes. Those problems are probably psychological. It may not be a mental illness; it amounts to a cult medical belief, because these folks have all the characteristics of cult members. They and their doctors get very pissed off if you disagree with them. It isn't scientifically valid; there's no medical consensus that it's true; it is controversial and not a conventional medical belief. The allergists say it doesn't exist. But a few very politically active people believe it.

In the absence of what they consider to be proof of exposure hazards based on human evidence, these physicians conclude that the workplace is safe.

Pressure to Reduce "Recordables"

Because OSHA requires businesses to keep records of their workplace illnesses that require medical treatment, other organizations can use those records to compare companies and give awards or demerits based on them. An important source of the conflict that corporate physicians experience between giving the ideal care to their worker-patients and maintaining loyalty to their corporate employer is corporate pressure to reduce the number of "recordable" illnesses. Incentives are strong for physicians and managers alike to make it appear that the company does not have health problems attributable to the workplace, particularly problems that the company must report. Many physicians and managers succumb to this pressure to downplay the occupational role in disease or to record fewer hazards—especially if they feel that their own position could be jeopardized if they do not comply or if their safety record is a performance criterion by which they are evaluated. If 10 percent of their annual financial reward is based on their safety record, it would scarcely be surprising if many of them feel motivated to do whatever they can to reduce those numbers. The people who cooperate with plant managers and safety officers to bring the numbers into line understand that their job performance is their bottom line. Management sometimes deputizes safety professionals to try to persuade the medical staff to reduce the number of occupational illnesses they record and treat.[19] As these physicians from a metals company and an oil company explained:

> The safety person lives—or dies—by the safety record, and some feel they don't want *any* lost-time accidents or illnesses. They'd go to almost any extreme to look for some non-occupational reason so they wouldn't have to count it in the safety record.

> We have to watch our safety numbers. Manufacturing companies tend to get very caught up in those numbers. It's an extremely perverse system. Management looks at it as, "The doctors aren't team players," unless we do

everything we can to classify things as not work-related and recordable so they wouldn't boost our safety statistics. Every day we have the Spanish Inquisition in here grilling the doctor, "Did you really think this injury was work-related? Did you have to treat it that way?" We can count on someone calling us up to question our judgment, and we have to summon a certain amount of patience to explain why we did it and not appear offended. Industries compare each other: "I have ten recordables in my company and you have eight in yours, so you must do better in your company than we do." The outcome of that process *ought* to be that "Yeah, we're doing something wrong. How do we analyze and correct the workplace so it doesn't happen again?" We may be telling the truth and the other company may be lying, because a lot of that goes on. My colleagues in some other companies juggle the figures or do less efficacious things for people or outright lie on their paperwork. The focus ought not to be on going to the clinic and convincing us to treat people less adequately and record it differently so our safety record will be better. These poor safety engineers come slinking into the medical department because management tells them they have to convince us, because they'll have to go slinking back to get chided and flogged if they can't.[20]

When doctors and managers aim to report less work-related illness, their focus is not necessarily on reducing the actual number of illnesses. A major reason for the underreporting is a subtle game that corporations and insurers play, in which physicians have an incentive to report everything that is not an injury to major medical plans instead of to workers' compensation. One surgeon expert in cancers of the head and neck, for example, said that over the years he had seen thousands of cases of cancer that he traced to companies' chemicals and yet had never reported a single case to the Bureau of Labor Statistics, never billed a workers' compensation carrier, and never made an employer pay for it. His explanation was largely economic. The companies had major-medical policies, they paid him more and faster, and he had never been deposed or dragged into a messy Manville-type of litigation, which doctors generally detest. Thus, none of the cases he detected were ever reported as occupational illness.

The result is a system that responds irrationally to health hazards: occupational health specialists deal with colds and minor injuries, while private practitioners deal with cases of occupational illness but do not report them as such.

THE MEDIA AND PUBLIC RELATIONS
ROLE OF PROFESSIONALS KEPT OUT
OF THE INFORMATION LOOP

Although many companies have processes that are highly toxic to workers and the environment, such as refining or manufacturing dyes, the doctors they employ often do not participate significantly in decisions regarding toxins. Doctors may understand company operations enough to recognize carcinogenic work exposures, and they may have the authority to participate in decisions, but in many cases they have little involvement in advising their employers on how to deal with such hazards. They do not have the authority to stop the diseases up front or the mandate to err on the side of safety. They have often been excluded from the earlier discussions on health issues to which marketing people and lawyers contributed; doctors are brought in late in the process, if at all.[21] Physicians in many companies are hired as medical technicians to do only clinical work, and employers essentially ignore them on other matters. One physician, who has provided health services to corporations and observed company doctors for years, said:

> Rather than get involved in toxic exposures, they just sit around listening to executives' hearts or chat with people about the employee assistance program. When it was discovered that one company's underground chemical storage tanks contaminated the county's water supply, the corporate physician learned about that from the newspapers years later like any other citizen. Yet for years people in the company had made decisions about how much leaking into the groundwater should be allowed. So the person best able to advise the company on how dangerous it is to poison the neighborhood is not a part of the loop. That company had made its medical director a vice president, so he was obviously a team player carrying a high rank in the company, sitting in on high-level meetings. There probably aren't a half-dozen vice-president corporate medical directors in America, but he was not there for things he should have known about and influenced. That characterizes the American attitude toward the corporate medical director. It's because doctors will tell them what they don't want to hear or won't keep a secret. Even when they are willing to hire a doctor, companies don't basically trust the medical person. That's because medical

people generally are trustworthy, and business isn't always a trustworthy activity.

Sometimes employers' concern with keeping information about health hazards from workers, the public, the media, and government regulators is so intense that they keep such information even from the physicians. A physician in a conglomerate described a case in which an employee working with plutonium in a hot cell embedded plutonium in his hand when his screwdriver slipped and pierced his glove. The physician found out about it five hours after a technical worker who measured exposures but was not medically trained had tried to handle the situation himself, quietly, rather than inform the company doctor and risk spreading the word that a worker had plutonium implanted in his flesh. The doctor objected to the incident being kept from him and the medical department:

> I treated this patient and was quite concerned. I should have been notified right away that we had somebody who had radioactivity in a wound and needed to be treated. Management just didn't understand that their role was to have me do something about it. They need to keep that out of the paper, for obvious reasons, because of a terrible public overreaction to the micro quantities they were dealing in. But they were overprotective *within* the organization, and that's absurd. It's an example of their blinders.

In a telecommunications company that OSHA cited and fined (for about $30,000) for carpal tunnel violations, the managers never consulted the doctors. The employer used a third-party insurer to handle its workers' compensation claims, and the division with the medical problem failed to seek the advice of company physicians. One doctor in the company said: "We were the last to know; I didn't even know about it until OSHA socked us with this fine."

Remarkably, a physician in a corporation responsible for high levels of groundwater pollution was never asked to evaluate the situation or advise the company. He said:

> I was disappointed that I wasn't more directly involved. Nobody ever talked to me or showed me any data about the bigger issues, except for one slip of the tongue. A high-level individual in the company reporting to

the CEO told me, "Yeah, in fact we have done all those bad things we're accused of," which was distressing. We were talking about somebody neither of us liked, so I guess we instantly formed a bond, and he wanted me to know what was going on. He described what the company had done and told me that this guy was trying to put a squeeze on him, and he said, "I know enough that we'd *all* go to jail if they knew." Those were his very words. I thought, Holy Christ! The walls have ears. Here this guy just blurted a secret out and told me that in fact we've done what everybody in the company says we didn't do. I was ticked off that my loving company would actually do what they were accused of in the pollution disaster and yet deny it in the press. I figured, "I hope they nail us, I hope they catch us," but I'm not in a whistleblower role.

A physician in a conglomerate described being kept away from information about cancer causation and denied opportunities to investigate workplace exposure risks:

People write letters complaining that they or their parents got sick from the emissions from the company. Those letters come in through an administrative channel and get to the legal people, and occasionally they inform the doctors of it. For example, an individual whose parents had worked at the company and died of cancer wrote a letter wanting information about what they were exposed to. The father worked there fifteen years ago, the mother eight years ago. Is their dying of cancer work-related or not? And what about other people? We could go back and look at what they were exposed to. I'd find that of potential value, so I said, "Let's dig into it and find out," but the attorney said, "Oh, geez, that was so long ago, we'll never get those records, we don't have time. I'll just write them a letter with our overall feel and just gloss it over and state that we haven't had any other cases"—just blow them off, as my kids would say. That would be it, and *I'd be totally out of the loop.* The legal department right next door to me was always involved in these cloak-and-dagger kinds of things, always arguing from the company's point of view.

One physician's employer had him reassure workers and the public about risks while depriving him of a potentially effective role in reducing hazards. He said:

I was concerned about people in one area having a certain kind of cancer, and I thought the data deserved further digging into, to see if we could go in and get rid of something that's causing a problem. But I was powerless to pursue it. Maybe I should have demanded further studies, but I was under a lot of pressure because management didn't want to acknowledge that it involved exposure to potential death, and nobody ever wanted to look into it. You're supposed to tell employees, "We looked into it, we've taken samples, and everything looks like there's no evidence of an exposure problem that will affect employees or the surrounding community, but we'll continue to monitor the situation and do this and that." That was always when I went from the headquarters to get involved out in the field. I'd hope that it would continue to be monitored after I left the field, just as we said it would, but I have no way of ensuring that, and the monitoring and safety people certainly weren't on *my* payroll. So it wasn't like I came in on my horse telling everybody everything was okay, turned around, and rode off. It was a group of people I was a part of allaying the fears of employees, telling them nothing is wrong, but not being careful enough with environmental concerns.

Physicians may discuss medical issues with management, but then, if the legal and marketing departments are involved in discussions about risk and toxic exposures, physicians are often left out of the final decisionmaking process. Often they are not informed of those discussions and find it difficult to determine how decisions about health risk were reached.

Ambivalence of Lawyers About Physicians Providing Information

Owing to threats of corporate liability, lawyers sometimes find themselves in conflict with doctors over whether to release health information. At other times—most notably on questions of labeling hazardous substances—litigation concerns lead lawyers to align themselves with company doctors.

Company lawyers are reluctant to have doctors disclose information about health hazards that could alarm people or be used against the company. Physicians in many corporations complain that lawyers do not want them to say anything about potential hazards because that would suggest that the company knew of problems but was not doing enough to solve them. Overall, increasing sensitivity to potential liability intensifies corporate pressure on professionals to restrict employee and public access to data. Lawyers, managers, and public relations people pressure physicians not to provide information that could increase their company's chances of being held liable for damage to workers or the public. They impose constraints on publishing and speaking, conducting studies of suspected exposure hazards, and drawing attention to problematic working conditions (see, for example, Dembe 1996; Sheehan and Wedeen 1993; Jasanoff 1995, 114–37; Sassower 1993, 76–99). Lawyers set up screening procedures out of concern over how professional staff members may use the company's name. They oppose doing studies or communicating possible health effects to workers and the public because the company might be held responsible for knowing but failing to do enough. They often cloak company reports on workplace and environmental hazards in confidentiality. They become particularly concerned when company studies involve notifying workers, government, or the media. One physician who conducted research and set up a cancer registry for his chemical company said:

> Companies run the risk of incriminating themselves and generating lawsuits when they do studies, no question about that. One time I was concerned when I got word that a lawyer didn't like the idea of our gathering all these data. He said, "You expose yourself to problems when you gather data." Lawyers would just like to burn whatever data you get—whenever you get information. Of course, I get disturbed by that, but I can understand their point of view, because someone can just find a rather innocent little piece of paper somewhere that an opposing lawyer could make look devastating in some way in a trial. That's the way things go in the courtroom.

A services company physician said:

> I was asked to give a talk to a trucking industry group on workers' compensation, and one question afterwards revolved around wearing lifting belts that protect your back. The questioner said his competitors all used them, and his lawyer said, "Don't use them because using them admits you have a problem." So I said, "Do you not give people hard hats in an area where you need a hard hat because it admits something might fall on your head? Your lawyer gave you that level of advice." But that's typical of some lawyers' advice: "Don't do anything. You'll admit everything if you say anything. So don't say anything to anybody."

In a major oil company, company doctors and scientists were refused permission to talk to the public about company health risks. A company physician said:

> We went to management and said, "This is why we need to say the following kinds of things." *We* would have put on presentations, but manage-

ment and company attorneys don't want anybody in medical or epidemiology to meet with the community because they're afraid we'll get caught with people asking us questions and our answer will adversely affect the lawsuit. So they hired an outside group to come in and do the community presentation.

Management and the legal department restricted what one pharmaceutical company doctor was permitted to say to employees and the public out of a keen interest in avoiding company liability:

> Our legal department won't allow us to study our own employees. Management and the lawyers want to review the way we say what we say. The lawyers exercise tight control over the studies and findings and information dissemination. They explain how we should describe situations to the workers and affected communities and public.

Former employees may be constrained from providing information by company severance packages that bar them from discussing company matters. In addition, contracts for new employees may include confidentiality agreements. A muzzle clause in the employment contract that an executive at a large international corporation was asked to sign stated that he agreed to "refrain from making any disparaging statements, either orally or in writing, about the company, its officers, directors, affiliates and officers, directors of any affiliates."

Court decisions that impede access to information are becoming more prevalent. For example, litigation awards for health damage may require that court records be sealed, and defendant companies often make confidentiality a condition of settlement.

Lawyers do not always favor limiting access to information. There is increasing pressure on company officials to speak out and provide information, thereby potentially protecting the company by making the public, workers, or other companies assume risks and responsibility. Lawyers therefore sometimes favor publicizing information about serious hazards. Hiding information from workers or the public can backfire, such that openness may be advantageous. A physician for a major computer company said:

Companies that are frank with their employees about problems do the best. You've lost the game when people get the idea you're hiding something from them, you're sneaky and not being open. They don't trust you, they're more likely to sue you, you're less likely to perform very well, and you're dead if you do it with the media.

Certain regulations and court decisions also drive corporations into more open communication.[22] For example, the assumption-of-risk doctrine maintains that if citizens are informed about possible health hazards, they may have assumed the legal risk such that corporations will not be held liable. Sometimes attorneys favor circulating risk information—even uncertain information that suggests rare possible hazards in the future—so that people aware of the possibility of harm will have assumed the risk themselves. Lawyers may therefore encourage written and verbal warnings to customers and citizens' advisory groups in communities where businesses are emitting hazardous chemicals. An attorney who litigates occupational health cases said: "The lawyers' assumption-of-risk argument is becoming more important than the marketers' fear of scaring people."

Marketers favor emphasizing the safety of using company products while withholding risk information from regulators, legislators, and the public. Similarly, public relations people want risk information to be understated and remote hazards not to be discussed. A corporate legal department thus comes into conflict with marketing and public relations officers about how to describe risks. Although attorneys often clash with or overrule physicians on questions of health hazards, doctors and company lawyers often find themselves allied against line managers concerned with sales, as this chemical company physician explained:

The lawyers are our allies in labeling. You make a hazardous product legally a *non*hazardous product just by labeling and warning people about it. If I responsibly tell you what this does and then you kill yourself with it, that's your problem. The lawyers are very punctilious about labeling, and we find ourselves clearly on the same wavelength about warning and labeling.[23]

A chemical company physician described the tension between physicians and managers concerned with sales:

The constructive tension between the health guys and the line guys is over labeling and sales. How you label the stuff and who you can sell it to are product liability issues. We could profit by selling you a chemical and then incur several million dollars in liability after you do something dumb because you don't know how to deal with it and your house is not equipped for storing it. The line people want to sell this dangerous stuff. I say, "Wait, you're selling to a small customer." We make a product that leaves some messy gunk that's an anticorrosion material you can add to well-drilling muds. The problem is, it's probably carcinogenic. We can sell it to drillers, but they are cowboys out there with mud on themselves, all over the equipment—it's a mess. We said, "We can just burn this stuff under boilers, just for heat, but we can't sell this stuff as a well-drilling mud edgement, because it's biologically active and carcinogenic." The line guys concerned with sales say: "Excuse me, but this doesn't cost us anything. It's pure profit. We'll sell it and label it and go talk to them a little bit."

A large oil company had a program in which doctors would examine chest X-rays of all employees in several plants who might have been exposed to asbestos since the 1940s to look for signs of asbestosis, although no law required them to do this. The company physician described the active effort to find the retired employees and notify them that their X-rays showed signs of lung damage, they needed more frequent medical follow-up, and they should not smoke. Subsequently many workers filed a class-action suit in a Texas industrial area against three or four other companies, but not this one, for failure to inform workers of their asbestos exposure and adverse health effects. A physician for the company that warned workers of asbestos risks—partly for defensive legal reasons—said this:

The other companies were successfully sued to the tune of several million dollars, and we were *not* sued because our employees had been warned. I don't mean to say we do great things worldwide, but this story makes a manager sit bolt upright and say, "You guys are earning your keep. I had no idea what the asbestos regulations and our liability were, but you guys ran a program, you informed workers, and the three companies across the street just lost millions of dollars. We didn't." Then the lawyers started asking, "Well, if this was so great here, are we doing it elsewhere?" So it caused a systematic assessment of our asbestos-hazard-warning procedures throughout the world. We did a major mail survey, assessed the results, and then issued new internal company guidelines to tell medical departments worldwide what to do with employees who may have been exposed to asbestos. It became legally driven as much as health-driven at that point.

Some physicians try to persuade employers to do health monitoring that statutes or regulations do not require, arguing that litigation over adverse health effects can be avoided through preventive monitoring. As an oil company physician explained:

We have successfully persuaded our management to do active, epidemiologically rigorous health surveillance. For instance, we have an ongoing mortality study—essentially a death registry of all our U.S. employees who ever worked for us more than a year. Periodically we do epidemiologic studies of the causes of death on that database, looking for jobs or exposures to certain chemicals that may indicate a problem. We are required to report anything suspicious to the EPA. That was a sales pitch to management. It's not something management would ever do on its own, and we sold that initially about fifteen years ago and need to resell it aggressively every two or three years. You have to sell the contribution of the medical department to them in tangible, bottom-line terms: this database is useful in supporting our legal defense and media and community relations and labor-management issues at the plant level. For instance, someone who drove a gasoline truck for two years out of his thirty-year career with the company sues us because gasoline has benzene. Our lawyers—usually outside counsel—ask us, "What data do you have about leukemia rates in the company relative to driving gas trucks?" So we go to the computer and extract leukemia rates of certain worker subpopulations, and it generally helps the lawyers in their defense.

A physician in another major oil company who identified cancer cases in company records used regulatory requirements to overcome management's opposition to informing workers and the government of the findings:

We analyzed our death certificates and found a fairly strong indication that we had an excess risk of leukemia and some related cancers among our oil and gas field exploration and production group. Management didn't want to hear that, but then we said, "You have to tell the employees and the government, and we have to study it further." They particularly didn't want to hear that we wanted to notify the employees: "Oh, they'll be outraged and will sue the company, and we'll have all these problems. We can't do that, and you haven't *proven* it yet," so that was a tough one. We had to point out the law requires us to inform our employees and the EPA about a possible hazard.

In this case, lawyers collaborated with the physicians, health educators, corporate communications personnel, and management on wording the answers the company offered to concerned workers. It was management rather than the company lawyers who most strongly opposed telling people about potential hazards, as the physician explained:

> Lawyers pushed for a full, open disclosure of what we had, but they looked to be sure we weren't saying anything inaccurate or inflammatory. Management looked at it in their traditional fashion: "Oh, my God! We don't want anybody to know what's happening until we're sure, until you've proven that something is there. We don't want the government to know. They might come and inspect us. We don't want the workers to know because then they'll be mad at us."

With the financial stakes in corporate liability cases rising, some corporations have tried to make other corporations responsible for health hazards. For example, asbestos and textile companies have provided data on the health risks of smoking in order to increase the liability of tobacco companies (see, for example, Brodeur 1985, 183). As with labeling, company attorneys in these cases have favored the disclosure of information about corporate health hazards so that other companies would be liable for them.

The Media Role of Physicians Reassuring the Public

Corporate officials worry that the media will assume an anticorporate stance on controversial issues. They fear that if media reports make disease rates appear to be substantial or growing, workers may protest or sue, stockholders may balk, the public may protest, customers may go elsewhere, and regulators or legislators may become more restrictive. They can attempt to control their images as thoroughly as possible and counter unflattering publicity by publicizing information favorable to the company. Public relations, of course, is not new, but its sophistication in many corporations has risen. Employers use the media to explain that exposure problems are either nonexistent or adequately contained and that employers are doing enough to prevent occupational disease, even as union officials and public interest groups call attention to its public costs.

Company doctors have an internal and an external role; that is, their public face differs from their private face. In their external role of speaking publicly to the media or testifying in lawsuits about working conditions, they generally downplay risks and keep their own doubts private. In their internal role within the corporation, they may acknowledge the ambiguity of the evidence when called upon to evaluate hazards and may sometimes argue for stronger exposure controls. Doctors who consult with management in-house about hazards do not necessarily believe what they say publicly about the low risk of substances when they give public reassurance through testimony or medical statements. Rather, they may feel pressure from their employer to keep their job and protect their career interests. A physician who has provided medical services to companies said:

> You see many chemical company doctors on television after a spill or an explosion, or reporting another cancer cluster. They're always reassuring: the data are inconclusive, the company's doing everything it can. That happens time and time again. They may have argued with someone before they accepted the job of going on the screen and saying that. You know that's what they have to say or they won't be there next year.

Increasingly, the public is informed by people without scientific expertise and by those whose job it is to quell any fears about occupational and environmental hazards. Companies generally channel public comments through their public affairs office. In the event of a major incident like an accident, public affairs deals directly with the media and the public and coordinates communication with those outside the company. They take that out of the hands of the physicians and researchers, who then do not have direct contact with the public on occupational and environmental health matters. An electronics company physician said: "Our public affairs department handles calls about suspected health hazards. People who aren't scientists or don't have a scientific background become involved because it's just too much to tie down a few engineers with doing that."

Doctors cannot make any statement about company working conditions or hazards without substantial planning and consultation beforehand. When employers bring physicians in to have them speak to the public, they typically advise them to take the position of top management and company attorneys: that no problem exists or that everything is being taken care of. Two physicians, for a conglomerate and a telecommunications company, said:

> People's health was being harmed, but they just said, "Here's what people are complaining of, and we've looked into it, and this report says this and this report says that, and there's not much to be concerned about." Basically we all sat down and looked at the stuff and talked, and it was like the feeling of a football team, that we'll go out and fight-fight-fight—for whatever. Then, at gatherings of employees, where we talked to the assembled people in a department or division, we would say, "Well, there don't appear to be any data that support this problem, and we're aware of your concerns, but the studies are negative, and we will continue to monitor it"—and so forth. That was the generic approach.

> Employees who contend that they got cancer because they worked in one of our buildings have gone to the newspaper with the allegation. Our lawyers were in on the front end of that before *any* statement was made to the newspaper. Any release in the company newspaper dealing with a potential health hazard—such as whether electromagnetic frequency radiation is a hazard—goes to the lawyers to read to decide whether or not it raises increased liability possibilities for the corporation.

Although company doctors do sometimes speak to the media about exposure hazards on the company's behalf, they play the role of company spokesperson less often than vice presidents of health, safety, and environment or company attorneys. Employers who feel under liability and public relations pressure generally do not permit doctors to describe risks to the public as they perceive them. A chemical company physician explained:

> Large companies want management skills from their doctors more than they want them to talk to the community about toxic air release. It's difficult for companies to be believed because we are a less credible source to lay listeners than our critics. The public may feel that we are tools of industry—owned people, kept men. I cannot undo that by being forthright, so I'm always at a disadvantage. I commonly edit stuff that comes out of our public affairs department, which tries to smooth out the corners of information by putting in modifiers like "only." I don't like to use terms like "only" or try to be cute with language to make a problem go away: "The benzene levels in the water supply are only this." But I can give them the risk associated with the levels of effluent and let them characterize it if they want. It's useful to compare the risk to other risks that people

might have: to say the carcinogen amount is similar to the amount in a peanut butter sandwich. It's important to put yourself forward as objective.[24]

Despite the advantages of having physicians appear to identify hazards objectively, few corporate managers or lawyers have allowed their physicians or company scientists—the employees most knowledgeable about hazards—to speak extensively to the community or the media about company health risks.[25]

USING HIGH-PROFILE CRISES TO COMPEL MANAGEMENT RESPONSES TO TOXICS

Company physicians who are aware of a chemical hazard may subtly use it to blackmail the employer by indirectly saying, "I'll keep your secret to myself, but I want more money for the medical function of the company." They can remind managers of the value of having in-house doctors manage risks rather than letting the hazard worsen or having outside consultants who are less likely to keep the information within the company so that government becomes involved. A chemical company physician explained:

> We had a whole set of male workers here who were rendered infertile from DBCP [dibromochloropropane], a few of them permanently, although most recovered. It first surfaced in another company, and then soon afterwards for us. The opportunity exists here for the medical department to remind management that an in-house occupational health service is able to manage what otherwise outsourced resources may not manage well. Management recognizes that as well as we do. In the case of aspermia in our employees, the company continued to follow the employees until the plant was sold to another company.

Doctors frequently cast health hazards in legal terms to get management to act. Although uncovering hazards may increase the chance that employers will be held liable, as many asbestos companies have shown, managers might believe that solving exposure problems will prevent future liability, as these physicians from an auto company and a textile company explained:

You're never welcomed as the bearer of bad news. You know by the body language they are disappointed. Then usually the questions start coming out: "That's not so bad, is it?" You have to do your homework to prove that it potentially could be bad and use arguments of what could happen if we don't change this or that. Sometimes it's useful to say, "See what happened at Company X, where this didn't get corrected." It's the big-stick theory. Management in general often knows that it comes back to bite them if they don't take care of it right from the start, so they usually are pretty receptive.

A lot of companies aren't sure that their physicians won't use that threat of a lawsuit and publicity as leverage against them, to blackmail them indirectly by saying, "You have a huge problem. You will get sued." I've seen that basic scenario of doctors blackmailing management operate so smoothly that the players hardly recognize that the game was being played. My chief medical officer at a textile company I worked for told me that a little mill back up in the hills about two decades earlier had manufactured asbestos into textiles. It could have been a bombshell for the company because they had never admitted it or done anything about it. We physicians said we ought to see what the liability was, and the company reluctantly agreed to let us go in and evaluate the worker population. We found out that several people who had worked for the company there had died of lung cancer, and it was almost certainly work-related, although no cases had been brought to the company. We also found older retired employees who were at risk. We convinced management to let us go in and identify people at high risk and at least begin to support them proactively, and bring down their liability by doing so. Management was convinced we wouldn't embarrass them in finding out what their liability was, and they were intrigued enough to want to know how they might minimize it.

Physicians often speak of cases like this, where they use management's fears of liability to bolster arguments for increased spending on research, treatment, or preventive measures.

Ripple Effects from Asbestos and Other Crises

The massive number of asbestos disease cases, along with the expensive and high-profile litigation over asbestos exposure, have had a ripple effect on occupational medicine in general. Asbestos litigation has also indirectly affected corporate policies toward exposures generally. It has sensitized companies to the economic threat that occupational disease can pose and alerted them to the trouble they could encounter from not giving out information. The asbestos record has deterred companies from putting products on the market without investigating associated risks of disease and warning people about potential hazards. Managers are afraid that an asbestos-like slew of lawsuits and adverse publicity could run their business into the ground. The Manville debacle has been so extensively publicized that few corporate officials who deal with medical issues are unaware of its magnitude. Managers and physicians have become more educated about asbestos, and lawsuits making lax handling of asbestos economically unprofitable have induced managers to change their practices.[26] The strong employee and government response to asbestos hazards has led some companies to provide better services to exposed workers and avoid repeating the errors and crimes of the asbestos companies.

Physicians sometimes push their health agenda by referring to the asbestos fiasco, and specifically to Manville's experience. Because the liability risks for corporations are so great, the ability of corporate physicians to identify a potential disaster has great strategic importance, and employers tend to listen carefully to their physicians in this area. Managers sometimes describe the asbestos cases as a prototypical example of something they wish to avoid in the future, but many also tend to see it as a special exception that they need not worry about, as these two physicians, from an oil company and a services company, explained:

> We've used the argument that, "Look, we have problems like benzene that could be the next asbestos problem, and we could get into the same trouble that Manville and the other companies did." That has a definite impact, but the managers still tend to dismiss it and say, "Oh, that happened to them, but it won't happen to us," or, "This isn't quite the same."

> Asbestos and tobacco companies' clear, purposeful misrepresentation, hiding, and lying was especially useful in court. And look what happened with A. H. Robbins and the Dalkon Shield—the company went out of business. But most companies feel that they don't have the same liability since they don't do *that*.

Asbestos has indeed been a dramatic and exceptional case in some ways: because so much money was involved; because high-profile litigation educated the public as well as corporate managers; because it has been much better researched and publicized than other occupational health hazards; and because of the military involvement in wartime shipyard exposures. In addition, jobs with heavy asbestos exposure—such as making asbestos or changing brake drums on cars—are extremely hazardous. Coal mining and lead are also exceptional because the evidence on black lung and lead hazards is overwhelming and because corporations have mounted stronger opposition in those cases than in others. Moreover, asbestos exposure is clearly linked with a disease, mesothelioma, that typically results from asbestos exposure. In contrast, other chemicals lack clear markers for disease causation, so that lung cancer or leukemia could be due to benzene, other chemicals, or non-environmental causes. These atypical features of asbestos make it especially uncertain whether occupational physicians, publicity, and the legal system will play as big a role in the case of other substances. Still, employers are motivated to act in those other cases to avoid the risks of effects parallel to the asbestos case. Asbestos litigation has created enough company expense and fear that preventive exposure-control programs appear more cost-effective to employers than in the past.

High-profile leaks and accidents have also affected corporate responsiveness to toxics and given rise to legislation requiring more protective corporate practices. For example, the Bhopal catastrophe of 1984 stimulated passage of the Superfund Amendments and Reauthorization Act (SARA) in 1986, which is partly directed toward controlling chemical releases, and the Santa Barbara oil spill in 1969 helped produce the National Environmental Policy Act and the EPA.[27] Environmental tragedies have made senior management aware of the importance of occupational and environmental health; they have provoked responsible behavior and helped to create an understanding that testing a product and doing studies in advance are a necessary part of doing business.

Although many companies have altered their conduct out of concern for future liability, stemming partly from the asbestos history, the effect of asbestos litigation on workplace health policies should not be overstated. Companies still sell materials that are inadequately tested and likely to cause harm. Physicians working for asbestos producers who have seen a suspiciously high number of lung cancer deaths and warned company management that a problem existed have had their advice ignored. Physicians in other companies, too, have been unable to convince employers to respond effectively to reduce health risks.[28] Although publicity about asbestos has encouraged large manufacturers to distribute more information in the hope of protecting themselves, many have masked the health effects of their products, as asbestos manufacturers have done and as tobacco companies have done with cigarettes. They have failed to warn employees and the public because doing so could lead to a loss of market share. A physician who provides medical services to companies said:

> Everybody knows you're sitting on powder kegs in this field if you make chemicals. Someone will come along with good information and embarrass you sooner or later—you can't be ahead of it all. Certainly lots of things are potentially serious carcinogens. Companies wait for the government to prove something with their epidemiological studies, or wait for doctors to report enough cases before they take it seriously.

As this physician described it, employers tend to be reactive, waiting for crises, clear evidence of damage, or obvious legal risks before they are spurred into action to mitigate hazards.

Physician Involvement in Asbestos Cases

The asbestos cases are legion, with many millions of dollars at stake. As workers and unions have applied economic pressure to companies with asbestos-exposed employees, a rash of asbestos lawsuits has spread over the last thirty years. Besides the many suits against manufacturers, a huge number of third-party suits have been brought by individuals exposed to asbestos by a party other than their employer. Some companies have declared bankruptcy or gone to great lengths to shield themselves from liability for asbestos disease claims. Although corporate officials have argued that they were unaware until the 1960s that asbestos was a health hazard, evidence indicates that industry officials knew it was harmful thirty years earlier and could have known about asbestos hazards forty years earlier had they acted on the evidence from the available medical literature.[29] Outside industry circles, asbestos hazards have been widely known since Irving Selikoff's scientific reports of the 1960s and 1970s.[30]

Physicians played a major role on both sides of a highly polarizing social controversy over asbestos. Doctors in universities and private practice have brought asbestos hazards to light and spoken out about disease patterns they have seen in patients. Authoritative physicians outside companies who have seen hundreds of cases of asbestos-related cancer have published their findings of a cancer epidemic originating in World War II shipyards. Doctors at the Mount Sinai occupational medicine program, following Selikoff's pioneering work, have testified widely in asbestos cases, relying on what by now is tremendous knowledge about asbestos-related diseases. Occupational physicians under government contract have provided medical evaluations for individuals exposed to asbestos and have done large-scale studies of exposed individuals. Having doctors in the middle of the asbestos controversy has in many ways strengthened the field of occupational medicine.

At the same time, and predictably, doctors employed by asbestos manufacturers have defended their employers (see, for example, Castleman 1996; Brodeur 1985). They have used research on asbestos diseases to attack testimony or medical records describing asbestos hazards. They have argued that company liability should be limited in many cases, as when workers show evidence of pleural plaque but no asbestosis. They also have testified that corporate officials and doctors in companies that used asbestos during World War II and through the 1950s did not understand asbestos hazards.

Doctors who worked directly for asbestos manufacturers that went out of business obviously lost their jobs, but others thrived. Paul Kotin, for example, was outspoken on occupational health issues during his employment as medical director of Manville. And doctors in other corporations have discounted evidence, suppressed studies, or argued that asbestos, along with other hazardous substances, presents only minor risks or no risk at all. A utility doctor said:

I'm concerned about the physician's position in the asbestos hysteria in society, in terms of the real risks in most settings and what it does financially to the economy. We overplay extreme cases of asbestos risk and don't concentrate enough on the real, core toxic areas. It ties people's hands so they can't do things they should do because of the threat of a minimal asbestos exposure.

A health official with the Union of Needletrades, Industrial, and Textile Employees, which represents workers at plants with high rates of lung cancer from asbestos, said:

> We've had run-ins with company doctors, at Raybestos and Turner and Newell out of Britain. My blood runs cold and I get shivers just thinking about these low-lifes. Our members over the years worked at some of the most heavily studied asbestos plants in the world, asbestos textile plants being some of the dustiest. A company hack in the asbestos industry in the 1970s and 1980s was very different from one in the 1960s or 1940s. They began to look more sophisticated. Just look at the tobacco industry; now they favor public health and education programs against childhood cigarette smoking.[31]

An official with the Oil, Chemical, and Atomic Workers International Union described physicians' participation in the asbestos fiasco:

> The asbestos story was probably company doctors' least glorious chapter. The stories are legion of doctors who examined patients and obscured the fact that the person's ailment was related to the plant environment. In Tyler, Texas, workers were being exposed to enormous amounts of asbestos, and the Public Health Service communicated with the corporate doctor about the nature of the problem, but workers were never informed. The record is replete with these instances.[32]

Employers increasingly recognize asbestos hazards and ways to reduce them. OSHA now mandates medical surveillance and protection requirements. Companies generally monitor exposed workers and hire specialists in subcontracting companies to do asbestos removal. Despite this increased vigilance, asbestos hazards remain. One oil company, for example, uses asbestos extensively throughout its refineries; it therefore does about 2,700 asbestos-related exams a year, following exposed individuals in medical surveillance programs throughout employment and into retirement. Having already caused over 200,000 deaths in the United States alone, asbestos is likely to cause hundreds of thousands more deaths worldwide, in addition to many more cases of chronic disease. For years to come, physicians are likely to continue their active involvement in defending employers, in mitigating the ongoing asbestos hazards, or in monitoring the toll in disease and death. With some notable exceptions, their involvement in responding to asbestos hazards from within corporations is in contrast to the roles that occupational physicians generally have played in responding to asbestos hazards from outside corporations in government and university settings.

POLITICAL CHEMICALS AND HEALTH DATA USED IN EMPLOYERS' INTERESTS

Debates in occupational medicine become highly political largely because the social and economic context politicizes corporate medical practice. An oil company physician offers a rosy view of science in corporations, claiming that major companies such as his own permit their physicians to use good scientific methods and findings:

> It's no easier or more difficult to do good science in large corporations than in academia or government. Good science depends on the investigators' motives and abilities to see their ideas through in any of these sectors. Nothing in corporations is intrinsically inimical to good science.

Corporations are political entities, however, and occupational medicine's capacity to have positive effects has to do with politics as well as science. For example, company doctors infrequently publish their research findings or give research presentations when they find adverse effects from company products, working conditions, or environmental contamination. In addition, employers typically challenge research methods only when the findings contradict their claims to be adequately protecting employees and the environment. At government regulatory hearings and before congressional oversight committees, corporate physicians testify that company conditions are safe. Their distorted use of statistics and research is not always deliberate, since physicians generally believe their own claims. Nevertheless, they have analyzed risk in ways that cause companies and government to disregard health hazards, as a physician who has provided occupational health services to companies explained:

Many companies contribute to the confusion over occupational carcinogens and other hazards by engaging in their own epidemiology and throwing their data in too. The more studies, the more equivocality and the more difficult to interpret anything. Risk analysis looks definite on paper: "The risk of your benzene exposure is one one-hundredth of your passive-smoke exposure." That causes people to say, "Then why should we spend time worrying about benzene?" The data are flawed, manageable, and misinterpretable. Risk analysis confuses environmental or occupational medicine and makes it impotent. It's a very manipulatable commodity—it's just a dream.[33]

Two doctors who work in a conglomerate and have provided health services to corporations pointed to the small amount of research and few published reports on workplace hazards that company doctors produce:

The paper trail is cleaned up quite a bit in the practice of occupational medicine. Our medical department would like to circulate reports of findings from health surveys, but our lawyers generally say, "Don't put anything in writing." Some of the operating officials also say, "Don't circulate that report," or, "Don't you know that if you find something, you have to fix it?" If we have a toxic spill, it's all dealt with on the telephone, so that there are no documents, no paper trail, if there is ever a suit. Sometimes I call a company lawyer and say, "Here's what happened," and the lawyer says, "Don't put it in writing." Companies refuse to give *us* written reports because they don't want to create a paper trail, especially on environmental things. "We had a spill of ump-tee-ump gallons, or a release of so-and-so into the atmosphere; we're just telling you about it. We have it taken care of. No need to report it." End of conversation. Then it doesn't get reported to the EPA.

Most corporate physicians go through their entire career without ever publishing a single paper. We give an award in the Western Occupational Medical Association for excellence in scientific writing, and only once did we give it to a corporate physician. It always goes to someone in an academic center. We bend over backwards to encourage these guys to write, but they're not at liberty to write or to speak. You ask them to participate in a publication, and they ask corporate medical and get turned down. There have been whistleblowers and heroes—people who have reported clusters of repetitive motion disorder or cancer or congenital malformation—but they're not around long. They sacrifice to do it. You find the same spectrum of whores to heroes in occupational medicine that you find in occupational toxicology and epidemiology, and companies know how to find whatever they're looking for.

The political aspects of the job of occupational physician include activities such as being the personal health advocate for executives or helping employers defend themselves against worker claimants. Occupational medicine has had overarching political significance, partly owing to the efforts of the American labor movement, the high medical costs of the privatized U.S. health care delivery system, and employers' aggressive stance toward employees and health regulation in the United States, especially when compared with their relationship to labor in other industrial countries.[34] The physicians' political role is magnified as they advise and testify about health and environmental matters. The scientific literature itself has been politicized. A university occupational physician said:

> Attorneys often know more about the scientific literature—such as on asbestos—than doctors do. It troubles me that you can't even have a scientific discourse about something without attorneys being involved in it. Doctors are expected to make important scientific decisions with insufficient information, and that puts a lot of pressure on people and discourages them from joining this field, because it's so very litigious.

Physicians encounter many forks in the road as they listen to arguments, evaluate evidence, and select which risk assessment calculus to use. Their individual decisions take place within a context that tends toward polarization. Health has been a significant bargaining issue in major conflicts between labor and management, and it also involves controversial social and legal questions, sometimes with huge amounts of money at stake.[35] The political requirements of a company physician's job are often indistinct and contradictory, but the need for a negative stance toward evidence of health hazards is generally clear.

The Journal of Occupational and Environmental Medicine and Peer Review

The *Journal of Occupational and Environmental Medicine,* as the official publication of ACOEM, exemplifies in part the politicized environment of workplace and environmental health data—as do other scientific publications in this area. The *Journal* has reflected changes in occupational medicine since its founding in 1959.

More articles are now directed toward clinical physicians—a growing proportion of the ACOEM membership. The original pro-industry orientation of the *Journal,* while weaker, remains. An editor of the *Journal* said:

> *JOM* was basically a place where members could send in almost anything and it would get published—more opinion, very little research being done. It was viewed as a biased mouthpiece for industry since it was the official publication—and still is—of the College [ACOEM], which was made up of just the industry docs—particularly in the old days. It's not surprising to find a lot of negative studies [showing no company health hazards], because that's what we were trying to show.

Peer review in publications and grants has its weaknesses in disputatious fields like occupational medicine—especially in its more contentious areas. A *Journal* editor said:

> The aura of objectivity in the *Journal* is in many cases just a facade. I know who the reviewers are out there. People say reviewers decide what gets published, but all this peer review we go through is an exercise not necessarily any less arbitrary than if I just sat down and read the article myself and said, "Okay, is this good or bad?" If I get a paper on a disputed area, I may want to publish it or to kill it because I totally disagree with it. A lot of things can be rigged, and journal editors know it's easy for them to rig an outcome if they want to.[36]

Similarly, most organizations that publish documents stating whether substances are probable carcinogens have a political dimension.[37] They bring together experts from around the world to discuss an issue and claim to seek input from a wide range of people before reaching a consensus. The list of participants, however, can easily be skewed. An occupational physician who participates in such research conferences said:

> The person who's in charge of deciding who gets to come to conferences that identify carcinogens clearly can slant that group however he wants. I know what the answer is as soon as I see the list of those invited. People have the sense that we're doing something objective and value-free or observer-independent. That's not true.

The fact that journals and research conferences tend to reflect the politics and controversy of the field, as well as of journal editors and conference organizers, is perhaps to be expected.[38] However, any public health field—including occupational medicine—lends itself to politics even more than private medical practice.

ACOEM AND AMBIVALENCE ABOUT TOXICS AS A CAUSE OF DISEASE

The main professional organization that company doctors belong to—ACOEM—reflects the preoccupations of its physician members. It also reflects company physicians' ambivalence about locating the cause of employee illness in workplace exposure to toxic chemicals.

Since the 1960s a field called "environmental medicine" has evolved. In the beginning, physicians began receiving training in the impact on human health of chemicals in the air, ground, water, and consumer products outside the workplace. Occupational medicine has been moving in the direction of environmental health and now considers the exposure effects of biological, chemical, and physical hazards outside as well as inside the workplace. Companies turned to occupational physicians to find ways to deal with pressing environmental concerns. The American Occupational Medicine Association's name change in 1992—to the American College of Occupational *and Environmental* Medicine (ACOEM)—reflected the public concern with environmental hazards (over occupational hazards) that has been closely tied to expanding environmental legislation.

ACOEM added the "E" to its name partly because of the growing influence of contractors who recognized business opportunities in expanding the domain of the organization and the profession. Bringing in environmental specialists would enable the organization to grow by branching out beyond the occupational medicine field, which was losing some of its in-house people.[39] A chemical company physician said: "The 'E' in ACOEM was a defensive thing to try to capture the market before somebody else did. We'll continue to see less in-house expertise and more from outside."[40] More bluntly, an occupational physician who has provided health services to corporations said:

That "E" got into the College name to keep the other specialties from walking away with a plum. That happened two years after we inserted it into
all the academic training program names in the country; it's just the run for
the money.

Occupational physicians recognized that the environmental
movement is huge, carries broad implications for medicine, and
has a potential audience of virtually the entire population. Although universities and legislatures provide money for environmental research, medical schools train few environmental health
specialists. For years people had complained to doctors about
multiple chemical sensitivity, airborne lead, and water contaminants outside their workplace—all within the purview of environmental medicine—but no professional group had addressed their
concerns. Entrepreneurs who knew little about environmental
health effects saw a growing niche and jumped in. And occupational doctors believed that their training and understanding of
workplace environments enabled them to assert their expertise in
the growing field of environmental medicine. Thus, adding the "E"
to ACOEM was partly a matter of filling a vacuum. Physicians
trained in occupational medicine can presumably transfer their
knowledge of biostatistics, epidemiology, environmental health,
and industrial hygiene to environmental problems.

Compared with most other specialty groups, occupational
medicine is a vast field in its areas of responsibility. Its reach now
extends beyond the factory fence to the environmental concerns
of the entire population, including infants and elderly people,
whose twenty-four-hour exposures are generally much lower than
those of employees who spend eight hours at one workplace. Occupational physicians have begun to deal with many newer health
problems, such as HIV, drugs, and a growing list of recognized
disabilities. Employees now tend to receive less attention as physicians increasingly turn their attention to illnesses caused by chemicals in the air, water, and soil. Moving into environmental concerns puts additional demands on occupational physicians, as this
chemical company physician, a longtime member of ACOEM, explained:

The major decision the College made to change its name to the American
College of Occupational *and Environmental* Medicine was a mistake,

because it will divert us and make it even more difficult for us to concentrate on the primary mission of occupational physicians, which is promoting worker health. It has moved us into an arena which literally comes to ignore workers, if we get heavily involved in environmental issues. That would be a shame and sad, because we don't have that many people trained in this field, and now we're taking on the whole country in environmental medicine, which gives us more of a power base by doubling our cohort population from employees only to all 280 million American citizens, but also dilutes our capacity to focus on worker health issues.[41]

Although ACOEM has expressed an organizational interest in environmental issues, the professional ACOEM meetings reflect the dominant concerns of its individual company physicians and consultant members: cost containment; smoking cessation, drug testing, fitness, and other kinds of wellness programs; and defending against government regulation. In contrast, government and university-clinic physicians generally are more concerned with ferreting out and preventing workplace exposure hazards, doing epidemiological studies, and discussing policy issues.

Whereas some academics sympathetic to industry also belong to ACOEM, occupational physicians in clinics and universities tend to belong instead to the American Public Health Association (APHA) or an organization that represents their medical specialty, such as internal medicine or surgery. The two organizations—ACOEM and APHA—reflect a significant divide; they have different concerns and give a different meaning to a preventive approach. Only a minority of the members of APHA's occupational health section are physicians; individuals can join the APHA if any aspect of their discipline and interest is in public health. Many industrial hygienists, people with a master's degree in public health, and epidemiologists join after they complete undergraduate or midlevel graduate degrees. Thus, the demographics of the APHA differ markedly from those of ACOEM. The APHA is further to the left on the political spectrum than ACOEM, with more worker advocates and university researchers in its occupational section. The concentration of APHA members in research, government, and university programs facilitates their interests in social and environmental issues beyond the workplace. A publishing company physician said:

The more traditional medical organizations like ACOEM are more reactionary, slower to respond to change, more cautious and skeptical of change than the APHA, which is more politicized. There's a good reason for it: the APHA is an all-encompassing organization, with a far larger segment of its membership in the twenty-to-forty age group than beyond it. Their activities and even their style of clothes are different.

Physicians from diverse backgrounds may attend ACOEM meetings and read the association's publications, but the way in which ACOEM raises issues makes its discussions most helpful to in-house physicians and to those who practice under contract to corporations rather than to researchers and clinicians outside corporations. Two physicians, in a major oil company and in a large medical center's occupational medicine program that treats workers, said:

ACOEM is valuable in terms of the contacts you make. It's more of a networking organization, with not many academics involved.

The ACOEM meetings are boring for anyone interested in scientific issues. Part of it is that they're interested in drug testing and health promotion, and I'm not. They're not interested in asbestos and occupational disease in their workforce, and they don't have the intrinsic interest in science.

In many respects, the organizational affiliations and approach to health concerns of company physicians differ markedly from those of occupational physicians outside corporations.

CONCLUSION

Occupational disease, unlike most injuries, presents many complex questions of causation, such as whether a person's asthmatic condition is in fact due to a workplace exposure. Questions about whether disease is traced to the workplace or to conditions outside the company often put management's interests in conflict with those of employees, especially in the areas of workers' compensation claims and lawsuits. The enthusiasm of company doctors for investigating occupational disease and their willingness to prevent it are uneven at best; any such reluctance is understandable given that company doctors draw their support from the corporations they serve. Constrained as they are by a complex set of pressures, they nonetheless influence corporate policies as well as the individual cases they diagnose or testify about. If employers defined the jobs of company physicians differently, these doctors certainly could do more to safeguard health. Company physicians find themselves in a difficult position when they are expected to protect the company's interest even when their professional interests and personal ethics lead them to want to advocate for employees or public health.

These observations have implications for how we study and understand the ethics of organizational actors. As the findings discussed here reveal, physicians would often like to see greater investment in preventive health practices. They may wish to conduct studies into the health effects of workplace chemicals. They might want to speak to the public, the media, legislators, or even juries about responsibility for hazards. But it is not insufficient appreciation of ethical principles, or even an inability to identify an appropriate course of action, that keeps them looking away from toxic hazards and instead focusing narrowly on the reportability of illnesses that occur, cooperating with others to deflect attention from workplace causes of disease, or stepping aside as others less knowledgeable about toxic hazards speak out on these matters. The social and political contexts of their employment, combined with their own career concerns, exert powerful pressure on the ethical framework of these professionals and on the choices they make, as well as on the daily pattern of their work lives.

Although the scientific knowledge of workplace toxins is growing each year, pressures on physicians to turn away from toxics are also generally increasing. These pressures intensify as work life becomes ever more corporatized, as employers experience growing competitive pressures to cut costs, and as the liability fears of managers and lawyers lead them to suppress information or avoid doing studies that could identify toxic risks in the workplace and the broader environment.

— Chapter 5 —

Drug Testing
in the Workplace:
The Allure of
Management Technologies

*The patient perceives that you can't be the helping and the
policing physician, so you have to decide which side of the
fence you're going to be on. Perception of conflict of interest is
a definite problem you have to look at closely all the time.*

—Utility company physician

Drug testing is not medicine.

—National health and safety official, AFL-CIO[1]

EMPLOYERS INCREASINGLY TURN to employment policies that focus
on drug users as a group that may pose a special risk in the
workplace. They have been concerned about the catastrophic potential of allowing workers with a drug use problem to remain on
the job. Drug testing in the workplace is an approach that conven-
iently sets aside any concern that repetitive or dangerous jobs may
be contributing to drug use.

Doctors employed by corporations have played an important
role in the use of medical technologies to test for drugs. They use
tests that they acknowledge are generally ineffective in detecting

drug use, or even harmful, while intruding into employees' private lives and falsely labeling individuals as drug abusers. In addition, a test of uncertain significance is given greater weight in making these evaluations than job performance. However, drug screening enables employers and company physicians to deter some drug use and to evade corporate responsibility for accidents and the hazardous working conditions that management has imposed. In examining how physicians and employers identify and deal with groups they consider risky, I focus on the social significance of drug screening and the ways in which corporate professionals and employers conceptualize its use.

DRUG TESTING AS A SUBSTITUTE
FOR PUBLIC HEALTH MONITORING

Drug use and wellness programs are part of the search for workers with individual health risks, as opposed to a search for occupational hazards from working conditions.[2] Companies identify users of marijuana, cocaine, opiates, amphetamines, and other drugs in their efforts to determine whether employees have health problems that would hinder their job performance or raise medical costs.

In the 1960s and 1970s the U.S. Department of Defense (DOD) began its drug testing of military personnel to address the problem of free access to a wide variety of drugs. It developed a punitive surveillance program, which led to cost-effective testing techniques that companies began to adopt. Many companies then initiated drug testing because of the Reagan administration's mandate and new regulation by the Department of Transportation (DOT) and the Federal Aviation Administration (FAA); the government was attempting to stop consumer demand after encountering little success in stopping the supply. Increased company drug testing emerged from the Drug-Free Workplace Act of 1988 and other congressional activity.[3] Companies developed the mandatory random drug-testing programs for people in safety-sensitive positions—such as interstate truckers and petroleum pipeline workers—that local, state, or federal regulations required (see Lieberwitz 1994, 192, 199–200; Normand, Lempert, and O'Brien 1994, 284–301). Management also carried out drug-testing programs because they saw other positive gains, such as screening out unproductive employees and avoiding adverse publicity.

Drug testing has now become widespread in the workplace. The American Management Association (2001, 1) recently found that 67 percent of its member companies in the United States conducted drug testing.[4] Large firms generally test all job applicants for every position and offer jobs only to those who pass the drug test. Testing is particularly common in companies where the work involves what managers perceive as special safety hazards. Most employers in the oil, chemical, and transportation industries, for example, test all new hires for all jobs.

Drug-testing statutes and case law tend to distinguish between job applicants and incumbent employees—generally allowing broader testing of applicants.[5] However, considerations of privacy, employment interests, fairness, and fundamental rights are not necessarily very different for applicants and incumbents. Certainly they have comparable interests in earning a livelihood and in avoiding tests that could deprive them of health insurance and employment opportunities. Nonetheless, the law especially encourages applicant drug screening.

Companies generally test all applicants for drugs regardless of their job level. White-collar workers such as secretaries or high-level executives recruited from other companies usually are tested along with production workers. The degree of sophistication varies. At one end of the spectrum are nuclear power plants, with elaborate government random and for-cause testing programs mandated by the Nuclear Regulatory Commission (NRC) and the Department of Energy (DOE).[6] Others, like banks and manufacturing companies, concentrate on for-cause and new-hire testing for drug use to evaluate whether workers are fit to do their jobs. Some companies only test for cause, after an accident or functional deficit creates the suspicion that an individual might be working under the influence of drugs.

Drugs and asbestos represent the two competing paradigms for explaining the major problem in occupational health. Drug testing is a significant concern for occupational physicians in corporations, just as asbestos may be the quintessential case for public health–oriented occupational physicians in universities and government.

Drug testing is a problematic screening approach for many

reasons. By seeking to identify individuals with specific risk factors such as vulnerability to drug abuse, company officials implicitly argue that all others are safe, that current levels of contaminants are not generally harmful, and therefore that changing company policies or supporting further substance regulation is unnecessary.

THE LEMMING EFFECT FROM EMPLOYERS' WISH TO DETER DRUG USERS

When drug testing was first introduced, some companies had 50 percent positive test results or even higher. Two physicians, one in a major pharmaceutical company and the other in an oil company, talked about those early years:

> I can recall some plants with incredibly high levels when they first introduced drug testing; a plant in Baltimore had a positive rate initially of 60 percent. In some areas the prevalence rate for drug use was just enormous.

> When we first started drug testing, we were running in one remote mining location 50 percent positives. During the hiring period, people in the parking lot were selling clean urines to the applicants to take in with them.

Corporations that test for drugs in an established workforce generally find that only a small fraction of workers use drugs illegally. Those that routinely test job applicants and use for-cause testing typically have a positive rate of only 1 to 5 percent—a significant decline from the positive test rates of 50 percent or even higher that certain companies initially had (see American Management Association 1996).[7]

Drug testing is time-consuming and not necessarily cost-effective. If drug use in a facility is relatively low—about 1 to 5 percent—companies can spend a great deal of money to avoid a single drug user.[8] The cost may outweigh the benefit for companies that identify few cases in expensive random drug testing. As a bank physician who conducts thousands of drug tests each year said:

We've been doing preplacement drug testing with the rate of positive tests at 1.4 percent. It costs a pile of money, about three-quarters of a million dollars a year, and they are looking for savings. So at one point I said to them, "Just tell them we tested them. We'll just pour it down the drain." It just didn't seem worthwhile to me to find that small percentage.[9]

Despite the high cost, even employers that detect only one or two cases a year worry that if they do not test, drug users will gravitate to them instead of to other companies after the community becomes aware of their decision not to test. Many employers therefore start drug programs to deter drug users from applying for jobs with them (see Normand, Lempert, and O'Brien 1994, 177–240). A telecommunications company physician and a chemical company physician said:

Pre-employment drug testing allows particular manufacturing locations and business units not to position themselves adversely in different communities where they need to hire. In some communities we were one of the last major employers to institute pre-employment drug testing, and we had a lot of active users who were selectively choosing to come aboard with us.

The reason we do drug testing on all new hires is not that it's good procedure. It is that it keeps us from getting a disproportionate share of junkies. If the word out there is that we don't do drug testing, then all the drug abusers would say, "Hey, let's go over there. They don't test us, but Shell and Monsanto and Westinghouse do." I suppose we are willing to take our fair share of abusers, but we don't want all the discards from everybody else.[10]

This practice creates a lemming effect, a rush to corporate conformity: when one company adopts drug testing, other companies quickly follow it, even without strong evidence that the tests accurately detect drug abusers. Although companies rarely test employees randomly, except in power plants and other safety-sensitive work sites, many employers announce that they are prepared to do random testing in an effort to keep drug users away from their company. This phenomenon is similar to the "bandwagon" effect seen among research organizations that rush to develop medical technologies that are not necessarily the most promising scientifically.[11] Thus, although some companies realize

that drug testing is expensive and not the panacea they had anticipated, they continue to test in part because other companies do.

THE TURF-EXPANDING FUNCTION OF DRUG TESTING

Drug testing is a principal way in which physicians define themselves as useful to management, even when they recognize that
testing has limitations or causes harm. A physician who has
worked in both corporations and government said:

> Drug testing is an incredible boon to company physicians. Management is
> interested in drug testing in order to purify the workplace, so drug testing
> is what the in-house corporate people do. The physician is the instrument.
> Management needs these physicians to do these damn tests.

Medical personnel advocate tests to expand their own resources
and power. Having drug testing under the purview of in-house
physicians expands the resources that employers provide to support substance abuse programs. Doctors who once complained
about the burden of drug testing now say they are grateful for it
because it helps them justify their time and their medical staff,
especially when their medical departments are embattled or shrinking; without it, they might lose the infrastructure now devoted to it
or even have their programs eliminated. In addition, medical units
within large corporations increasingly have to defend how they
serve their company's customers. Drug testing helps them do this
because it is popular and has customer appeal.

A company's medical department conducts placement exams
after applicants get a job-offer letter and reviews each positive
drug test result to make sure that the use of a legitimate prescription drug or other excusable substance did not cause it. For example, doctors sometimes use cocaine when they sew up lacerations,
deaden eardrums, or insert tubes for bronchoscopies. The use of
Tylenol-3 with codeine and various prescription drugs can often
result in a positive drug test. Federal regulations require that medical review officers (MROs)—who are licensed physicians knowledgeable in substance abuse—review the paperwork and give
those who fail a drug test an opportunity to explain the result.[12]

However, a safety or human resources unit may carry out the actual mechanics of sample collection, packaging, and shipping the test, since it is not an inherently medical procedure that requires a doctor or nurse. As an oil company doctor said: "It's not like we exercise a tremendous body of knowledge. The test is negative or positive, and if it's positive, you can go on to investigate some other things in order to reach a judgment."

Rather than have internal drug testing, many companies hire contracting companies or outside physicians who do drug testing for many companies. In-house physicians oversee contracts with external laboratories to ensure that testing meets government certification and licensing requirements. Workers generally are less opposed to drug testing when companies pay outside doctors and testing firms to conduct the tests. However, the prospect of outside testing intensifies the efforts of company physicians to defend their turf and resources. An aerospace doctor who charges the government for the drug testing it requires of its major contractors
· said:

> A VP said, "Y'know, this is going to be so difficult, we might be better off, for accounting purposes, to have an outside firm come in and do nothing but the urines for us." Of course, as the person running the medical department, I didn't want an outsider coming in and taking work away from us.

In the late 1980s and early 1990s legislators and government officials advocated eliminating physicians from drug testing, on the grounds that employers and government should not incur the cost of having physicians perform a function that lesser-paid employees could handle. Company doctors and their major professional organization, ACOEM, successfully fought this effort by opposing bills that would have eliminated the physician's role in drug testing.[13]

DRUGS AND THE MEDICALIZATION
OF MANAGERIAL PROBLEMS

Employee intoxication is a valuable defense for employers because it can shield them from financial responsibility for injuries.[14]

Management may also be able to escape corporate liability by holding workers responsible for their behavior when in fact it may be partly induced by a stressful job and a dangerous work environment. For example, when an employer finds drugs in a worker's blood or urine after an accident, it may conclude that drugs were the cause. It is increasingly common to use drug testing as a way of blaming workers for their own injuries and illnesses. A physician who conducts drug testing and participates in workers' compensation cases explained:

> Sometimes a claimant's urine or blood will be tested, and if they are definitely intoxicated at the time of the injury, we can get out from under the responsibility of paying for it because intoxication is a defense. So if you are intoxicated on the job and you get hurt, the employer is no longer liable for it.

Supervisors refer individuals they suspect of taking drugs to the medical department for testing and an evaluation.[15] They also require employees who return to work after a treatment program to submit to unannounced periodic drug testing. Companies that have a policy of drug testing every time an injury occurs may selectively choose which employees to test—for example, shop-floor workers but not managers. A physician who supervises employee drug testing said: "Except for safety-sensitive positions, we don't do drug testing unless there is some indication, like a history of use. That can be pretty arbitrary and minor, but it isn't done routinely."

Drug testing is a shortsighted approach to factors that contribute to drug use, such as work overload, repetitive jobs, and job insecurity from downsizing.[16] Although drug testing is irrational as a solution to reducing employee drug use, it serves other managerial goals.

POLICING DRUGS

Although drug testing does not eliminate drug users from the workplace, corporate America has adopted what is essentially a police position: drug use must be stamped out. Drug testing is not necessarily a medical endeavor. It is designed to promote workplace safety and the ability of workers to do their jobs, to protect employers against theft and embezzlement, and to safeguard the company's reputation for not hiring drug addicts. Corporate officials' interest in drug testing conflicts with the traditional medical priority of providing health care and rehabilitation; it puts physicians in the awkward position of policing workers rather than extending help to them.

An important reason many doctors running corporate medical programs support drug testing is their military background. It shapes their expectations about what a corporate doctor should do and makes drug testing and its related heavy paperwork requirements more palatable. Unlike medical training, military experience also prepares doctors for simply carrying out orders, such as performing the tests requested by management. A physician from the auto industry said: "I don't have a problem with drug testing. That might be just coming from the navy, because our mandate was just to go ahead and do that, so it just came along pretty naturally." Two other company doctors with a military background, one now employed by an airline and the other by a telecommunications company, expressed a similar attitude:

> My role in drug testing is completely specified by the regulations, so I can just do what's in the book. I'm not interested in doing something for the sake of being punitive against an employee or making myself more powerful. I just do this because it's a job and they pay me, so I read the book and follow the guidelines. Sometimes it allows me some discretionary latitude and some ability to be a human being, but sometimes it doesn't.

> Drug testing is part of being a corporate doctor. If I wanted to be out doing clinical practice, then I would see this as terrible. But for me, drug testing is fine. This is part of my job and what I was trained to do. It goes with the job. To me, it's like scalpel and sutures.

On the other hand, many company physicians harbor strong objections to the drug testing their employers require them to conduct. They say that drug testing should be relegated to the security unit or the human resources wing rather than the medical department because it puts physicians in the awkward position of policing workers rather than extending help to individuals. A physician who has provided medical services for several companies and a utility company physician whose medical department conducts drug screening said:

> Drug testing is the best example I can think of, of how corporate physicians ultimately get used; they're turned into policemen. Very few have the temerity to say that they just don't agree with the concept and won't do it. Occupational physicians shouldn't have anything to do with police activity—ever. It's just a manipulation of our training.
>
> Drug testing is a policing function. The responsibility should be outside the health department. To me, random drug testing is the most invasive of all the things that the company does. I don't want to be in that business. It's detrimental to our relationship. You actually create a situation where people get more clever about hiding it and pushing off getting help. You should just be totally focused on helping and prevention.

A doctor who does drug testing for a chemical company said:

> I find random drug testing in an employment setting reprehensible and absolutely offensive to people: guilty until proven innocent, pee in a bottle with two people looking. I didn't go into medicine to be a security guard. The primary purpose of drug testing ought to be to detect the problem that is treatable, that you can do something about.

Company physicians often say they are not responsible for termination decisions, because they deal only with the technical aspects of running and interpreting tests correctly. They maintain that their job is to make the worker fit to do the work, and that drug use is one reason people may be unfit. Some corporate physicians try to disengage their clinical role of diagnosing and rehabilitating drug users from the corporation's policing function. A physician with a retail sales company said:

> We did not want to be stigmatized as cops, detectives, snoops, and so we divided up the responsibility into two pieces. We are the professional staff reviewers for any positive test results. We try to exculpate the offender, if indeed there's been an offense. But if I cannot find any legitimate medical basis for a positive test, the hiring group deals with it. The medical department is not involved in suspending or firing them.

Being charged with managing drug testing, however, makes it more difficult for doctors to separate their clinical drug-testing role from the corporation's policing function. One utility company physician reported directly to the medical division, which had an annual drug-testing budget of over $1 million. Despite his clear role in advancing management's drug-testing goals, he still argued that doctors serve only as technical advisers to verify that the tests are valid:

> I try to make it very clear to employees what role I'm in. The drug-testing role has no doctor-patient relationship. As the company's technical expert in drug testing, I go to arbitrations and legal proceedings as the company's witness and "hired gun." Management decides what happens; health care does not discipline or sanction anybody. We serve as the technicians to make management's policy work, and we're not the enforcers. I've tried to keep us in that technical role. Dealing with the perception is a frustration. It's clear in my mind what I'm doing when. Once it leaves this office, people get confused.

While managing the drug-testing program, this doctor tries to hide that responsibility from the employees:

> I distance myself from the cop role. I have a capable manager to handle drug testing who has been the visible one running around doing the actual administration and management, and I've tried to keep a very, very low profile. A lot of people outside of this department don't know that this man reports directly to me and runs the program. I've just been uncomfortable with that role; I don't advertise that one at all. I protested vigorously saying, "It is not appropriate for me and the medical department to administer drug testing. It is a safety and management issue, not a health-care issue." I lost. I have to administer most of it.

Although doctors who conduct drug testing within companies may personally oppose it, particularly in the case of random testing, their opinions generally do not persuade companies to abandon testing. They work for the employer and generally carry out company policies—which in the area of drug testing are more an extension of law enforcement than a true effort to identify people who have problems that affect their ability to work.

THE FAILURE TO DETECT WORKER IMPAIRMENT, PRESCRIPTION DRUGS, AND ALCOHOL

Companies test for substances that can affect perception and judgment and increase the risk of accidents. If company policies were truly consistent and focused on major problems, they would discourage the abuse of any substances with these effects, including alcohol, prescription drugs like Valium, and over-the-counter non-prescription medications like antihistamines. But employers have not been nearly as concerned with prescription medication and alcohol as with illegal drugs.[17] A physician in a chemical company with a drug-screening program that virtually ignores prescription drugs said:

> We have workers and executives taking far too many prescription medications, many of which affect the central nervous system. In the 1970s and 1980s corporate American leaders focused on marijuana and in some cases became single-issue people. While they and their families were popping pills like they were going out of style, somehow marijuana was the problem in America. They have become much more conservative and punitive in their approach than they should be.

Nor have managers focused on fatigue as a major cause of accidents. Although faulty technology, poor work organization, and excessive overtime all contribute to accidents, management relies on drug use to explain injuries and fatalities. But studies do not correlate the concentration of drugs in the urine—whether cocaine, marijuana, or barbiturates—with impairment, whereas blood-alcohol levels do correlate with behavioral abnormalities. Controlled studies indicate that illicit drugs in general are a minor contributor to work-related accidents and fatalities, especially outside of motor vehicle–related deaths, which are a significant part of overall worker fatalities.[18] According to two union health officials:

> Drug testing was created to put workers and unions on the defensive, to distract people from the real issues in employee health and safety, and to give management the right to go after people individually. Drug use, as bad a social problem as it is, is not a significant contributor to workplace safety and health.[19]

> A lot of employers think that one big problem in workers now is that they're all on drugs and that's why we have so many accidents. One company that said many accidents are drug-related had evidence on three out of the thousand or so, so they illegally put into effect a policy of testing after every accident, no matter what. Somebody got drug-tested if they got a cinder in their eye from walking across the parking lot. The company had an overbroad program.[20]

Drug-testing evidence is often misleading. It does not necessarily say anything about how long employees may have used the drug, whether they are chronic users, or whether they are addicted to it. It does not measure a person's character, morals, or work performance.

Drug testing by hair sample raises special problems. A hair is similar to a growth ring in a tree trunk, because its growth marks can show that someone used drugs several months ago but not necessarily very recently. However, more specificity about the time of use is important in identifying real substance abuse problems affecting work (see Durbin and Grant 1996, 2.21–2.22).[21]

Two purposes of an employment exam are to identify persons who have a health condition (such as asthma) that working conditions could exacerbate and to screen out applicants for positions (such as forklift operator) in which drug use could place others at risk. Drug testing, however, typically serves neither purpose. Even when a drug test is reasonably accurate, employers often handle positive test results in ways that are ineffective in preventing impaired work performance and in ways that are punitive—as when a person is disqualified from a desk job because tests show urine metabolites of marijuana smoked a few days or even weeks earlier.[22] People are often denied jobs even though a drug is not necessarily affecting their health or performance or even their behavior at the time of the exam. Most drug tests diagnostically do nothing positive for employees, except perhaps for those individuals who are in such severe psychological denial that they have no idea they have taken drugs or become intoxicated. Moreover, many employers who test for drugs do not offer treatment programs or intervene beyond terminating the employee, while others offer only one chance at rehabilitation. An airline physician said:

> The random drug-testing program is a sword and a velvet glove. For many companies it's a sword: when you're positive, you're terminated. The FAA's drug-testing program does not require the employer to treat the individual; the employer must remove the employee from a safety-related job. If I'm a pilot or a flight attendant and I test positive for cocaine, I can't do any other job, so if I'm removed from a safety job, that means I'm gone. If I'm a mechanic that worked on airplanes, I'm history. In our company we use the glove first: we say to the employee, "Rather than just throw you

out the door and lock it, we're going to help you overcome this addiction by having you treated and monitoring you and letting you return to the work site." The sword is: we make them sign a statement that says if they are positive again, they will be terminated immediately with no recourse.

CONFIDENTIALITY AND WORKER TRUST

In private practice, doctors see dealing with drug use as clearly within the medical model of diagnosing and treating individuals. In contrast, when drug-testing information is passed directly to management and used in ways that affect employment, it becomes part of a policing function that precludes any confidential doctor-patient relationship.

Drug-testing records are often not confidential. People can be fired for positive test results and then experience long-term difficulty finding other work. Physicians regularly report drug-testing information to management, and many feel intense pressure from management to divulge diagnostic information as well.[23] Doctors often cooperate with managers who send employees to the medical department by giving them "confidential" information. One doctor in a major computer corporation justifies this practice with a minor caveat:

> If a manager sends somebody over for problems of absence, performance, or behavior, they would be informed that the person has a substance abuse problem without any specifics—we don't tell them whether it's alcohol or drugs.

For doctors to be able to detect disease that could be due to the work environment, employees should be able to come to the medical department in confidence, knowing they can safely provide information. Some doctors protest that corporate drug testing undermines whatever credibility and employee trust they have been able to cultivate. Workers may fear that the medical department secretly does drug tests and become less likely to cooperate with the medical department's other programs when physicians are responsible for drug testing. A chemical company physician said:

We've had people wonder if we're secretly doing drug tests on them, so we have to make it known that we don't do that. They come in and get their drug test and then they come in for their physical and give a urine sample, so they wonder: What's the difference?

A doctor in a major oil company that secretly did drug testing said:

When drug screening started, it had an immediate impact on the willing-ness of people to participate in our preventive medical examination pro-gram because they thought we did drug screening during that exam. We never did. But the company did a pilot study once that did include anony-mous drug testing. That was a fatal misstep. It was eventually publicized, and people realized that they *were* tested even though their names and any identifying data were separated from the sample and there was no way to match that up. People felt that was breaking a bond of trust, and *I* would have felt that. After that, our participation rate in our preventive medical examination program dropped for about three years, and the unspoken comment was, "You're going to do drug screening."[24]

Workers develop ways of evading tests. For example, em-ployers typically do not require them to undress for testing, so employees can carry clean samples with them (see Drury et al. 1999; Durbin and Grant 1996, 6.1–6.18). They also can briefly stop using drugs to circumvent specific tests, thereby rendering the tests useless. By promoting employee subterfuge, drug testing in-tensifies managerial problems.

An individual doctor's intent may be to help employees by pointing out their problems and sharing evidence with them in the hope that they will take action. Nevertheless, concerns about the use of medical information in companies are legitimate. Manage-ment asserts a need to know whether an employee or potential employee has a substance abuse problem. Physicians regularly re-port drug-testing information to management and many feel in-tense pressure from management to divulge diagnostic informa-tion as well. A major oil company physician said:

Our drug policy requires that employees disclose any drug problem and that the medical department inform management if they know about it. Employees sign a form that says that they will inform management them-selves, which authorizes the medical department to inform management. Then when I tell employees they have marijuana in their urine and that I'd like them to report this to management, if they say they won't, then I say I have to. In fact, they gave me permission when they signed the informed consent form and took the job.

Certainly employees tend to be reluctant to describe a history of drug use to someone who works for the company. The drug testing and intrusive medical services that employers unilaterally impose contribute to their suspicions. The records are often not confidential, people can be immediately fired, and the company's approach may not be toward rehabilitation.

New employees typically have to sign a statement when they join the company saying that they realize they may be subject to drug testing as a condition of employment. Two physicians, at a metals company and an oil company, respectively, said:

> We had for-cause alcohol and drug testing for people whom management suspected were under the influence. We didn't have mandatory testing. Well, it was called voluntary, but it was really mandatory: you didn't have to take the test, but you'd get fired if you didn't (*laughter*).

> If you want to work for us, you have to pass the physical, part of which is the drug test. It's not a surprise. People are told about it up front: "If you don't want to take a drug test, then you have to go someplace else to work." We do random testing here every day, day shift and night shift, so every time someone comes to work, they know that they're subject to random drug testing.

In many cases, companies will not hire contractors or allow them on company premises unless the contractor has a drug program. The government, as a big purchaser of services and goods, mandates drug-testing programs but without specifying exactly what the drug policies must be. A physician who does company drug testing under contract said:

> A lot of our clients say that we can't send any person on their property unless they had a drug test within the last thirty days; we have to have a random program for some of them. But drug testing is a clear violation of some people's civil liberties in the way it's done.

Company attorneys generally favor drug testing as a means of protecting the company from liability and ridding the company of drug users by terminating anyone using illegal drugs. The legal department defends companies against the invasion-of-privacy argument—that people who are not drug users should not be sub-jected to involuntary drug testing. In some cases, however, com-pany attorneys oppose drug testing in the wish to avoid lawsuits. A newspaper company physician said:

> I was the primary actor that put in the corporatewide drug-testing program here. We insisted on auditing the program to see that it functioned as it was designed. Legal people often present the argument: "We don't want a smoking gun. We don't want to have a report on our own program, be-cause if that report comes back negative, it's a matter of record, so at some future date we can be hung with our own audit." The legal department opposed drug testing to avoid the legal conflict that they could envision taking place from a public and an employee force that's antagonistic to drug testing. We had to get past that initial hurdle.

In view of these problems, employees and unions have re-sisted drug screening that presents problems of confidential infor-mation and inappropriate safeguards, especially when employees as well as applicants are screened. They have generally opposed random testing and said there should be a reason to conduct a test, especially when employees rather than applicants are screened.[25] Still, government-mandated workplace drug policies exist whether employees oppose them or not. According to a la-bor official:

> Companies have won the right to do drug testing most times. We've re-sisted it and lost that fight essentially. We say there should be a reason to conduct a test. No one wants someone who's driving a bus to be under the influence of drugs. But random drug testing is something else. The idea of everybody being guilty until proven innocent is ridiculous.[26]

Employees have argued—largely unsuccessfully—that drug testing violates their constitutional rights and that companies must have valid reasons to test, such as poor job performance. Al-though laws vary by state, courts have generally upheld the right of employers to drug-test both employees and applicants if they have a written policy and have informed the employees of it; in these decisions the courts have considered safety and cost along with privacy rights.[27] Courts take the position that employees relin-quish their privacy rights when they agree to work for employers that must protect safety. Employers may test for cause, test classes of individuals, and randomly test employees in dangerous jobs for which the federal government requires random testing, provided that they apply rules consistently to categories of employees without singling out particular workers solely for personal reasons. Employers may refuse to hire applicants who fail the drug test if drug use seems to account for their failure. Employers have wide latitude to do drug screening within these broad boundaries (see, for example, Willborn, Schwab, and Burton 1993, 175–98; Rothstein 1994).

Physicians carry out the corporate mandate to test even though they may disagree with company attorneys about the circumstances of testing people, the handling of test results, and the consequences of positive tests. The lawyers often prevail in such in-house conflicts because they address the employer's major concerns—the costs of litigation and adverse publicity.

CONCLUSION

Unfortunately, management has embraced a generally punitive approach to drugs. Drug testing often takes on momentum in corporations after senior officials hear about other companies' testing and initiate a company program, even when valid data do not justify it and drug screening does not necessarily indicate impairment at work.

Except when there is reasonable cause, or for certain occupations such as airplane pilots and truck drivers, employee screening for drug use generally is unnecessary without evidence of inadequate work performance. Employees tend to find drug testing a demeaning procedure that intrudes upon their private lives and unjustifiably treats them as guilty until proven innocent, even if they have a decade's experience with the company, rarely miss work, and have never had an accident (see Normand, Lempert, and O'Brien 1994, 215–40; Macdonald and Wells 1994, 125–27). Companies need a working personnel function that successfully monitors employee performance for behavior changes within an initial employment period. Employers ought to look first for behavioral abnormalities, such as absence or poor performance, and consider drugs as only one possible explanation, along with family problems, physical or psychological illness, and management practices. Then, depending on the job's safety risk and how severe the problem appears to be, they could consult with occupational health professionals to determine whether there is a medical problem that requires intervention.

It is important, of course, to be able to run an airline without drug-abusing pilots, but employers have oversimplified a complex issue. Reducing the frequency of drug use among workers instead requires a multifaceted program that includes rehabilitation. Employers who do drug testing often lack nonpunitive employee assistance programs that could play a valuable role in prevention and treatment. Essentially, companies reject people without helping them recover from their drug problems.[28] Rather than terminate an employee who tests positive and spend thousands of dollars training a new person, an employer could offer treatment to its employee with years of company experience. Supervisors and worker representatives need to be trained to detect substance abuse problems, and company programs should address alcohol as well as drug use.

Concern about drug use by employees does not in fact require widespread drug testing. Even for the drug-testing programs that the government requires, companies should provide strong evidence for the effectiveness of their program, as well as rehabilitation and prevention programs, confidential services separate from the workplace, and effective preventive health and employment policies. Investing in improved management policies, work organization, and employee assistance programs could deter drug use more effectively than broad testing.[29]

Corporate enthusiasm for drug testing is part of a broader pattern of workplace screening, to which we turn in the next chapter.

—— Chapter 6 ——

Workplace Screening

It's in the individual's long-term interest to make an adjust-ment to the workplace.

—Metals company physician, justifying his
company's screening practices

FACED WITH RISING health costs and an increasing threat of law-suits stemming from worker disease, many employers have adopted health screening policies that focus on individuals who may pose a special risk in the workplace. The prospects of higher costs for insurance and workers' compensation, along with law-suits and further regulation, keep employers interested in any means of identifying those with threatening medical conditions or personal habits. In recent years employers have screened workers for genetic predisposition to disease as well as for a broad array of health risks related to smoking, reproductive hazards, the AIDS virus, and biological traits (see Schafer 2001; Andrews et al. 1994; Draper 1993a; Schiller, Konrad, and Anderson 1991).[1] Company doctors say that they test for several reasons: to protect the safety of employees, products, and property; to save money that high-risk employees would cost employers; and to shield companies against liability. Employers now collect extensive medical infor-mation on a wide range of risk factors in an attempt to prevent on-the-job health damage to especially vulnerable individuals. De-spite legal developments—such as the Americans with Disabilities Act (ADA) and the ruling in the Johnson Controls case, which

156

barred fetal exclusion policies—employers still focus on identifying high-risk individuals.[2]

Professionals occasionally are in the public spotlight for the tests that they give employees to detect drug use, genetic abnormalities, AIDS, psychological disturbances, or dishonesty. More often, company screening is low-profile, but it still effectively shifts the focus of concern away from working conditions and toward the vulnerabilities of individual employees.

Doctors and managers obtain medical information in a variety of ways, including questionnaires, coworker reports, and insurance records. In other words, they need not actually conduct their own testing programs. They can determine the employability, job placement, insurability, or general treatment of workers by using information gathered from outside sources. They may also use this information to hold workers responsible for problems that corporate officials themselves have created, such as dangerous jobs.

In this chapter, I examine three major examples of the screening approach: companies' use of genetic information, fetal exclusion policies used for reproductive hazards screening, and stress programs. In each case, company physicians' identification of workers they perceive to be high-risk shifts attention away from working conditions.

SCREENING OVERSHADOWS MONITORING

Employers and company physicians favor screening as a way of avoiding hiring or retaining workers who may pose the greatest threat to the company's financial health because of personal characteristics or biological traits (see Normand, Lempert, and O'Brien 1994; Draper 1991; Hanson 1993).[3] In contrast, companies that take the monitoring approach examine environmental contaminants to determine whether workers' exposures are too high.[4]

During World War II companies did preplacement health evaluations to place the limited number of available civilian workers in the right job while others fought the war. Although such a shortage of workers can encourage employee screening, high unemployment and widespread hiring cutbacks are more conducive to it. When labor is plentiful, companies can screen to hire only the healthiest applicants. Hard economic times also tend to increase employee testing because companies can more readily find replacements when they use testing to avoid workers with problems.

The important question here is: Do we focus on the individual or on the environment? In fact, a certain percentage of people may develop diseases and others may not, but in most cases the idea that workers' own biological traits cause disease is unproven. Proponents of screening generally assume that factors other than workplace exposure are responsible when individuals become sick. In their conviction that only a small percentage of the workforce is at risk because of these individuals' genetic predisposition to disease, employers imply that the workforce is safe once that group is removed. Furthermore, people who believe that current levels of contaminants are harmless and overregulated are more likely to believe that something is wrong with people who get sick, so we should try to identify them and screen them out.

Employers and corporate physicians who favor a screening approach often see those who oppose it as technophobic and antiscientific. However, opponents of screening typically favor other advanced technologies and scientific developments and in fact do not oppose science and technology generally.[5]

Employers have been much more likely than workers to locate risk in individuals rather than in the conditions affecting workers in general.[6] The corporate practice of screening out workers tends to expand as labor's power declines and corporate managers gain more power to define risk in their own terms. Those in a position to be harmed by medical screening are far less likely to support it. Labor unions generally oppose screening out individuals, arguing that problems of risk should be defined in terms of hazards to all workers—hazards that should be reduced through engineering controls, product substitution, and vigilant government regulation (see, for example, Samuels 1999; Alvi 1994, 305–11; Otten 1986; U.S. Congress, Office of Technology Assessment 1990a, 33). Thus, people's position in the labor force has a strong effect on how they perceive the possible benefits and dangers of medical screening. The belief that high priority should be given to information about which individuals are riskier to employ is not universally shared.

The public health orientation toward eliminating workplace environmental hazards such as asbestos has now largely given way to a search for workers with a biological predisposition to disease or inappropriate lifestyle, and corporate professionals have been a central part of this shift in emphasis. Over the past ten years many corporations have reduced or eliminated their health and environmental staff. In addition, corporate medical personnel who could be working to prevent illnesses and monitoring the health effects of work are instead collecting genetic information and testing for drugs. This focus on identifying individual workers at risk rather than on locating the hazards to which all workers are exposed has intensified as employers have been held responsible for the effects of chemical hazards. Corporate support for genetic screening, though understandable as a business interest, has had a destructive effect on employees and the public, and it has diverted attention from pressing environmental health hazards and problematic management policies. Concern with identifying uncommon biological traits has replaced efforts to prevent more pervasive health risks.

GENETIC INFORMATION

Employers use genetic information to assess an individual's predisposition to disease. They have screened for genetic traits such as G-6-PD deficiency and sickle cell in attempts to prevent on-the-job health damage and to avoid declining profitability due to spiraling health-care costs and litigation. Employers can remove expensive people from their payrolls or make them pay a higher share of the cost. Company lawyers argue that if employers fail to use genetic information to prevent health problems, they will leave themselves vulnerable to lawsuits for health damage. In addition, insurers argue that they must be allowed to use genetic information in their decisions to offer coverage and set premiums so as to eliminate uncertainty in underwriting, protect their profits, avoid overly high rates for lower-risk individuals, and charge people rates that accurately reflect their risks.[7]

Diseases with a genetic component are prevalent. For example, color-blindness and diabetes have a genetic component, and employers have screened for these conditions for years. Heart disease and breast cancer are also in part genetic, as are many other diseases (see Schulte et al. 1999; U.S. Congress, Office of Technology Assessment 1990a, 77–95, 128–29).[8] An important example is possible genetic predisposition to beryllium disease. Beryllium is a metal that has been used in the manufacture of nuclear weapons, brass fixtures (as a gilding material), ceramics, aerospace products, and chips for electronics. Although beryllium is highly toxic, employers have suggested that workers should undergo genetic tests for susceptibility to beryllium disease to identify those who are more likely to develop clinical chronic beryllium disease (see, for example, Maier and Newman 1998; Kreiss 1994).[9] This is only one of many examples of how genetic information has been used in the workplace over the past thirty years. The American Management Association found in its 2001 survey of large U.S. corporations that hundreds of them test for susceptibility to workplace hazards, collect family medical histories, or conduct specific genetic screening tests, such as for sickle cell anemia and Huntington's disease.[10]

Employers claim that sophisticated screening enables them to continue to offer a major medical policy and distribute risks and costs fairly without being burdened by individuals with an adverse genetic profile. The burden on small employers of having employees with high medical costs can be especially heavy. A large company can more easily support high-risk employees, but an employer with twenty or fewer employees is less able to maintain several employees with high health costs.[11] Genetic information is thus part of a major focus on screening out high-risk individuals of all sorts, as opposed to a search for occupational hazards from working conditions.

Stigmatization

The use of genetic information to assess an individual's predisposition to disease is similar to drug screening. Physicians and employers acknowledge that the tests they use detect few problems and result in few positive test results. They nevertheless have advocated ineffective screening policies—which impose heavy social costs as well as economic costs to corporations—in order to accomplish various non-health-related goals.[12]

People perceived as having a medical "disorder" find themselves considered a poor risk for employment or insurance. These individuals can also be stigmatized in their personal lives and may find it difficult ever again to be perceived—or to perceive themselves—as normal (see Gostin 1995; Holtzman and Rothstein 1992; Brock 1992). Genetic information about individuals can affect their family members' access to insurance as well. The social stigma of disease can limit the ability to marry and impair family relationships. (On the social stigma of disease, see Wilfond et al. 1997; Healy 1992; Nelkin and Brown 1984; for a classic analysis of stigmatization, see Goffman 1963.) It is a primary driving force behind workers' concern about company testing and privacy in medical records. A national labor official described the stigmatization of employees who have been labeled high-risk:

> Recently in Oak Ridge, Tennessee, a company took four men without any clinical manifestation of disease off the job because they supposedly "flunked" a test used to detect risks of chronic beryllium disease.[13] They wouldn't have had to worry about it if they had a decent exposure standard. It's cheaper to move the men. There is a very destructive shunning effect that creates family stress. I've seen it destroy families among shipyard workers who have been diagnosed with bad X-rays but have no other manifestation of disease. Also, after we finally got a good vinyl chloride standard to clean up the PVC industry, the pallet plant and warehouse at a Goodrich plant in Louisville, Kentucky, became known as the leper colony, because that's where they sent you to get you out of the exposure if you flunked your liver function test. The other workers understood that that is where sick people go, and sick people do not do well socially or psychologically.[14]

He gave an example of employees barred from employment through employer screening of high-risk workers—including low-tech screening for nongenetic risks:

> We already know and have documented that anyone who worked for the Rocky Flats nuclear facility will not get a job easily with any other employer that does any kind of screening. For example, a machinist voluntarily left the DOE facility at Rocky Flats—because he wanted to get out of DOE—and applied for a machinist job at the brewery nearby. He wasn't even permitted to fill out an application form; the receptionist was told that

anyone from Rocky Flats is not eligible for employment in the company. They are at high risk, no question about it. We now have fifty thousand former DOE workers from these facilities. We don't even have a system to take care of their medical care. They can't get medical insurance or a job.[15]

As genetic technologies develop, assisted by the $3 billion Human Genome Project to map the human genetic structure, employers have increasingly been able to identify genetic predispositions and diseases.[16] Physicians will be able to target many more individuals as high-risk for a widening array of diseases as a result of this research.

Companies that screen will inevitably get some positive results, with adverse consequences for individuals who are labeled high-risk. Unintended social consequences will proliferate as "predisposition" becomes understood as "defect" and as physicians and employers perceive an ever-increasing number of people as biologically flawed. As individuals are identified as high-risk for a widening array of conditions, the burden and social costs of screening practices falls on workers, their families, and the public (see Geller et al. 1996; Billings et al. 1992). Employers nonetheless have shown great faith in the powers of new medical screening to identify "problem employees." Without additional social and legal safeguards, many individuals could become virtually uninsurable or unemployable because of the use of genetic information.

Social Stratification and Discrimination

Corporate professionals, employers, and insurance companies claim that genetic information enables them to identify at-risk individuals in a nondiscriminatory way. However, job discrimination and exclusionary policies can be based on genetic information even when workplace screening has been ineffective as preventive medicine. The placement of employees stemming from the application of medical information can be discriminatory, sometimes with grave economic consequences for employees and their families.

Social stratification and discrimination are major problems with genetic information, in part because the layering of our society by race and ethnicity, gender, and social class affects the ways in which such information is used. Many genetic abnormalities are disproportionately found among specific ethnic or racial groups. For example, G-6-PD deficiency and sickle cell trait are found in high proportions among blacks, so employers who screen out people with those traits screen out a disproportionate number of blacks. These groups then may experience discriminatory practices by employers and insurers.[17] Through information access rules, insurance company policies, and employers' hiring and testing practices, medical information can be used in ways that deepen racial and economic inequality (see Gostin 1995, 320; Duster 1990; Bowman and Murray 1990; Reilly 1992a). Thus, in airline, chemical, and steel companies, blacks who have only recently entered relatively high-paying production jobs have been identified as high-risk (see Draper 1991, 65–96; U.S. Congress, Office of Technology Assessment 1990a). Excluding racial minorities from relatively high-paying jobs penalizes economically disadvantaged groups and deepens divisions in society based on race and ethnicity. Making it even more difficult to recognize the social dimensions of screening is workers' lack of access to the aggregate medical data that may show specific ethnic groups being disproportionately screened out. These distortions go beyond issues of medical risks to individuals.

Employers often initiate screening programs without adequate scientific evidence to justify them. Many screening tests not only suffer from narrow applicability and limited predictive value but also promote a false sense of security by suggesting that the screening out of some workers eliminates the health risk to all others.[18] Moreover, some diseases are called "genetic," and screened for as such, despite evidence of important environmental causes for them.[19]

Besides their suspect validity, screening tests and questionnaires calling for medical information are generally voluntary in name only. Some individuals are pressured to take tests and provide medical information, some are threatened with losing their employment or insurance, and some find that the truly voluntary and independent counseling recommended for private patients is unavailable to them (see Davis 2001; Mehlman et al. 1996; White 2000; Walters and Palmer 1997).[20] When individuals with few job alternatives and little information on workplace hazards are offered "voluntary" tests or opportunities to divulge health information, their choices are limited indeed. Those who refuse to be tested are simply not considered for positions.

One approach employers and physicians continue to pursue is to inform workers that they face special genetic risks on the job, then let them choose whether to endanger themselves or their children for wages. Employers overlook the restrictive conditions, however, under which choices about health and employment take place. As with drug testing, rhetoric about informed consent and voluntary testing has tended to mask the coercive context of screening in the workplace. It is not merely an individual and welcome choice when workers are told they may be at special risk and they have a "choice" to stay on or quit their job. People who take dangerous jobs are not freely making an "individual" choice.

Antidiscrimination and disability statutes are countervailing forces to employers who locate blame in employees through screening because they limit corporations' traditional stance of at-will employment.[21] The Americans with Disabilities Act curtails employers' ability to restrict people—such as diabetics on insulin—from certain activities. Rather than blanket restrictions, limitations are to be tailored to the individual. Employers are not supposed to screen out disabled individuals unless it is for a job-related disability that cannot be accommodated (see American Management Association 2001; Rothstein 1997b, 281).[22] Although under the ADA employers cannot test people before offering them employment, that does not eliminate the problem of job discrimination, despite new laws and political developments.[23] Disability and discrimination laws still allow employers to use screening to locate blame in employees' individual risks and predispositions.

The Social and Legal Context Affecting Genetic and Drug Screening

The legal and social environment is generally hostile toward genetic screening and comparatively favorable toward drug testing. These different attitudes reflect the broad social context, which includes such issues as racial and class stratification, controversy over genetic technologies, and political rhetoric about crime. Although society and the law generally view genetic testing less favorably than drug testing, it would be easy to overstate the differences. Genetic screening shares many problems with drug screening, some of which are different from those featured in the public view. Advocates of both types of screening make claims and favor policies that shift the burden of workplace hazards from management onto individual workers and the public. Here I briefly consider several aspects of the legal and social framing of genetic screening in employment as it compares with drug screening. Such a comparison points to social misconceptions about risk and social factors that help explain the strangely distinctive treatment of genetic screening, even when it shares important characteristics with drug testing and other types of screening.

Statutes Mandating Testing The common view is that genetic testing is less prevalent than drug testing because it is not required, unlike drug testing.[24] It should be noted, however, that drug testing is not universally required in employment, and its use far surpasses mandated screening (see American Management Association 2001). Moreover, employers say that they are also required to screen workers for genetic susceptibility; over twenty years ago employers claimed that OSHA regulations required them to conduct genetic testing.[25] More recently, employers have argued that the threat of employee lawsuits over workplace illness requires them to know who is at special risk so that employers can avoid being held liable for damage to employees whose vulnerabilities they know or should have known about through testing. However, becoming aware of an employee's special risks is quite different from denying that person a job.

The popular view that the law requires employers to do drug testing but not genetic screening ignores the complexities of the legal requirements and the way employers have interpreted them. Significantly, the Americans with Disabilities Act requires employers to provide reasonable accommodation to people who are—or are perceived to be—disabled;[26] employers are under no such obligation in relation to drug users.[27] In addition, while the ADA arguably prohibits employers from excluding workers through genetic screening unless they have a legitimate defense, employers may still collect genetic information after they have made a conditional job offer.[28] A close analysis shows that the current law may actually encourage employers to use genetic information about employees.

Culture and Politics   A partial explanation for why the legal and social response to genetic screening is so different from the response to drug screening is cultural. The general U.S. culture tends to be suspicious of genetic screening, associating it with eugenics, Nazi oppression, and brave-new-world fears of cloning and Frankensteinian nightmares (see Marks 1995, 148–51; Kevles 1985; Gould 1981; Kraut 1994). In contrast, the tough-on-crime rhetoric that pervades our political culture supports the punitive approach toward drug testing that employers generally support and the unfavorable reception given to rehabilitation and prevention programs (see Shain 1994, 257–60).

It would oversimplify, however, to argue that U.S. culture and politics oppose genetic screening but favor drug screening. In some respects, the general culture is also conducive to genetic screening. The great enthusiasm for genetic technology in areas as diverse as pharmaceuticals, agriculture, forensic medicine, and prenatal health screening—as well as the investor excitement generated by biotechnology stocks—has produced a "halo effect" that makes genetic screening in employment appear unduly promising (see Nelkin and Lindee 1995). New genetic discoveries and the favorable public response to them improve the prospects for workplace medical screening (see Buchanan et al. 2000; Walters and Palmer 1997, 44–49; Kevles and Hood 1992; Pennisi 2001).

The general culture is also, in some respects, profoundly ambivalent about drugs. Social attitudes do tend to favor employer drug screening. However, aside from a recent toughening of drunk-driving laws, the culture in many ways supports alcohol and drug use: the culture promotes prescription drugs intensively; intoxication is indulged or encouraged by positive associations in the media and social environments conducive to it; and the favorable images of drug and alcohol use that pervade the culture, depicting it as adult or manly, facilitate drug and alcohol use by children. These drug-favoring aspects of the culture encourage employee subterfuge in response to drug tests and lax or uneven employer enforcement of drug policies (see Durbin and Grant 1996, 6.1–6.18).

Common cultural ground underlies both genetic and drug screening. American culture and politics are generally unsupportive of prevention, a fact reflected in the law. This accounts for various antiprevention phenomena that affect both genetic and drug screening. There are three notable examples: refusing to provide employees and the public with more useful information about risks (see, for example, Beamish 2000; Bird 1996; Jasanoff 1995; Short and Clarke 1992; Freudenburg 1992); funding research on unlikely "magic bullet" cures rather than the preventable workplace and environmental conditions that produce disease (see Bayer 1988; Epstein 1979; McCaffrey 1982); and resisting programs designed to reform the workplace practices that contribute to drug use and disease and to reduce drug use through rehabilitation and education (see Blackwell 1994, 327–31; Ashford 1976).

Thus, the argument that genetic testing will not become as widespread as drug testing because it lacks popular support is unfounded. Genetic screening may become more prevalent as employers widely adopt drug testing to combat the consequences of a so-called permissive culture. Favorable publicity for genetic technologies and research may further reinforce that trend.

Immutable Characteristics Versus Lifestyle Choices   Another partial explanation for why the legal and social response to genetic screening is so different from the response to drug screening is that in matters of employment, the law and society tend to oppose as discriminatory or unfair any differentiations among people according to immutable characteristics while supporting any selection among individuals according to "lifestyle" choices, such as drug use (see, for example, Conrad and Walsh 1992; Annas, Glantz, and Roche 1995b). However, to some extent, both genetic and drug testing screen for people whose characteristics are at least partly beyond their control and who are socially disadvantaged. The public, courts, and legislatures are learning that drug use—including illegal drugs, cigarettes, and alcohol—may not be entirely volitional, given the addictive properties of the drugs themselves, deliberate company policies of increasing the drug content of products, and mass media advertising designed to encourage addiction. In addition, the fact that unnecessarily high-stress or high-exposure work environments—the result of certain managerial choices—may produce drug use and disease weakens the argument that drug use is simply an employee "choice."

Genetic *monitoring* also weakens the case for an immutability-versus-choice distinction between genetic and drug testing. In contrast to genetic screening, genetic monitoring entails periodically examining the effects of environmental contaminants on workers to determine whether exposures are too high. In this type of testing, employers use genetic information to detect the effects of workplace exposures rather than to detect the inborn traits that genetic screening seeks to identify.[29]

The Turf-Expanding Function of Testing   Another partial explanation for the less favorable response to genetic screening compared with drug screening concerns its relative inability to boost corporate medical departments and the physicians who work in them. Although company physicians and others in corporations occasionally see genetic information as a means by which they might expand their turf and resources, this is a relatively minor factor spurring on the use of genetic information in corporations compared with the major turf-expanding function of corporate drug screening. Unlike genetic screening, drug testing is subject to aggressive advocacy by company physicians who use it to increase the company resources devoted to screening (see, for example, American College of Occupational Medicine 1991, 652; Swotinsky and Chase 1990).

However, genetic screening could serve a function for in-house physicians similar to that of drug testing, albeit on a smaller scale. Unfortunately, such an outcome would make it less likely that a company would eliminate genetic screening if it realized that screening had only limited effectiveness.

Social Stratification and Class Distinctions   A fifth partial explanation for the different legal and social responses to genetic screening and drug screening concerns social stratification and class distinctions. The law and U.S. popular culture tend to interpret genetic screening as something that affects broad social groups and to justify drug testing by associating drug use with "low-lifes" (see Nelkin and Lindee 1995, 13, 163–68; Annas, Glantz, and Roche 1995b, i–ii). The social reality is somewhat different. Alcohol, prescription drugs, and illegal substances are used and abused by middle- and upper-class people, and employers have focused on screening for genetic risk in jobs where a lower-status group—such as blacks or women—is a relatively new minority in an occupation (see, for example, Samuels 1995; Draper 1991, 65–96; Reinhardt 1978). Thus, genetic screening, like drug testing, has an important social class dimension.

Title VII of the Civil Rights Act of 1964 provides limited protection against genetic discrimination by making it illegal for employers to limit, segregate, or classify employees in any way that would tend to deprive individuals of employment opportunities or otherwise adversely affect their status as employees, where screening programs disproportionately affect a class protected under Title VII (such as race, sex, or ethnicity) or treat a protected class differently.[30] Prime examples of disorders that could give rise to disparate impact claims are sickle cell trait, G-6-PD deficiency, and hypertension, all of which are found among blacks at a higher rate than among the rest of the population (see U.S. Congress, Office of Technology Assessment 1990a, 41–45).

As with the ADA, employers may be able to defend a policy that discriminates according to protected status only upon presenting a valid business justification.[31] Also, testing and finding a risk factor in employees does not in itself require exclusion from the workplace. Employers can choose to treat such employees in nondiscriminatory ways or to make reasonable accommodation for them in view of their special health risks.

Furthermore, Title VII reaches genetic testing and discrimination only if the genetic trait at issue traces gender, race, or ethnic lines. A limited number of genetic traits meet this qualification. And even if an employer's genetic policy discriminates on an impermissible basis, an employer would have to satisfy only the less rigorous business necessity defense if the discrimination is unintentional, making it more likely that the policy would survive judicial scrutiny.[32]

One would hope that genetic claims of discrimination that do not fit the Title VII model would have a place under the ADA, but the status of such claims is uncertain at best. As discussed earlier, it is unclear whether genetic predisposition for a disease is a disability covered by the ADA. Even if it is, employers still enjoy potential defenses under the ADA similar to those available under Title VII (see Andrews, Mehlman, and Rothstein 2002; Marks 1995, 148–51; Kevles 1985; Gould 1981; Kraut 1994; Shain 1994, 257–60).[33]

Thus, most genetic discrimination claims have, at best, an uncertain status under federal employment discrimination laws because genetic predisposition is not necessarily a disability and only occasionally follows race or gender lines. Genetic predisposition defies simple categorization, yet employment discrimination laws require categorization as a prerequisite to relief. In addition, employees with health risks tend to underutilize Title VII protections, in part because employers screen for many risk factors using tests that appear to be nondiscriminatory.

Genetic screening is not unique in raising Title VII issues. To depict genetic screening as less common than drug testing because it uniquely runs afoul of discrimination laws is to ignore the Title VII issues that drug testing may raise. For-cause testing can be a pretext for discrimination, as when employers test minority workers rather than predominant groups, or the screening may have an adverse impact on specific racial or ethnic groups.

Privacy and Discrimination Effects We can solve the puzzle of why genetic screening is treated so differently from drug screening in society, despite many commonalities, by looking to the social, cultural, and legal factors I have discussed here that explain the different treatment. Nonetheless, genetic screening and drug testing share some comparable privacy and discrimination problems that are often overlooked. The law tends to emphasize employer prerogatives in both types of screening in its continued support of at-will employment, the wide latitude it grants in medical tests after conditional employment offers, and the almost complete employer latitude it permits in applicant and for-cause drug testing.[34] As noted earlier, the confidentiality of medical information is weaker in the employment context than in private medical practice; employers routinely obtain information about employees' health and fitness to work, and they may successfully defend screening of high-risk workers with business justifications.[35] Beyond employer testing, insurance records and data banks such as the Medical Information Bureau pose substantial opportunities for discrimination and threats to privacy (see, for example, Capron 2000a, 2000b).[36]

In addition, our discrimination laws are not capable of dealing with the disadvantages of social class that screening policies intensify.[37] Our laws now recognize race and sex distinctions as discrimination, but our society generally has failed to recognize discrimination in the deeply entrenched disadvantages of social class, which screening policies both reflect and exacerbate. Thus, a close examination of the screening that company physicians conduct offers a critique of discrimination law and its limitations.

REPRODUCTIVE RISK

Employers became interested in reproductive hazards because of lawsuits over fetal risks,[38] media coverage of corporate practices, and the efforts of company physicians who urged employers to take steps to prevent reproductive effects. Many companies have followed fetal exclusion policies, by which fertile women have been barred from particular jobs because of possible fetal damage. These policies, most pervasive in companies in the 1980s through the early 1990s, are an important example of a discriminatory screening approach. Despite the limitations of such policies, the social trends that have encouraged worker screening generally have encouraged reproductive hazard screening as well.

Reproductive Risk After Johnson Controls

In the 1991 Johnson Controls case, the Supreme Court ruled that the corporation's policy of barring fertile women from exposure to lead because of possible fetal damage unjustifiably discriminated against women.[39] However, the Johnson Controls decision addressed companies' vulnerability to third-party suits in a limited way.[40] According to physicians and others in corporations whom I have interviewed since the Johnson Controls decision, this has left many companies that formerly had fetal protection policies in a quandary as to what they should do instead. Some employers have continued their policies of barring workers they consider high-risk—even in the face of discrimination suits—because they continue to fear costly third-party suits on behalf of those damaged by work exposures. An oil company physician, for example, stated that his company's fetal exclusion reproductive policy from before the Johnson Controls decision remains in effect:

> It's been a little nutty, frankly, and we're still operating under the old policy. If the woman can't be protected, we would designate places that she can't work. There's been some internal debate about whether what we're doing actually is legal. But we're still doing what we had been doing.

Other companies, like Johnson Controls, had policies that their managers knew were exclusionary, but they saw no other way to protect people they considered at risk. Some companies simply ignore reproductive hazards; others have no consistent policy and handle reproductive issues on a one-on-one, ad hoc basis.

Employers have argued that excluding women from exposure to lead and other toxins protects fetuses from harm and protects women from reproductive damage.[41] Fetal exclusion policies have been selectively applied, however, and overbroad in excluding women. Most of the jobs barred to women have been relatively high-paying production jobs in large companies like General Motors and DuPont—jobs traditionally held by men. And significantly, the question of special risk and exclusion has emerged only when women were relatively new to an occupation and a minority—as women are to the chemical industry and lead battery plants—not where women are in a majority, such as low-paying electronics jobs that involve exposure to powerful solvents, or hospital jobs that entail exposure to ionizing radiation (see Draper 1993a).[42]

Health screening information in the workplace is inappropriately applied in the case of fetal exclusion, as well as in the case of genetic screening and drug testing. For example, under fetal exclusion policies, employers and the doctors they employ have often barred women from jobs that entail exposure to lead, but the men who hold these jobs, as well as the children they might father, remain vulnerable to damage from lead (see Lemasters 1998; U.S. Congress, Office of Technology Assessment 1985).[43] Although individuals in a particular group—such as fertile women—may be considered high-risk because of their biological or personal characteristics, many others may also be at risk. Focusing on the hazards to one potentially high-risk group—in this case, the fetal hazards posed by maternal exposure—can supplant concern about reducing the more general health hazards of employment. The purported discovery of a high-risk group thus diverts attention from the remaining individuals. Policies of banning women from jobs fail to protect workers and the unborn from job-related harm, in part because they leave remaining workers exposed to substances that can cause sperm damage and other reproductive effects, along with genetic damage and cancer.[44]

Employers resist broadening their understanding of reproductive hazards beyond women and are reluctant to focus on men even though there is little evidence that the risks are confined to direct exposure of the fetus. Although the scientific and policy aspects of reproductive hazards continue to be complicated, research now sometimes involves male reproductive toxicology, so employers are more aware of reproductive hazards to men than before Johnson Controls (see Lemasters 1998).[45] Nevertheless, employers still focus on the risks to women in part because male reproductive hazards are relatively unfamiliar to them and in part because women and motherhood fit together ideologically in a way that makes the evidence for excluding women more compelling than it might be if employers examined these assumptions critically. Employers suspect if they focused on male reproductive hazards, they might have to exclude men from jobs. In addition, they know that broadening their concern about reproductive hazards beyond women might lead to further pressure to clean up the workplace if both women and men were known to be at risk. A medical researcher in a major oil company said:

> The health people in the company want to change the policy to be consistent with the Supreme Court decision [Johnson Controls]. We also talk about expanding it to become a reproductive policy, but there's a lot of fear that the employees will get all upset, partly because it will get into men instead of women. If the policy targeted men, that might raise additional concerns. We might have places where men wouldn't be able to work. Then we'd have to change the procedures and change the process to make it safe.

The physicians permitted a nonphysician manager to overrule them on a medical matter. One physician in the company who regrets his stance stated:

> Well, (sighs) we just decided then that it wasn't something we felt strongly enough about that we wanted to push it very hard. We may have just dropped the ball on it by not doing anything after that.

In many companies, physicians expect that when they or other health personnel inform women that a job is hazardous, the women will simply quit the job. An oil company physician said:

> The company has an industrial hygienist or a toxicologist review how the chemicals are handled, classify the hazard, and inform the person in advance where there is some exposure. It's common that a woman quits when she is informed of this, because she doesn't want to take any chances. If it's a fetal toxin, the woman in most cases is transferred for a period of time until the baby is born.

Individual Choice and the Use of Waivers

Both before and after Johnson Controls, employers have argued that they must have the choice of how best to protect people's health when they deem it advisable, and they have used powerful choice rhetoric to legitimate their policies.[46] For example, the Johnson Controls company's chief counsel, Stanley Jaspan, asserted that an employer must not be "required to expose the individual, to expose the child" (see Supreme Court 1990, 36). He said some women had acted irresponsibly in ways that could endanger a fetus when the company tried a voluntary approach allowing pregnant workers to change jobs. He argued that employers rather than women workers ought to be able to choose what is safe or hazardous for the fetus.[47] This corporate perspective on reproductive risk draws on the decisionmaking models favored by free-market economists and rational choice theorists, who maintain that individuals are fairly compensated for dangerous work and freely choose it (see, for example, Viscusi and Moore 1990).[48]

Significantly, employers' stance regarding individual choice about reproductive hazards at work closely resembles the pro-choice arguments that equal rights advocates use against fetal exclusion policies. All highlight the right to unrestrained decision-making and the freedom of choice. Opponents of corporate fetal exclusion policies typically argue that women should be given health information and be able to choose for themselves with minimal interference whether to take the risk of possible fetal harm rather than be excluded from jobs. Thus, both employers and critics of their policies share certain misconceptions about the social context of risk: both overestimate the extent to which individuals can freely choose risk in the hazardous workplace.

Although the Supreme Court decided in the 1991 Johnson Controls case that employers could not choose to exclude women, the rhetoric of free choice remains strong. Since that decision, employers have often taken a new approach to choice. They concede that women may choose to remain on the job but insist that in doing so women must accept responsibility for any damage that may result. Some large employers require women to sign a waiver—essentially an agreement saying that they choose to risk their reproductive health and will not hold the company liable if they want to stay in jobs that may be hazardous to fetuses. These employers switched to using waivers soon after the Supreme Court decision in the belief that continuing their fetal exclusion policies would leave them too vulnerable to lawsuits for discrimination against women. Employers maintain that they are giving women the choice by having them sign waivers and that women themselves assume the risks, similar to the notion of "informed consent." Women may be denied jobs, however, if they refuse to sign away their rights. A physician who works for an aerospace company said: "We ask the person to sign a waiver to indicate that they prefer to stay on the job even though they recognize a hazard to the fetus."[49] A chemical company physician who supports having women sign waivers if they remain in jobs with toxic exposures, and whose company uses waivers for reproductive hazards, put it more bluntly:

I'm a great believer in freedom of choice, so I think people should be permitted to kill themselves. I feel that we have to give women the choice as it relates to desiring to stay in the workplace. I'm a pro-choice person, and that extends to the workplace. I think individuals should have the freedom to expose themselves to toxic chemicals if they choose to do so.

Generally it is not permissible to exclude women from exposure to lead or other toxic substances because of possible fetal hazards. But employers who instead have their employees attempt to sign away a third party's rights—such as the incipient or potential rights of the fetus—may not actually protect themselves from lawsuits on behalf of damaged fetuses.[50] The medical evidence that low exposure levels are hazardous to fetuses is complex, but accumulating (see Mattison and Cullen 1994; Bellinger et al. 1987).[51] By using waivers to respond to reproductive hazards, employers continue to leave themselves vulnerable to lawsuits for fetal damage and to cause workers and others to risk reproductive damage.[52]

One reason employers are so concerned about liability for reproductive hazards is their anticipation, based on the background rate of birth defects in the population, that the children of a certain number of female employees will have birth defects from various causes.[53] Though some miscarriages and defects are inevitable, they could lead to lawsuits on behalf of a damaged child. Two physicians, for a chemical company and a consumer products company, said:

> The only thing we can do is advise all employees that a material in their work area could have an adverse effect on the fetus. Either their supervisor or the site physician counsels the women about reproductive hazards. In the vast majority of cases, women have decided they would go ahead and work at the job that they were already assigned to. So far we haven't had any adverse effects, but we don't know. Our warning of the women certainly would help us in defending, but our lawyers have said that it probably would not be a legal defense because we are obligated to provide a safe and healthful workplace.[54]

> Fertile women who choose to stay on in jobs that may be risky for them are of concern, of course. The outside lawyers would have a field day—all you need is a miscarriage, which could happen to a third of the pregnant women *anyhow* in quote "usual" circumstances. If it's a jury case, which it usually is, you would be up the river without a paddle.

Besides trying to transfer responsibility for hazards to workers through waivers, many companies try to shift the responsibility for hazards to private doctors outside the company. Physicians employed by corporations send women to their personal doctors for their judgment about risk and ask them to certify that they believe the working conditions are safe for the fetus by making statements such as: "I guarantee conditions would be safe for her to continue working," or, "I approve having this woman remain at work." This happens in a wide range of companies, including computer, defense, printing, airline, and chemical companies.[55] Requiring that private doctors sign agreements permitting environmental exposures represents another defense mechanism through which employers attempt to shift liability. By using waivers from private physicians, employers believe that the outside doctor may then be held at least partially liable for any reproductive damage or for encouraging women to continue working if damage results.[56] A physician employed by a major airline said:

> In the medical department we provide a rather elaborate job description of work-site exposures for a pregnant woman. She then takes this to her obstetrician, who looks at it. That job description describes what they do physically, whether the job involves heavy lifting and pushing or changes in temperature, environment, barometric pressure, biorhythm, or time zone. Then *he* will sign yea or nay that this person can work for the next thirty days. The private physician may be reluctant to sign, but nevertheless we insist that the employee get that document. We will not put employees back into their work environment without it.

A chemical company physician emphasized the advantage of shielding the company from liability by relying on private physicians' opinions, saying, "We tend to accept the treating physician's opinion. It's cheap liability insurance."

If private doctors sign a paper stating that fertile women cannot work, those women may be fired. Moreover, women are excluded from jobs if their private doctor will not sign such a letter, even when the job does not present health problems.[57] The company policy leads some women to believe that they are excluded because their doctor will not cooperate.

Requiring that private doctors permit exposures is similar to requiring that women sign liability waivers, in that in both cases responsibility for adverse outcomes may rest with someone other than the employer.[58] We can expect this pattern of requiring waivers from employees and private doctors to become more pervasive as employer concern grows over the costs that reproductive risk may present.

When employers respond to chemical hazards by excluding fertile women or by allowing employees to risk reproductive damage in full awareness of the risk, workers are faced with truly difficult choices. Despite variations in the arguments about fetal exclusion, the rhetoric of choice that both sides used in Johnson Controls reinforces the fundamental notion that women should be able to assume the risks associated with hazardous conditions. Since the case was decided, employer strategies toward workplace safety have solidified that notion through everyday employment practices. However, because of limited information and job alternatives, individuals cannot freely choose risk in the hazardous workplace, and as a matter of social policy they generally should not be able to choose jobs with avoidable life-threatening hazards, since employment hazards in fact are broad social problems rather than simply matters of personal choice.

WORKPLACE STRESS CLAIMS AND
PSYCHOLOGICAL TESTING

Some companies also do psychological testing to reduce theft, pilfering, absenteeism, and safety hazards—some of the same reasons they use for drug testing. Employers often direct psychological testing at particular groups, such as security officers and employees with access to restricted areas. They also may test those they consider "problem" employees. A union health official said:

> As a union, we've encountered psychological testing for hiring people that they know are not going to be pro-union. One mine instituted a very sophisticated policy of screening applicants in an area of the country where the union historically is very strong. They screened people out using psychological testing, and they brought in families for interviews. They just wanted to make certain that people were not going to be voting for the union. It has been very successful. They have kept the union out.[59]

The evidence for being able to identify accident-prone or expensive employees through psychological testing is not strong. But even though psychological test results are of uncertain value, employers sometimes use them to detect drug abuse.[60] As a physician for a major oil company said: "We don't use psychological testing for preplacements because it's not been shown to be sufficiently predictive. But we have uncovered chemical dependency that way."

Employers also use psychological analyses to deflect attention from workplace exposure hazards. An example of the *de*-medicalizing of health hazards is the dismissal of workers' complaints from medical symptoms of chemical exposures as merely "psychogenic illness." Here is how an airline physician psychologized workers' medical complaints:

> Many times the employee and company disagree on whether the worker can go to work because of an issue that is not even related to their job that they are unable or unwilling to deal with. It may be a very significant personal thing in their lives or in their past history that may never have surfaced before. We're trying to make a better person. Then they will automatically become a better employee because they become more productive and dependable, whereas in the past they may have hidden behind a lot of medical disorders.

Rather than consider the workplace as a source of problems that affect health and productivity, management will generally look for problems that employees supposedly *bring* to the workplace, such as drug or alcohol abuse, depression, marital troubles, or financial difficulties. Although stress and wellness programs have become major concerns in occupational medicine, company programs tend to ignore workplace factors, such as occupational stress, that contribute to employees' behavioral problems and illness. They treat work stress as a controversial area that is best avoided because it places too much responsibility for worker problems on employers. Yet substance abuse may be a way in which workers cope with a stressful work environment that management has imposed; in this sense, the abuse is management-driven rather than a problem that workers bring to the workplace. Work-related stress can come from a supervisor yelling at employees, work overload, poor air quality, repetitive motion at machines or computers, and broader issues such as anxiety over job insecurity and economic restructuring. Also, job satisfaction and control over work processes are critical factors, because people who are dissatisfied and have less control over their work suffer greater psychological strain, chronic disease, and substance abuse.[61] As a result, drug testing is often a shortsighted approach to work environment factors that contribute to drug use.

Another reason companies avoid the work-stress issue is their desire to minimize workers' compensation claims. Stress claims in many companies are hotly contested, and employers often assert that they are illegitimate on their own merits. Work stress has become a major cost concern—particularly in California—with many people filing stress claims and suing corporations (see, for example, Willborn, Schwab, and Burton 1993, 813–22). Companies that draw workers' attention to problems of work stress could thereby encourage claims against themselves.

Stress management programs in corporations often suggest that stress is highly subjective and that individuals respond to stressful stimuli very differently. A company's focus on worker health promotion can to some extent "blame the victim" insofar as it tells people that they alone have full responsibility for their own health (see Ryan 1971). Their behavioral problems and illnesses are seen to stem entirely from personal limitations, which they can remove with guidance from counselors and therapy programs.

Employers who do recognize worker stress generally argue that personal and emotional problems are far more threatening to employees' health than work exposures. These physicians from a chemical company and a pharmaceutical company said:

> Stress is the most important epidemic that we have in occupational medicine today. From the standpoint of the sheer numbers of people that it's affecting and the impact on numbers of workers, stress has a far greater impact than any other issue, including the chemicals in my own company. The stress issue makes the toxic-chemical issue look like Bambi.

> We started doing health surveillance to make sure that we were not exposing our employees to problems in our chemical plants. We found out we weren't, and the biggest problem was lifestyle: cholesterol, blood pressure, drinking. So we added a lifestyle component and exercise facilities to our health surveillance.

Private life is interpenetrated with the occupational life. Employees do not just leave all their health problems at home, such as stress at home and their kids on drugs. Their personal life affects their work, just as their work affects their personal life. People going home do not leave their work environment behind when they close the door at their workplace. The work environment can contribute to spousal abuse and other problems at home. Asbestos is a good example. Men have contaminated their wives with asbestos because it was on their clothing.

Company employee assistance programs began dealing with drug dependency and alcoholism in the 1970s, then broadened to encompass other factors that affect worker health and productivity, such as depression and family problems. Many companies offered incentive plans for wellness, such as additional benefits for employees who stopped smoking or lowered their cholesterol levels. Other companies established fitness facilities and no-smoking policies. The shift has been toward screening and wellness programs and away from routine care of the sick and injured.[62]

Some employers have treatment programs to retain workers with problems, partly to reduce the expense of turnover and training new employees. But such programs also cost money, and companies in financial trouble are likely to abandon them. Moreover, not all employers give employees who test positive for drugs an opportunity to rehabilitate themselves before being terminated. An aerospace company physician said:

> When you had a robust economy, it made both economic and medical sense to put forth a significant amount of effort to get people with drug problems and alcohol back on the job; when you have good people without alcohol and drug problems also being put out on the street, it sometimes becomes very difficult to rationalize why you would continue to put out that effort for those individuals.

Even well-intentioned employee assistance programs still serve the employer's interest by screening employees. An occupational health specialist who screens workers for drugs as part of a large medical surveillance program said:

> Employees have some concern that we are the people with the big bat who can take away their jobs. My emphasis is more on this wonderful thing we're doing for them, and how we will make them healthy. But a lot of employees look at this from the standpoint of, "If I go there, they'll find out I don't see as well as I used to, so now I can't drive a forklift anymore." You can't get around that because that *is* one problem with medical sur-

veillance. Employees are mandated to come to the clinic; they're not like sick people who come on their own volition.

CONCLUSION

Employees who are screened have few options aside from finding another job, because the decision to screen workers is a management right, provided employers do not break the law while screening. According to statutes, private labor relations law, and arbitrator rulings, employers are not required to bargain for the right to screen even in unionized settings unless employees succeed in making screening a subject of collective bargaining. In addition, labor unions tend not to cover preplacement screening for genetic susceptibility in their policies and collective bargaining agreements, just as they tend not to cover preplacement drug screening. They typically focus instead on the member employees they can legally represent.[63]

As medical information about high-risk individuals accumulates, more people will find it virtually impossible to obtain health insurance and more will be stigmatized as bad risks for employment. Furthermore, when new medical information makes individuals appear to be high-risk, they are likely to experience as personal what is in fact a social problem that reflects stratification in the broader society.

Chapter 7

Information Control and Corporate Professionalism

I tell the workers when I meet with them, "Your records are secure, we have locked cabinets, and nobody has access to them." I tell them they can feel at ease that privacy of their records is not being violated.

—Metals and mining company physician

Management definitely pressures in-house doctors for information on individual workers—no question about it. Doctors are told, "If you don't give me that information, I'll find somebody who will." With the growing number of doctors, they will find somebody who will. I'm sympathetic to doctors trying to make a living, and yet I feel that if we lose the confidentiality of medical information, why bother to call ourselves doctors?

—Chemical company physician

Management looks at medical records if they want to. Nothing stops them. The doctor can go find a job somewhere else if he objects. What's he going to do? It's economic power. This is employment.

—Union official[1]

A S NONMEDICAL PERSONNEL increasingly gain access to medical information, the privacy of medical information and records is a growing social problem, with adverse consequences for patients and the public. In nonmedical corporations doctor-patient confidentiality tends to be even weaker than in private practice (see Snyder and Klees 1996; Rischitelli 1995). Employers use medical information

183

in their decisions regarding hiring, firing, transferring, insuring, and compensating people (see National Academy of Sciences 1997; Draper 1991; Etzioni 1999).[2] Such information helps management to become aware of potential health hazards and to lower costs related to employees' disease. Encroachments on confidentiality and privacy in nonmedical corporations are a precursor of declining medical privacy in society generally, in that the growing influence of non-medical personnel on health matters in corporations is an even more advanced version of similar processes in the broader society.

Medical information that employers and physicians obtain in the workplace affects individuals as workers and as public citizens. Some physicians describe the testing they conduct as a service to employees, but any medical testing on the job is problematic because of the uses to which the results will be put. Medical information has harmful or unjust applications as well as beneficial uses in the workplace. Job applicants who are considered high-risk for future illness often have trouble getting work and many find it virtually impossible to obtain health insurance (see Capron 2000a, 2000b; Andrews et al. 1994; Billings et al. 1992).

New scientific, legal, political, economic, and cultural developments have significantly changed the social arena in which medical information circulates. These changes affect the use of medical information by corporate professionals and employers as well as perceptions of its possible benefits and dangers. In this chapter, I focus on how physicians use medical information and strategize about giving such information to management; how the major social issues concerning the privacy and confidentiality of medical information affect employees and the public; and how individuals respond to such issues differently, depending partly on how the uses of medical information affect them. There are at least two important overarching questions: Who should control medical information? And who should bear the burdens that arise from the uses of information about health risks?

PRIVACY, CONFIDENTIALITY, AND MANAGEMENT ACCESS TO HEALTH-RELATED INFORMATION

The professional stance of the occupational medicine field is that the general medical ethics principles of confidentiality apply in corporations. The ACOEM code of ethical conduct, for example, says that records should be kept confidential.[3] Company doctors also state that records and the doctor-patient relationship are confidential. Corporate physicians or their employers may be legally liable as well as in violation of professional ethics if they breach confidentiality.

Despite ACOEM's ethical guidelines for its members, breaches of confidentiality do occur. Physicians contribute to the leakage of medical secrets in numerous ways. They frequently pass on to nonmedical managers the results of medical tests required by employers. They yield employee medical records to third parties, including company lawyers and benefits administrators. These physicians from an oil company and a chemical company point to ways in which company medical staff circumvent medical confidentiality, whether or not they do so deliberately:

> We would never release any information in company medical files without the employee's permission, except in the overriding interest of public health, or if a local or national regulation requires us to do so, or if the employee has a drug or alcohol problem, or if the employee is suing a company. Other than that, there is no breach of medical confidentiality.

> We have had some clerical people [in the medical department] who get a little gossipy. They sit in the lunchroom talking. We've had to swat them down a little bit and say, "Look, you have information about Mary and Fred that you might find interesting, but just keep it to yourself and don't talk about it, particularly out in the cafeteria."[4]

A mining labor official said:

> The prospects for keeping the records confidential are not good as long as the health facility is part of the management structure. All miners have been through a chest X-ray surveillance program. The mine operator selects the local clinic to do the X-rays, but the company is not supposed to get a copy of the film or the results. In one case the local hospital took films and regularly made a copy that went to the company. The hospital said these folks paid for the film, so they should get a copy of it. It went on just as standard operating procedure, and nobody questioned it—not the hospital doctors or staff, not the company doctors involved—I know what their backbone is worth. This is in a program that is explicitly regulated as being confidential.[5]

Because medical information in the workplace is unlikely to be kept confidential between physicians and patients, health risks raise issues of privacy and control. An important case in point is genetic screening, discussed in the previous chapter. Whereas doctors in private practice view genetic susceptibility within the medical model of diagnosing and treating individuals, genetic information that is given to management and used to affect employment becomes part of a policing function that precludes any confidential doctor-patient relationship. In addition, employees often are not informed of their employers' use of medical information. For example, for thirty years Lawrence Berkeley National Laboratory tested its employees for sickle cell trait and disease, as well as for syphilis, without employees' knowledge; moreover, the testing was not reasonably related to job performance or to a likelihood of harm to the tested employees or others. Management gained access to this medical information even though employees were unaware of the testing or of the employer's uses of the test results.[6]

Managers Pressure for Information

Employers and insurers have access to vast amounts of information about the health history of individuals and their use of medical services. Employers who provide health services themselves or pay contractors to provide services for them generally argue that their need for reliable and low-cost employees entitles them to information about health risks from employee medical records. Most of them also maintain that existing laws, such as OSHA's access-to-medical-records rule, adequately protect the rights of employees to privacy and access to medical records.[7]

Physicians often speak of being pressured by managers for information on individual workers. In private practice, physicians are to treat medical information in their charts as confidential unless patients consent to the sharing of that information by signing a release, but in corporations physicians have less control over records. Plant supervisors, personnel directors, safety officers, and lawyers inside and outside the firm ask physicians for details about a person's medical condition. They often work closely with physicians because many job placement issues—such as absenteeism because of sickness—involve medical opinion.[8] Some doctors complain that at times they are inundated with requests from managers for a broad range of detailed medical information and test results. A physician in a services company said:

Usually the personnel people have the attitude that they want to know everything about everybody who works for them, so they want to see everything that was ever in the medical record about everybody. Somebody's grandmother had cancer—they want to know about that. It's a control game almost like blackmail: the more information I have about you, the more control I have. It's mostly a power game.

Doctors say managers persist in calling to ask for information, indicating that they expect eventually to wear a physician down into submission; the frequency of their calls suggests that they often succeed. Many physicians feel intense pressure from local managers to divulge information about a person's fitness to work, including diagnostic information. An oil company physician and a conglomerate physician described management pressing doctors for medical information:

The confidentiality of medical records erupts as a perennial problem because employee records very often become the focus of a conflicting, adversarial situation. Employees leave, have injuries and diseases, and make accusations of negligence or improper behavior. Managers want to do everything they can to assure that they have all the data from the medical records.[9]

The supervisor or personnel director or safety officer typically wants to know the diagnosis or treatment: "Why is so-and-so out sick, and when will he get back? Give me that record because I think he's malingering." You ultimately have to decide whether you will give them the information or get fired or quit if push comes to shove. It rarely comes to the firing and quitting part. In most cases it's resolved with only a residual continuing resentment. If the local physician says, "I'm a doctor, and you can't have these records, they're confidential," and draws a hard line like that, his job is at risk. That's the way it is.

Local company doctors sometimes call in the corporate medical director to adjudicate their disputes with supervisors who demand information that the physician believes is confidential. As a medical director in a chemical company explained:

Physicians get pressure. I got pressure when I was a plant physician. They work for the plant manager, reporting to the plant manager's organization if not directly reporting to the plant manager. But we try to make sure that our physicians have enough backbone and know what their professional and ethical obligations are so they don't have to succumb to that pressure. I have heard occupational physicians say they felt that they were being needlessly or excessively pressured for diagnostic information. The biggest issue is when you have medical information about an employee that could significantly affect their ability to work the job longer-term.[10]

Nurses who run medical programs are even more vulnerable than doctors to pressure from supervisors and personnel directors to turn over confidential medical information. A physician in a financial services company explained:

> Maintaining confidentiality is very much of a problem where employee health services employ nurses with an on-call or consulting physician, and the nurse reports to a low-level manager, who insists on access to all the information. As a company doctor, I inherited a nurse who was a close personal friend of the personnel manager and a direct conduit for all sorts of problems. Nurses are at too low a level to withstand pressure from personnel directors or local managers.[11]

Supervisors lean on nurses with greater success because it is more difficult for nurses to keep information within the medical department.

Data Banks and Search Companies

Electronic record keeping and the growing sophistication of health data banks exacerbate problems of access and privacy. For example, employers and insurers can obtain employee medical information from the national Medical Information Bureau (MIB), the genetic data banks operated by various biotechnology companies, or the DNA forensic banks of state governments. (See Capron 2000a, 2000b; Medical Information Bureau 1998; National Academy of Sciences 1997; Marshall 1993, 75; Reilly 1992b, 1169–70.) They may use this information for employment-related reasons that go beyond insurance underwriting. The industry-sponsored MIB has medical information for about 15 million people in the United States, and these records include information about genetic and family diseases. When people apply for insurance, they sign a waiver authorizing the MIB to have the data and permitting insurance companies to obtain whatever records the MIB has. However, the MIB can incorporate inaccurate data that can lead to discrimination against individuals seeking life insurance, health insurance, or employment. Serious injustices occur when the information in data banks and credit companies is incorrect.[12]

Employers can hire computer-search companies to investigate a pool of prospective employees and get a great deal of information about them that may help predict future medical costs. Credit reporting agencies like Equifax and TRW can do low-cost searches that give companies valuable information about a person's health risks, prior exposure to health hazards, employment, medical history, past workers' compensation claims, felony reports and legal records, driving records, insurance history, drug treatment reports, and use of medications. In many cases search companies provide employers with health risk information about employees and job applicants that is even more valuable and cheaper than the employers' own questionnaires and in-house screening program, and they can provide this information without the knowledge of the employees or applicants.

These background checks often mix personal, medical, and financial information. A physician who has provided medical services to many companies received a call from a major search company asking for personal and medical information on a recent graduate of an occupational medicine residency training program in which the physician had taught. He said:

> She started asking me over the phone, "Have you ever been to dinner with him? Does he drink much? Does he talk about the Communist Party?" And then she got into more and more personal and medical stuff. They're one of the three largest credit reporting agencies in the country, and it's the most incredible invasion of privacy you've ever imagined. For less than twenty dollars, they'll give you a person's last ten years of major medical and workers' compensation charges and, from RVS codes, essentially tell you what diseases they have. They'll do sub-rosa investigations to find out about alcoholism, drugs, troubled teenagers, bad marriages—the laundry list just goes on and on. You just figure out how much you want to spend.

In their promotional material, the search companies portray their background checks as useful to employers in evaluating the potential costs that an employee might represent. Company human resources offices have been besieged with such material. The sales pitch is that having a corporate doctor conduct preplacement exams, even including a drug test of the urine, cannot begin to match the potential cost savings offered by the search company.

Concern about medical data has usually focused on employers' own screening tests, but company testing is in fact an issue of minor importance compared with the flood of information coming from search companies, data banks, and credit reporting agencies—information easily abused by employers and largely beyond the control of medical professionals. Such disclosures of medical information may have serious repercussions that become increasingly important as medical data continue to proliferate.

STRATEGIES FOR SUBMITTING MEDICAL INFORMATION TO MANAGEMENT

Physicians develop strategies for submitting medical information to management. For instance, they withhold diagnoses from managers; they keep confidential information in separate employee assistance files; they give managers information when employees file compensation claims or lawsuits or when managers perceive that they may do so; and they advise employees not to reveal information about their health that they wish to keep confidential. Although physicians use these strategies to help them determine how to provide medical information to managers, they also use them to help justify conduct that they might otherwise perceive as violations of medical confidentiality.

Doctors Withhold Diagnoses When Management Demands Information

Doctors say that when personnel directors and supervisors ask them for medical records, they simply report whether the worker in question is fit for work, without divulging specific diagnoses.[13] Doctors sometimes defend giving information to management by arguing that they protect doctor-patient confidentiality when they give managers just enough information to understand that the employee has a medical condition requiring specific work restrictions—for example, that he or she cannot drive, lift more than thirty pounds, or sit for more than six hours per day. Management then makes hiring, firing, and job assignment decisions based on physicians' advice. For example, a physician in a manufacturing company and a doctor who provides health services to companies, said:

> Management tries to tell employees, "The physician told us not to hire you." No. Our job is to explain to the supervisor that employees meet or don't meet the medical requirements for the job or can meet them with certain accommodations. The personnel department and not the physician has the responsibility of hiring and firing. Management doesn't like to say to people face to face, "I'm not hiring you," so they try to shift the blame onto the medical department. It is *so* true.

> It's out of my hands after my physical assessment finds something that tells me this person shouldn't be a clerk-typist. My recommendation says, "This employee does not meet the physical qualifications of the job." What will the employer do with that information? Many doctors are skittish about providing specific diagnostic information, but we're playing games when we try to avoid saying the word if it's something like your safety concern with epilepsy, and instead give five pages of restrictions of what is necessary to accommodate the patient; when it would work much better simply to tell personnel, "Joe Smith has a medical problem of seizures. It appears to be controlled, but you have to be concerned about that." Or, "The employee has diabetes and is on insulin. They'll need food if they experience an insulin reaction, and you need to know the patient's not drunk or having an epileptic seizure if the patient suddenly falls out or acts a little weird. Now let's resolve the problem and not try to hide it behind things." It's sensible to do that, very practically.[14]

Such a straightforward explanation comes through at times. Doctors may not have a great deal of time or desire to beat around the bush in pages of notes to supervisors.

When physicians say they withhold from management only a precise diagnosis, they imply that it is easy to draw a clear line between confidential and nonconfidential information, and that most information about the fitness of an employee for a job can acceptably be given to management. Then clearly on the other side of the line is confidential information that they cannot by any means give managers or company lawyers. As a utility doctor said:

> A supervisor might question a work restriction, or whether I let somebody come back to work. I tell them that management is never entitled to specific details of the diagnosis. They are entitled to restrictions and limita-

tions, and I will define those and we can talk about those in great detail—
and that's where I draw the line.

But in fact, the line between confidential medical information and
work restrictions information is indistinct and difficult to draw.
Doctors are expected to provide management with information to
allow them to decide whether the person is fit to work, but it is
often hard to determine how much management should know
about fitness to work.

In many cases company physicians convey important medical
information about a person's condition without revealing a precise
diagnosis. From the work restrictions alone, one could infer a
medical condition and the presence of other information in the
confidential medical records. For example, from restrictions on
lifting, squatting, and stooping, one can infer that a person has a
musculoskeletal problem. Even simply telling management a person is temporarily unfit to work or has specific work restrictions
because of a medical condition divulges significant information.
An aerospace company physician said:

> I've been putting one limitation on people who have heart disease or have
> a heart attack and come back: no excessive overtime. Most of the super-
> visors now know that means the person had a heart attack or heart dis-
> ease. Ninety-nine percent of the time they already know it, and I *want*
> them to know it.[15]

A physician who has provided medical services for electronics
companies and an airline physician acknowledged the way in
which doctors reveal medical conditions without explicitly stating
a diagnosis:

> There's supposed to be, at least in theory, confidentiality for recommenda-
> tions from the examining physician in a corporate setting. The person has
> no right arm; he can't do certain things. But you're not supposed to talk
> about the diagnosis of no right arm, so you say, "Find a job placement for
> this person where he can function only with the left arm." And everybody
> knows the diagnosis—there's no right arm—and yet that satisfies every-
> one's ethical notion of living with the code of ethics.

> We merely tell the employer they are fit or unfit to work, and we may put
> restrictions on them if they are fit to work. You can guess what the prob-
> lem is from reading into the restrictions, but it's not specifically stated. We

may say that someone who just recovered from a bad back injury as a result of a motor vehicle accident should not lift or bend repetitively, day to day. It doesn't take too much intelligence to recognize that those restrictions are probably there because this person has a back problem, but the problem is implied, not stated.

Thus, despite their efforts to distance themselves, doctors become involved in decisions about hiring, firing, and transferring employees and sometimes at least indirectly reveal diagnostic information along the way.

Doctors Keep Medical Information in Separate EAP Files

In companies with an employee assistance program for workers with substance abuse and psychological problems, EAP records of tests and communication with counselors are supposed to be kept separately and treated more confidentially than the company's general medical records. Some physicians deliberately put information they do not want management to see in the EAP file, in the hope that they will not have to give it to company lawyers who ask for medical information. As a physician with a large oil company explained:

> Employees' drug and employee assistance records for sexual-psychological or substance abuse problems are kept separate from the main chart. They can be subpoenaed, but only if the lawyers specifically ask for an EAP or psychological record, and most lawyers are not smart enough to do that. We tell employees that we won't let anyone see these records unless they say it's okay.

In addition to EAP records, detailed questionnaires can identify a wide range of health and behavioral problems.[16] A health official with the United Steelworkers union said:

> We've seen a lot of people subjected to so-called medical histories where the clear intent is to find something in somebody's background that explains a disease they might have in the future—for example, two pages on all the ways they are exposed to noise: Do you hunt? Do you listen to rock music? If you answered yes to one of those questions, and file a claim for hearing loss ten years down the road, they will come back and say, "This guy shot skeet, so obviously he's deaf. It had nothing to do with work." We've seen extremely long and invasive so-called basic medical his-

tory forms that ask, "Did you wet the bed as a child? Did any of your relatives have psychological problems? What age did you first menstruate? Have you ever had an abortion? How many pregnancies have you caused (in the case of a man), and what was the outcome of each one?" Companies we've questioned on it have always said they need this to establish a good medical history for this person.[17]

Remarkably, company physicians refer to records that have drug, alcohol, and psychological information in them as "confidential." Doctors often tell managers of an employee's drug or alcohol use after managers who perceive a conduct problem have sent that employee to the medical department. In one company with an EAP and drug-testing program, for example, a doctor who did the company's drug testing said:

The confidentiality *we* imposed on drug testing was completely lost because it was personnel's job to call EAP and set up the appointments with people the urine screening picked up. There might have been some question about which drug it was. It's just such a long history of sharing all information, it's just a joke.

Although company physicians claim to tell workers that no one will see their employee assistance records unless they expressly permit it in writing or it gets subpoenaed, they also point to ways in which they breach confidentiality of these records along with other medical information.

Doctors Give Information with Compensation Claims or Potential Suits

If you file a claim, there is no confidentiality.

—Railroad physician

When it comes to confidentiality, physicians describe their stance like acrobats walking a tightrope, desperately seeking ways to avoid clearly failing on ethical doctor-patient relations. Records may be largely confidential only until an employee's health is contested for some reason—exactly the time when a worker might most want confidentiality. Any employee could someday be a workers' compensation claimant, so in that sense employee records—including EAP records—are vulnerable. In the event of disputes with management or lawsuits, employee medical records typically become available to management and company attorneys. For example, in any kind of litigation, both sides are entitled to the medical evidence if health becomes a source of contention. Physicians and managers often extend this access to circumstances where managers simply anticipate that employees may file claims or lawsuits. Thus, by trying to persuade employees to cooperate and confide in them, doctors may be encouraging workers to act against their own interest. Doctors usually give managers and company lawyers the entire medical record, not only the parts of the medical record related to the case. Two physicians, one in aerospace and the other employed by an oil company, said:

> Our workers' comp people might review the records if there's a problem employee or they anticipate someone's about to file a claim or sue. They are allowed to look at the whole record.[18]

> When people accuse us, saying they were mistreated or fired, the lawyer for the company will knock on my door and say, "I want *everything* I can get to protect the company's hide. We want to know everything about their record."

Rather than subpoena medical records, company lawyers or workers' compensation officials often review records if they pertain to a claim or suit against the company. Company attorneys prefer to get medical records without subpoenas, partly because when companies create a subpoena and communicate it to the plaintiff's attorney, they may also telegraph how they will handle the case.[19] Instead, internal attorneys often simply look at the whole record to see whether anything might relate to the legal dispute. An oil company doctor and another from a computer company said:

> I try to be very compliant in providing the information the lawyers working for the company want. It rarely takes a subpoena. I don't try to posture or prevent them from getting it. Some of my colleagues do, but I always felt that I'm willing to provide information and my opinion on it so long as I could be assured that someone made a legal claim and their health has been made a legal issue.

> We give the lawyers handling suits the whole medical record. They don't have to subpoena it. They are entitled to see whatever it says. In

every company I've worked for, legal can get whatever records medical has and may show managers records; that is their prerogative.[20]

The subpoena serves individual employees by forcing attorneys to focus on the precise records they want. The legal department can subpoena an entire medical record if a person's medical history is being questioned for a disability. But usually employee claims are more focused, such as those regarding injuries to a particular body part. At least formally, the medical department only needs to communicate the specific information in the record that the subpoena requests.

Although in-house lawyers and outside counsel are all attorneys the company has hired to protect the corporation, physicians are more likely to ask outside counsel to produce a subpoena.[21] About inside counsel they say, "We work together and understand each other; we need to be team players." Partly this is a matter of the social relationships in which physicians are involved: they may be on the same floor in the same building with company attorneys; they may participate in other activities unrelated to a specific employee. Doctors who give in-house counsel more information than outside counsel do it in part because it is like horse-trading: they believe they may need the inside lawyers for help with something else. As a physician who provided services to corporations said:

> The in-house legal counsel is a co-employee you see in the cafeteria. You may be on committees on medical-legal questions and interact with the legal department on many other issues, like acquiring real estate you want to put a clinic on; whereas it's a different environment when the counsel is outside. A lot of companies use in-house counsel for screening malpractice claims, so they will be the physician's defender at some point—the first line of defense that does the initial screening and makes an initial settlement offer before it gets to an outside malpractice firm. I'm not sure that *I* would want to alienate the legal counsel if that person was going to defend me.

Workers' compensation records and doctors' reports are available to the employer, insurance companies, potential employers, and even the public. Employers seek these records in their attempts to demonstrate that employees had a preexisting disability or impairment before their subsequent injury. Two doctors who provide medical services to companies said:

Workers' compensation claims are basically in the public domain; you can go down to the Workers' Compensation Appeals Board and have the file pulled if you know the claim number. Access to them is easy. You can actually obtain the physical file—whether it's documents in the file or a judge's determination that indicates what the injury and award were.[22]

These [ACOEM] ethical statements are just enormously hypocritical, given the fact that government, the insurance industry, and the medical industry all know that there's absolutely no confidentiality in workers' compensation—absolutely none whatsoever. Some people still have that misperception. The minute that record is finished, it's mailed in its entirety to an insurance company; it's read by secretaries, lawyers, and other doctors. I've seen complete medical records at the conference tables of supervisors and comp carriers going over all these troublesome cases. The doctor and the nurse and the safety people—everybody's all there picking through it. Workers should be told that.

In some companies the group that handles workers' compensation benefits actually resides in the legal unit rather than in health care or human resources, which tends to make their relationship to doctors more adversarial. Especially in self-insured companies, the claims litigation group reviews the medical records, decides whether to accept or deny a claim, and pays the medical benefits. Rather than use subpoenas and have patients sign releases, claims managers and lawyers simply review entire medical records. A utility company physician who resists sending employees' full records to the claims group said:

This corporation views workers' compensation as a legal issue, not as a medical one. The workers' compensation benefits group here is under the legal department, which has the attitude that when an employee files a claim, the legal group can insist on getting the entire medical record without signed patient authorization or subpoena. The general counsel finally decided we should send the patients a little information brochure to tell them we'll get their records. I send what is pertinent, without telling them it isn't the entire record, and generally they're so confused and overwhelmed they don't realize they don't have the entire record. One doctor who's been here close to fifteen years routinely gives claims litigation people the entire medical record and feels that's his role as a physician here. He was hired to support the company and turn the records over; the company wins in any conflict between company and employee. He's in his midfifties and has not been through a formal training program or become board-certified in anything. He is in an insecure position and feels vulnerable.

Workers generally do not know that their test results and other medical information in their records can be circulated to managers and lawyers on both sides if they file a workers' compensation claim, if the records are subpoenaed, or if doctors cooperate with managers' and company lawyers' demands. Workers who like the doctors may believe that they would not give records to management unless they are subpoenaed. They may admit something to physicians because they want their help, but later learn that a potential lawsuit precludes confidentiality.

Many employees lack faith that the corporate physician keeps their records private. Much mistrust of company doctors comes from the belief that if workers become sick or injured, their medical files will be used against them to deny them compensation. Doctors' involvement in drug testing, their testifying for the company in workers' compensation hearings, and their cooperation with company lawyers and personnel managers in disability claims further undermine trust in the doctor-patient relationship. Employees who know their records are readily available to management and can be used against them if they file a claim or suit would be especially reluctant to put sensitive information, such as a family history of heart disease, into the record. A services company physician and a chemical company doctor said:

A lot of people don't understand that litigants basically give up their rights to confidentiality when they litigate a health-related case, whether it's workers' comp or a health-related third-party tort case. They get surprised and say, "Wait a minute! All these people have all my medical records!" You have no privacy to medical records if you enter into a lawsuit that revolves around a health issue—other than for certain psychiatric records, which varies by state. You are not supposed to print them in the paper, but the idea that they are somehow sacrosanct is just not there.

When workers file a claim against a company, they should know the company will defend itself. But I don't think workers understand all the ramifications. They should become educated consumers and learn what the reality is.

Management is entitled to look at medical records when employees sign waivers of confidentiality. Unionized employees who bring grievances and salaried employees filing workers' compensation claims sign waivers saying that the company can look at their medical records. Employers who investigate workers for security reasons also have them sign a release of all records. Although employees theoretically can refuse to sign releases for their medical records, their refusal is likely to result in loss of their claim. A union official said:

> The confidentiality business is a hoax, because companies will be able to get records if it's important to them. If a miner files a claim for black-lung compensation, the attorneys first subpoena the chest X-rays from NIOSH in Morgantown, West Virginia, where miners end up with a file of X-rays as part of the black-lung program and chest X-ray surveillance program— one about every five years after the one when he's first employed. The miner has to produce these films because it doesn't look good on his claim if he decides not to release them. The judge will sit up there and say, "Look, you had five films taken, and we can't see them. What's going on here?" That won't be terribly persuasive to the judge. Therefore, when the subpoena comes, the films go right away.[23]

Concerns about the corporate use of medical information are warranted. Employees who reveal a medical or psychological problem to physicians are more likely to confront breaches of confidentiality in corporations than in private practice. Whether a corporation hires doctors in-house or uses physicians in contract firms, managers often get the information they request. Employees may reasonably fear that adverse medical findings could jeopardize their job or be sent to third parties for use against them. Some employees would feel safer seeing an outside fee-for-service or preferred provider rather than their company's doctor. However, employers may not pay if an outside doctor provides the services, and state laws may restrict employees' ability to see outside doctors for work-related illnesses. Thorny problems of confidentiality arise even in companies where employees trust the physicians and find company programs to be low-cost and convenient.

Doctors May Advise Workers Not to Reveal Medical Information

Doctors may want the employees' trust, but they recognize that they must report medical information to management for fitness evaluations, security clearances, and other managerial concerns, and that any specified piece of information can be subpoenaed in future legal disputes. Hearing unsolicited medical or psychological information—such as successful earlier treatment for depression or drug abuse—might put the doctor in a bind because adding it to the medical record could harm the employee's job prospects. Doctors handle that kind of situation in different ways. They can record the information on a separate page or otherwise enter it into the medical record in a way that reduces the chance of its going to the corporate legal department. Alternatively, they may advise the employee that what they reveal will go into the company's records and may go to management.[24] Although physicians generally do not take this approach, a utility company physician who does said:

> I explain the situation to patients and let them help me decide how they want to deal with it. The patients have to be educated and told. Some patients say, "I don't care if you put that in my medical chart," and others say not to. They also have the option of not discussing it with me. I do it differently than everybody else because I'm so concerned about this issue, and I probably err a little bit on the side of putting less instead of more in the chart; it isn't necessarily the best way to do it.

It can be hard for company physicians to decide when to recommend that an employee consider withholding information because of its possible consequences. They must judge whether the person truly represents a safety hazard; and in the case of office workers they may choose not to probe into their medical and psychological past because of the low risk that they would hurt themselves or others. An auto company physician said:

> Sometimes things get blurted out too soon. I sometimes try to stop them from telling me things that could hurt them and just let them know up front. I say, "Your behavior has been kind of strange. I need to ask you a question, and you realize of course who I represent." Sometimes I give them alternatives: "These are the consequences if you don't say or if you do." I make a judgment call and try not to probe too much, unless somebody has a safety-intensive job: "You can withhold what you need to withhold, but I need to have at least enough information so I can decide whether it's safe for you to go back to work."

A doctor who does medical evaluations of workers at an employer's direction—and who supervises other doctors who evaluate workers for employers—said that since he was hired to give employers his medical opinion, he tries to make it clear to employees that he is not their regular doctor, and that the same confidentiality rules do not apply. He then talks openly with the employer about the employees' cases. He said:

> People come in for a onetime visit or are seen over two or three sessions over several months. They provide information to us in meetings with them, we review records sent to us, and we consider psychological testing and all the other evidence. Confidentiality is limited. We tell people up front that our opinions based on the information they provide us will be put into a written report and sent to the employer or other referral source, who will use it for administrative decisions about such things as treatment, temporary or permanent disability benefits, vocational rehabilitation, or some accommodation at the workplace. We try to avoid having the person say halfway into the interview, "But, Doctor, I want to tell you something off the record." I encourage doctors to say, "Nothing is off the record. If that's the only way you can tell me, then don't tell me. If you do tell me, chances are it will be in my notes and the report, and we can report anything we find to the employer or their insurer. So knowing that, it's up to you how to proceed." In fact, there is no off-the-record with employees we see.[25]

Doctors who warn employees of management access to records are not providing for "informed consent" in any meaningful sense, however: the worker's refusal to cooperate with a medical examiner may invalidate his or her claim for compensation.

THE INDEPENDENCE OF PHYSICIANS SUPPLYING MEDICAL INFORMATION TO MANAGERS

The extent to which physicians give nonmedical managers access to medical information depends in part on three structural factors: whether physicians report centrally to corporate medical directors or to local managers, whether the company is self-insured, and whether it is contract physicians rather than in-house physicians providing the information. Paradoxically, the independence of physicians from a centralized medical department, from a separate medical insurance company, or from direct corporate employment can make them more dependent on managers who pressure them for medical information about employees. These types of independence make physicians more vulnerable to managerial demands and influence their perspectives on divulging medical information.

Central Reporting Versus Reporting to Local Managers

The type of medical department structure exerts a major influence on physicians and on how they handle disputes over medical information. Most big companies formerly had a centralized structure with individual physicians reporting to the medical director. Although at Mobil Oil and a few other large corporations medical departments remain centralized, company doctors now typically report to local managers rather than to a centralized medical division in company headquarters. This is a significant structural difference, because doctors in decentralized structures are under greater pressure to please nonmedical management and nonmedical considerations become more salient in their decisions. Local plant managers are emboldened in their efforts to influence company doctors by the fact that they have more control over doctors' budgets, salary increases, and promotions. A medical director from a conglomerate and a physician from a consumer products company—both in decentralized structures—stated:

> If you as medical director don't control the doctors and the company's purse strings, if you aren't involved in giving them raises and bonuses and meting out punishment and discipline, then doctors could care less because they report at the local level, not to you. If managers don't want to have a medical department they don't have to, and nothing says they must always consult the corporate medical director. That is a weakness with our corporate structure, but many companies are like that.

> Docs are under pressure if they have to report to a plant manager who has a workers' comp or disability problem and wants to get so many widgets on the line by such and such a time. It is a tough issue, and doctors feel a lot of pressure.[26]

Doctors who work in centrally organized medical departments report that they experience less pressure to comply with managers' demands. They say that local managers generally lean on them less for information about specific employees than in decentralized companies, where local managers pressure them more often to handle illnesses and injuries in certain ways. They also describe greater company support for their decisions as medical professionals. In such an organization, the boss they must please, and the one who knows and controls their budget, is typically a fellow physician. Central reporting, besides shielding doctors from some managerial pressure, allows them to appeal to the corporate medical director up the line when problems arise. Two physicians who report centrally in oil companies said:

> If I had to report to the human resources manager here at the plant, I'd quit. That would be just rife with opportunities for attempting to influence things inappropriately, particularly in our current environment, with so much emphasis on making the plant productive, making it earn money, and reducing reportable injuries.

> It's a lot easier to protect the confidentiality of records in this centralized medical department, because plant managers don't control my raises or promotions. I can always call my boss and say, "I'm getting a lot of pressure to turn over records on XYZ case, and you may hear about it, since I'm not doing it." The medical department reports high up in the corporation, with the medical director's boss one level down from the CEO, which helps. Reporting to the plant manager at the site where you work rather than to the medical director is a prescription for disaster. I'd never work for a company that was set up that way, though most are like that.[27]

Medical directors as well as local company physicians strongly prefer centralized control. They argue that in decentralized organizations, local managers may be running individual plants without realizing that the lack of uniformity among the widely varying medical programs makes them more likely to be out of compliance with OSHA directives and to bring legal liability to the company. Allowing doctors to have centralized control can threaten management, however. The fact that centralized medical departments shield physicians from the local management is one reason managers oppose such a structure. A medical director in a conglomerate said:

> I would prefer more centralized medical operations, far and away, because we would have a lot more medical facilities out there if I called the shots, because the medical director is more enlightened than a lot of plant managers are. The downside of central reporting is that the plant manager often tends to be more demanding and expects more of the medical department because he pays for it anyway in an overhead charge that goes to headquarters regardless of whether the medical department performs. He also tends to keep doctors out of the plant because they don't work for him: "You guys work for that doc in New York. I won't tell you what I do in the plant." So it cuts both ways.

Physicians in centralized corporations, with a higher wall around the medical function, may feel that because they work for the corporate medical director they need not listen as closely to local managers. Those managers then claim that they need control of their assets and that the medical director does not know their problems or the resources they need to do their jobs. Having doctors work for them, they argue, would make them a more profitable business unit.

Insurers and Self-Insured Companies

Although company doctors do physical examinations that generate information, health-screening information also makes its way to managers after employees go to their private physicians and file claim forms that insurance companies administer. Insurers then report to the employer on the workers' medical treatment. Periodically, insurers send to the benefits or human resources manager a report giving detailed medical information on the people whose claims they paid. In this way, managers learn about the predispositions and diseases of individual employees, as well as who has been treated for anything from venereal disease or psychiatric problems to heart disease. Even when employers are reluctant to use medical information to exclude workers, insurance companies may pressure them to collect medical information and to identify higher-risk individuals. Employees who want to get reimbursed must fill out a claim form that asks for the diagnosis. Although occupational medicine's ethical guidelines and ADA rules instruct doctors to give managers a report on an employee's fitness to work rather than a diagnosis, the employee's third-party health insurance will not pay without a diagnosis.[28] Employers get records showing the third-party payer reimbursement for procedures performed on employees. Health-care providers and insurers build a record on the tests they conduct, doctors' visits, and hospital stays for employees. Information ends up in the human resources department if the health care is reimbursable. The company gets a coded printout if the employee's health care is covered by a third-party payer such as Blue Cross under a fee-for-service plan. A utility company physician and a union official said:

> The reality now is I could go up and pull anybody's claims in health care without looking at a medical chart and be able to tell you their whole medical history, just by looking at their claims that have been paid for.[29]

> Companies know if you or a member of your family go to a psychiatrist and you have psychiatric coverage—or if employees go for an abortion—because it shows up on the insurance reports; they know every bit of it.[30]

In some cases the insurer is the employer. Self-insured companies have access to vast amounts of information about a person's health history and use of medical services.[31] Confidentiality problems for self-insured companies are generally more severe than for companies with outside insurance coverage, since claims processing and risk information are readily available in-house. A physician who has provided medical services to many companies said:

> I've never seen a company that went self-insured that didn't seriously compromise whatever little bit of corporate confidentiality of medical records existed. They become intensely interested in medical records. It is in corporations' self-interest to screen workers out and violate the confidentiality of employee records, rather than take measures to reduce exposure hazards. You could argue that they won't be here if they don't. The insurance industry is the model for corporations. Its ability to screen and deny service has made it the one solid, profitable industry forever in this country. And it has never respected medical confidentiality.

Insurance companies and self-insured employers have a long history of screening, charging different rates according to risk, denying service to high-risk individuals, and failing to respect medical confidentiality (see, for example, Smith 1994; Hudson et al. 1995;

National Institutes of Health/Department of Energy 1993, 792; Pear 1997a, A1, A16).[32]

Contractors and Confidentiality

The lack of confidentiality of employee medical files increases as employers turn to outside contractors to conduct tests and provide screening data. Employers who contract with outside physicians expect to get some information back. Many contractors who are under competitive pressure to keep a company's business will send management entire employee medical records, believing that other contractors are doing the same.[33] They may readily submit employee information to the companies that hire them, despite professional standards that regard this information as confidential. Small clinics that contract to provide health services to a company may be unaware of the regulations and ACOEM's code of ethical conduct concerning medical records. Contract physicians are less likely than in-house physicians to be active members of ACOEM, the relevant professional medical association; they are often eager to keep their contract with the employer and will therefore send records back to whomever they are told to send them back to. They often assume that since the company pays for the medical information, it is entitled to all of it, rather than just aggregate data or a determination that specific individual employees are fit to work. Employers without in-house doctors may then keep the medical records that contractors send them in the personnel files. Two physicians who have worked as contractors, one now with a financial services company and the other with a services company, said:

> Companies that do periodic examinations and surveillance exams are obliged to send detailed medical reports to the personnel director. You know it's wrong, but you don't get the contract if you don't do it, so that puts the burden on the integrity of the vendor. Service providers breach confidentiality and won't even go through the formality of having the employee sign a release. I fear the changes going on will produce more of that. That bothers me.

> Basically you sell your availability if you provide services. You can say, "I'm going to put a wall up and won't do something," but your competitors down the street do it. It would all stop if all the doctors together said,

"We won't do it," but you can't get them all to say that. They feel they don't have a right to keep the records confidential. Some practitioners are good about saying, "No, we won't show you these records, and here's what we'll give you," but they run the risk of being blackballed out of business, and they probably run a bigger risk than does the corporate physician.

Although contract firms may in some respects be more independent, they may also experience greater pressure to submit records to employers and thus violate confidentiality more often. Managers do not gain access to medical records simply by walking into a health-care facility and looking at them, but outside contractors can pass test results along to them. Full-time company physicians may be better able to withstand pressure to turn over records. Some contractors I interviewed who were in-house before their corporate employers laid them off said they are under more pressure now, as contractors, to submit information about workers. One doctor who has been an in-house company doctor, a hospital occupational medical doctor, and a part-time consultant to a corporation said:

Providing information to the employer is clearly an ever-present challenge for outside consultants. Looming over us is the threat of losing business. One company that had some serious health risks from chemicals they were using, and ergonomic problems, wanted all the medical records on a certain employee. We sent the company a letter saying that based on our evaluation, the patient is fully cleared for all responsibilities of this position, but that wasn't good enough. We had a battle back and forth for about eight months. Finally, the employer just walked because we wouldn't dance for them.

Another employer wanted all the records of exams and wanted to know whether people had previous back injuries. They pressured the contract physician to accommodate beyond ethical restraints. A resident we had working at this facility said he couldn't do exams for this company if all the medical records went to the employer, so the VP of the hospital fired him.[34]

A doctor who provided services to corporations and trains occupational physicians said:

The medical exams have developed a *little* bit of confidentiality over the years I've been in the field, but precious little. When I was just coming into this field twenty-five years ago, 180 of the 200 client companies that had me do physicals had a corporate policy that their personnel departments got the records of my examinations. So I sent a thick letter with all the supporting information to what's now the College [ACOEM] and said, "Please explain to me how I'm supposed to live by this code of ethics when this is what *I* do and what all the other practitioners in my neighborhood do, and if I were to stop I would lose about 180 of my 200 clients." They never answered that letter. If some young doctor does the same thing today—I'm sure he does—and writes in, he'll go twenty-five years too without hearing from them.

Employers are legally required to maintain records in many instances. They have argued that OSHA requires them to keep records for at least thirty years, so they must control the records to avoid an OSHA violation. However, OSHA regulations do not require that the records be kept on-site; they simply say that employers must have access and be able to get to them quickly.[35] Major confidentiality issues arise in companies that have off-site doctors who have records in many widely dispersed sites, when no one knows where all the records are and what the procedures are for protecting them.

Companies with no physician or medical department may instead have twenty file cabinets of medical files that the companies' own safety managers and other on-site personnel do not have the expertise to interpret or handle properly. These records—containing records of people's blood pressures, family histories, and test results—could become a legal liability if somebody unauthorized to see them put them to improper use. For this reason, companies that generally handle their records in-house may nevertheless want outside contractors to deal with their medical records.

When physicians are employed by corporations, their legal responsibility to keep test results confidential has historically been quite limited. Although few legal provisions currently restrict the distribution of employee medical information within companies, case law and state statutes shape physicians' professional judgment about what constitutes proper confidentiality within companies.[36] In addition, the Americans with Disabilities Act specifies certain confidentiality protections and limits what employers can ask on preplacement examinations to questions relating to the job the person would do.[37] However, the law governing medical confidentiality is murky in many respects and very much in flux, particularly concerning employer medical programs. The extent to which medical information must be kept private—and not revealed to employers, insurers, or others—is currently being redefined. Physicians therefore face uncertainty in developing strategies for providing medical information to managers, whether or not they report to centralized medical departments, work in self-insured companies, or work in-house as company physicians.

EMPLOYEE ACCESS TO INFORMATION

Employees typically have limited information about medical practices and health risks in corporations, though state and federal right-to-know laws now dictate that workers be permitted to review their own medical records and certain records pertaining to exposure hazards.[38] These laws certainly have had a major effect on health practices in companies: employees can use OSHA access rules to obtain medical records from supervisors and doctors and to obtain the information about health hazards that employers must record for OSHA purposes, such as material safety data sheets. However, employees with access to their individual medical records may still lack information on employers' medical practices.

The Toxic Substances Control Act (administered by the EPA) has requirements for keeping records of medical tests and diseases that are generally more stringent than OSHA's. Employers who record such information for the EPA must give it to employees who request specific portions of it, but employees generally are unaware of what kinds of information employers record for the EPA and may not know what information to request.[39] Employees miss an opportunity to get a great deal of data if their request is not specific or does not deal adequately with the EPA recording requirements.

Employees who obtain medical and exposure records do not necessarily know how to interpret the medical information and scientific evidence that right-to-know laws have allowed them to acquire. Physicians may or may not cooperate in helping them understand exposure conditions, and safety officers or others—rather than company physicians—may have that responsibility.

Employers also control access to the information about company resources that they could use for preventive measures. Employers may say they have done extensive monitoring and know that the work environment is safe; employees often do not have access to long-term monitoring data so that they can see whether a pattern of disease exists. Employees also have difficulty evaluating the validity of employer threats that stronger toxics controls would run them out of business.[40] An airline physician said:

> There's always a hidden agenda, and the reasons for things are frequently not obvious. I used to write propaganda in the military, so I recognize it when I see it. Every time we come up on a contract negotiation period, the company publications start talking about how much money we're losing, and then the day that's over they start talking about how great we're doing, because the next thing is they have to convince the stockholders that management is doing well.

Doctors who have evidence about testing programs, diseases, or company negligence that is likely to help employees in compensation claims and lawsuits against the company conceivably could disclose it to those employees. However, the balance of power between management, labor, and the medical staff impedes physicians who might otherwise wish to share such information openly with workers. Employers recognize that physicians providing information to employees from medical and exposure records could reveal working conditions they wish to keep secret, lead workers to file claims, or encourage union officials to turn a potential hazard into a cause célèbre. A union health official said:

> We see physicians who are open and willing to share information from medical records. The problem is usually that the physician has been told to check with the lawyers, who go crazy when they hear that anybody wants any kind of information. We've had cases where employers wanted people to sign statements that they won't use the information against the company if it's released.[41]

When physicians lack strong evidence that an exposure hazard is significant, they may resist telling workers about it or doing anything about it themselves. As their patients have become better informed, doctors have become both more open with them and more careful at the same time. Two doctors, one employed by a conglomerate and the other by an airline, faced the dilemma of determining how much to tell employees about exposures and what other actions to take with exposed workers. They said:

> We had a foundry with an awful lot of pulmonary problems. These guys had worked there all their lives, and it was the only plant in town. Do you race in and say, "Everybody whose pulmonary function is down 20 percent is out of here?" That would mean virtually the entire plant.

> The company did a study to determine how much methylene chloride was present in the work site, and some numbers were pretty high on people who basically took mops and buckets and sloshed the stuff on airplanes. It's a carcinogenic solvent we used for decades as a paint thinner to strip airplanes. Unfortunately, it has poor "warning properties" because it's not irritating and you don't smell it when it begins to get through the respirator. So the dilemma was how much to tell people who worked with methylene chloride for many years. Should we educate those who've been exposed? They'll freak out if we tell them it's a carcinogen. It was unpleasant because of the inevitable union reaction to anything like this. They tend to disbelieve anything that any company person tells them about it, so when I try to do my best to give them honest and tempered medical judgment, they say, "Yeah, you're just a company hack. What do you know?" And management becomes alarmed if some of my medical staff say inflammatory things about toxic exposures gratuitously. It's a good example of the crunch I get into.

Certainly companies differ greatly in how they deal with employees on health issues. Some widely announce studies they are planning before they do them and inform employees about exposures.[42] Others conceal or lie about risks. Some company physicians who have uncovered chemical hazards have given the facts to unions, while others refuse to help unions get such information. Contract physicians typically send medical information directly back to the employer, who often decides to share very little or none of it with employees.

The best information often comes from employees who work with health hazards and are concerned about protecting themselves. Employees have frequently uncovered exposure risks on their own and asked OSHA to come in and do something about it. Using epidemiology as a method of detecting hazards involves counting the bodies—or victims—affected and then tracking diseases back to a cause by comparing the disease rates of groups in the population. An official with the Oil, Chemical, and Atomic Workers International Union said:

> Medical departments and corporations did not expose problems before the unions pushed on occupational health questions. It's always been us discovering hazards using the body-in-the-morgue method, as we like to characterize it. We say, "There's a problem. We just have to work back and find the cause." Companies were aware of dibromochloropropane [DBCP] because a contract doctor had told them it was a problem. One doctor told us, "I told the company it was a problem. It wasn't my job to tell *you*, the union." That's how they construe the doctor-patient relationship. We are able to work cooperatively with the company doctor in situations where we confront a problem head on and the company's aware that we will pursue it. But everyone knows it's a confrontation. It's easier to reach a compromise with a company where the union has power and is willing to mobilize behind an issue. Then the company docs are instructed to be responsive, to be helpful. Sometimes companies want to resolve a problem when the fight is public. They hire more sophisticated docs and tell them to get rid of that problem, after they just waved off the ninety-nine other problems we had discovered before.[43]

A labor official with the United Steelworkers of America said:

> Most actions from company doctors fall on the side of not doing enough as opposed to doing too much. That's a problem in malpractice cases: you go after them for what they *do*, not so much for what they don't do. Physicians are pressured to understate medical information to patients. Doctors I've worked with also suffer from a paternalistic attitude, where they feel they know what's best for their patients and make decisions for patients who should have a choice.[44]

Organized labor has played an important role in expanding employee access to health and exposure information, although its influence is diminishing along with the steadily declining percentage of the workforce that is unionized.[45] Unions in some cases have essentially forced companies to pay attention to health issues by publicizing hazards or by setting employers up so that they end up with large fines if they do not remedy hazards. Unions have in some cases successfully pressed for more access to medical information and greater independence of physicians from corporate control.

CONCLUSION

People with no access to medical records have no way of knowing whether they contain inaccuracies, and yet misrepresentations of information can have devastating consequences in terms of employment, insurance, and stigmatization, especially with the rise in the number of computer searches of employees and job applicants initiated by employers. The greatest threat to privacy is not necessarily from company doctors but from contractors, the MIB, and managers who review company medical information. Too often, test results that should be considered confidential in fact are not. Since employers and agencies can ask people on questionnaires about their health—and since medical information is entered into data banks when individuals apply for insurance or third-party reimbursement—having private physicians perform tests does not solve the privacy problems.

Balancing the employer's right to know against the employee's right to privacy becomes more complex when the distribution of medical information affects pending litigation. Employers often want more information to defend against employee claims and lawsuits than doctors can provide without violating professional standards of ethical conduct, undermining their professional credibility, and exacerbating their conflicted relationship with patients. We next consider several other legal dimensions of corporate employment that exert contradictory pressures on physicians.

Chapter 8

Preventive Law by Corporate Professional Team Players: Liability and Responsibility in the Work of Company Doctors

For health professionals, just getting on the business-meeting agenda is an achievement, and you're always last if you can get on the agenda.

—Chemical company physician

The other name for occupational medicine is legal medicine. It is political and legal because doctors are looking over their shoulders in everything they do in occupational medicine. Corporate physicians are not the leaders of the band; they inevitably comply with company requirements. They do what the company or its lawyers tell them to do and are unlikely to buck the official company policy. Their jobs depend on it.

—Physician in a national occupational health agency who works with physicians in corporations

OVER THE PAST several decades law has dramatically altered the relationship of professionals to colleagues, clients, and the public. It shapes professionals' judgment about what constitutes appropriate professional conduct in many areas, including medi-

214

cal screening, employee placement, chemical emissions, medical malpractice, and responsibility for the costs of disease. Professionals follow news stories about litigation involving corporations and talk with colleagues and fellow workers about the meaning of court cases and statutory requirements. They tend to cast social questions and moral quandaries as legal matters, and their interpretations of the law have important effects on their decisionmaking. The prospect of a massive lawsuit or a jury trial with a multimillion-dollar award to the plaintiff often affects their work far more than one would expect from the slight probability of such a suit.

Corporate professionals undergo powerful contradictory legal pressures. Company doctors point to the adverse effects of the legalization of their field, as attorneys and the law increasingly direct their work. They focus less on preventive health than on preventive law—and especially on practices designed to avoid company liability and reduce the costs of compliance with government regulation. However, litigation and regulation also have positive effects in requiring risk reduction, compensating individuals for harm, and providing incentives for corporate management to curtail hazards. Doctors' perception that they could be sued individually for failing to protect employees and the public can positively influence their conduct and reinforce professional standards in corporations. In fact, the legal structure has been both beneficial and harmful for occupational medicine. Lawsuits are good to a point, beyond which they waste money on litigation that could be put into health programs. Moreover, it is not the legal requirements themselves that constrict corporate professionals the most; rather, it is the ways in which corporate management has chosen to respond to legal and economic pressures that put the greatest constraints on professionals in corporations.

THE EFFECTS OF THE LAW ON CONCEPTIONS OF PROFESSIONAL BEHAVIOR

Laws relating to professional work have changed radically over the past forty years, notably in such arenas as physicians' standard of care and workers' assumption of risk (see Rosenblatt, Law, and

Rosenbaum 1997). The threat of lawsuits against companies and the growth of legal departments within corporations have had major effects on the work physicians do. Physicians are sensitive to the legal implications of medicine and the role of lawyers in complicating medical practice, at times to the detriment of employees' health.[1]

Lawyers have risen in the corporate structure and now work in bigger and more heavily funded corporate legal departments. They have a major corporate role in interpreting the Americans with Disabilities Act, OSHA standards, and hiring and firing regulations. Many company lawyers handle medical-record information requests, grievances over benefits, and workers' compensation claims. They advise doctors on how to structure programs and review contracts and personnel policies. They also become involved in lawsuits after individuals are injured or die. The corporate legal department tends to subcontract litigation and all extraordinary events to outside attorneys and firms, leaving the internal staff to deal with routine matters.

Physicians in large corporations have extensive contact with lawyers who call them about pending suits or about what doctors should do in their practice. In-house counsel asks physicians to review specific cases and to evaluate whether claimants have a case or not. Corporate attorneys advise doctors on how to testify and deal with the media or opposing attorneys in depositions. Some companies instruct physicians not to respond when outside lawyers contact them, advising them that all responses must come from the legal office. Lawyers argue that certain information should be provided, and certain tests be conducted, in order to avoid company liability. In many cases—as when it issues directives regarding the handling of records or the diagnosis of certain illnesses—a legal department sets policy for the medical department. In other cases it persuades, as when it tries to get the medical department to provide information in ways that may reduce future employee claims.

Both the attorney and the doctor work for the company to protect the company's interest. When I asked company doctors about potential areas of conflict with the legal department, many said there really is no conflict because they run things past the legal department and do what the lawyers tell them to do. One longtime company physician said he did not need to run things by the legal department as much anymore; he already knew what they would say and therefore could do exactly what he expected they would tell him to do. Company doctors who testify on the company's behalf sometimes give the sense that the lawyer is standing next to them as they do their job. Rather than clash with lawyers, physicians sometimes incorporate the legal defense into their work, experiencing little sense of conflict. One doctor employed by a major consumer products corporation described the closely affiliated goals of company physicians and lawyers and said that when lawyers advise physicians, their major concerns are "avoiding lawsuits, hefty fines for noncompliance, and bad publicity." He explained:

> We work closely with company lawyers trying to anticipate what will be an issue rather than wait for somebody to file a suit. We're all singing from the same hymnal, and that's what I like to do. We can call up legal and say, "Look, I have a concern that this will pop up, and can you help me dress-rehearse this and prepare our case in advance." Crisis management takes an inordinate amount of time once something has happened. You're much better off if you can prevent it and reach an accommodation with the other person, so that's why we choose to call legal.

A chemical company physician said:

> There's mutual respect between medical and legal. I assist attorneys in the company in medical-record review, toxic tort cases, and workers' comp review. I give them straight medical information. They ought to know their case will not fly, and the sooner they learn the better, even though they may not want to hear it. We also have a few Superfund hazardous waste sites they are responsible for, and I've reviewed health risks for them on materials that might be at the site. They review medical publications that emanate from our department. We publish a health and environmental guide on a product, and the lawyers look at it to make sure we won't say something that means someone will sue them later.

Sometimes it is difficult to sort out how much time doctors spend on legal issues because they deal with worker surveillance, placement exams, and regulatory matters—all of which have a strong legal component. In fact, so many medical matters are becoming legal matters that it is hard to think of an occupational health issue that does not have legal ramifications. As a telecommunications company physician said:

> Virtually every decision is subject to review in court, which didn't used to
> be the case. Issues used to be decided pretty much on a straightforward
> medical basis; today very few medical issues are straightforward. Almost
> all of them have legal overtones.

Some physicians have told me they have almost constant contact with the legal department, which is many times larger than their medical department. Physicians generally spend far more time on legal matters than they did decades ago. A corporate medical director of an oil company, for example, said that he usually spends four hours a day on medical issues with legal implications or actually meeting with lawyers, whereas he used to spend about an hour a month. Two physicians, one at a computer company and the other at a telecommunications company, said:

> I spend at least one to two hours a day consulting with lawyers or review-
> ing briefs and other legal documents. This firm has one hundred times as
> many lawyers as doctors.

> The medical people in a corporation even ten years ago might have spo-
> ken with a lawyer once a month on a very complex case. Today virtually
> every day every physician in the company spends at least an hour and
> sometimes three or four hours with attorneys, because almost anything
> that comes along has legal ramifications.

A national labor official said:

> The major occupation of occupational physicians is being involved in liti-
> gation, whether it is administrative or tort. They spend more time and
> money litigating than treating or doing research or anything else. It's multi-
> ple testing, writing testimony, and keeping records for going to court. Most
> corporate physicians I know are very uncomfortable with this.[2]

The amount of legal involvement increases dramatically when environmental and safety issues are part of occupational medicine. Physicians increasingly have been drawn into litigating environmental health problems. In the asbestos industry, for example, many in-house and consulting occupational physicians advise companies on setting up procedures and exposure limits, and as the basic liability problem has shifted from manufacturers—primarily Manville—to companies that remove asbestos, they work with attorneys defending against suits. That growing arena involves translating issues of toxicology and epidemiology into terms that lawyers can use in defending against lawsuits. An airline physician complained that adversarial legal cases threaten to overwhelm him:

> The company has defined my role completely differently than I thought it would be. I hardly ever get a chance to just treat people who'll get better, which is what I used to like about occupational medicine. Now everything adversarial that involves the medical department comes to my desk: workers' compensation, contested cases, grievances, and lawsuits. Then I wind up dealing almost always with adversarial cases, where somebody is really angry no matter what I do. The administrative aspects and the adversarial-political aspects are wearing thin, and I'm tired of anger and criticism and lack of appreciation of the complexity and difficulty of what we do.

Despite the fact of frequent doctor-lawyer cooperation as fellow professionals and corporate employees, medical and legal priorities may often clash. Physicians feel torn between what their own medical judgment would lead them to do and what the lawyers want them to do. Many times when the company doctor believes an individual should return to work, the lawyers see a liability. Some public health–trained physicians resist when lawyers tell them to provide employee files or to describe risks to workers in specific ways. Many company physicians say they are bombarded with requests from the legal department for medical records. They describe their ongoing frustration over their conflicts with in-house lawyers. The in-house legal counsel can perceive the physician who advocates for the patient as an adversary, as someone who needs to be controlled or contained.[3] The medical department sometimes has been able to prevail in conflicts with company lawyers, but lawyers tend to be more aggressive in asserting how the company should act in internal disputes. They tend to be given precedence over physicians when they take a stand that doctors oppose, as these two physicians, from an oil company and a publishing company, explained:

> Lawyers are viewed as saviors and protectors from threat. That's a powerful position. Often they are perceived as the organization responsible for

professional expertise in a situation of threat or attack, so that is a very powerful place to be.

Clearly the legal department's interpretation of observing regulations and laws will carry the day when a company that must observe those laws employs you. The legal counsel is essentially present to keep the company from getting in trouble, so a compromise or concession must be sought if the legal department feels a particular action or process that medical people want would legally endanger the company.

A national health and safety labor official said: "Litigation and liability has become such a major part of the operation of many companies that it indeed becomes a final word or a final screen for everything, which is unfortunate." A physician for a bank stated: "We don't have any conflict with the attorneys. They tend to be on our side." But this same physician displayed on his office wall a framed quotation from Shakespeare's *Henry VI* in calligraphy: "The first thing we do, let's kill all the lawyers."

According to doctors, the fear of lawsuits against the company distorts the practice of corporate medicine, putting it on the defensive. As a physician for a major oil company said:

A corporation spends a lot of money unnecessarily on preventive legal medical practice. Sometimes the lawyer doesn't want the doctor to do something the doctor wants to do because it might show something the lawyer doesn't want to show. Let's say a former employee is suing the company for a bad back, and the doctor thinks another test would be good to make sure that he doesn't have something else, and the lawyer asks the doctor, "What if that test is abnormal? Then what?"

Lawyers and medical malpractice carriers often seek to settle cases with the least amount of loss even when physicians protest that they have done nothing wrong. In certain situations the company chooses not to fight employee claims because doing so would either cost more than settling or raise other issues that could harm the corporation, as this chemical company physician explained:

I mainly have conflict with our law department on settling. It's painful to me to settle and give away the store when I want to dig in my heels and defend a case that the lawyers tell me is expensive and stupid to defend. But it's crazy to go through this big ceremonial war to carry out my principles and still probably lose in front of a jury even though we're right.[4]

Many physicians in corporations say they dislike lawyers, objecting to what lawyers want the doctors to do and describing tension between them. Some physicians say lawyers tend to be trained in amorality: they do not see problems in moral terms, these doctors believe, in stark contrast to their own training and orientation. A metals company physician said:

The corporate legal profession influences outcomes by shading the truth. To be a successful lawyer, one characteristic you must have or acquire is amorality. It's win-at-all-cost, which has nothing to do with justice. The lawyer's foremost responsibility is to the company, and it's fine if the employee happens to benefit from that. The doctor will favor the employees even if their needs conflict with the company. The inability to differentiate right from wrong morally goes totally against the grain of a physician and his upbringing, training, and relationship with people. Physicians with the best intentions in the world can be destroyed by the way the legal system deals with them. Boy, I'm dead if they hear this! I dislike lawyers, and I blame them for a majority of our social and medical ills. But if the other side called me as their witness, it would create a problem, and our lawyers would say, "That's conflict of interest and you can't do that." I've never testified for the other side in my many years here.

This observation is common—and significant. Doctors may clash with attorneys for the company, but in contested cases the "other side" usually consists of employees. Like this physician, doctors generally cooperate with company attorneys in defending cases, whatever their sentiment about the attorneys involved.

PERCEPTIONS OF VULNERABILITY TO SUITS AGAINST DOCTORS

Physicians in private practice, whether or not they are in occupational medicine, often complain that the high price of malpractice insurance and the threat of lawsuits by patients place an unfair burden on their practices. But in the case of company medicine, employees generally have been unable to sue company physicians, in part because they have been considered fellow servants or co-agents (see Boden 2000; Willborn, Schwab, and Burton 1993, 709–19).[5] In addition, workers' compensation is the traditional and exclusive remedy of workers who get hurt; they generally cannot sue physicians who fail to diagnose diseases or to inform them of risks before they are injured.

Doctors generally have their employers' backing when they are named in a suit. Their companies answer the complaint and defend them when they testify. Because companies carry insurance for doctors and have the support of a corporate legal department, physicians who work for them are less concerned about lawsuits and malpractice insurance expenses than physicians in private practice. As these physicians, from a publishing company and an oil company, said:

> My friends say, "What happens if you get sued?" and my response is, "If somebody wants to sue, fine, but that's what they pay our lawyers for—to keep me and the other managers in this company out of jail." I just refer outside lawyers to my lawyers and let them hassle it out. They talk to our workers' comp people on workers' comp cases, so I don't get caught with that. They handle it lawyer to lawyer.

> This is a very big company with very deep pockets and a lot of smart lawyers that work for them. They don't want to sue me when they sue the corporation. When they look at the company, there's no way they can see me. The company says they will stand behind us if we use good judgment, so I don't think about being sued very much, though we are constantly involved with the legal system.[6]

Many company doctors are further protected from lawsuits by patients because they treat only minor injuries and illnesses. Much of what they do consists of giving physical exams rather than delivering primary care to people with serious diseases. They may diagnose health problems as part of the medical monitoring required by government regulation, but they send people to private physicians for treatment rather than treat employees themselves. Thus, they do not bear the same risks as private physicians. A telecommunications company doctor explained:

> There have been employee complaints of malpractice by our medical staff, but very few relative to the volume of clinical services. What we do is relatively low-risk anyway—mostly evaluations and no surgery. Doctors in this corporate environment don't feel the great malpractice issue.

Nevertheless, vulnerability to lawsuits is growing within corporations. Whereas professionals forty years ago could expect the law and their corporate employment to shield them from legal action, today physicians and other company personnel are experiencing an increasing liability for workplace hazards (see Tebo 2000; Plater et al. 1998, 869–904). Legislatures and courts have created exceptions to the exclusive-remedy provision of workers' compensation under most state law. They have allowed tort actions against company physicians and employers in limited circumstances, such as for intentional torts or suits against employers and their doctors serving in a "dual capacity" as employer and provider of medical services, as well as third-party suits against manufacturers based on negligence and product liability.[7] Citizens from the community have sued company physicians in third-party suits, and employees have alleged that individual professionals intentionally put workers at risk, withheld information, or failed to warn people.

Increasingly, company physicians find themselves in what must seem the worst of both worlds: they work in a corporate structure and need to be team players, but they can still be individually sued and even made criminally liable for their performance in a corporation. Many occupational physicians who seldom worried about liability in the past now fear being held personally liable for corporate decisions to which they only contributed.[8] Doctors become more attentive if they think they are individually responsible because their employer may not necessarily stand behind them or continue to cover their malpractice insurance if problems arise. A manufacturing company physician said:

> You can be sued in a corporation, and it can cost the corporation millions, though the corporation generally covers and insures you. But a physician in a corporation could be sued and even end up in jail for serious malpractice of occupational medicine, such as a misdiagnosis of asbestosis during medical surveillance or another medical mistake that would require gross negligence. These things happen where physicians found something and didn't inform the patient. The condition progressed and led to more problems. Not informing was the mistake.

A factor that intensifies doctors' concern is their belief that a manager or company professional such as a doctor is more likely to be sent to jail than a CEO. As a physician with a major computer company said:

Most of the time employers respond to hazards because they genuinely care or they're afraid of lawsuits. With criminal lawsuits in the last few years, a lot of employers have had their antennae out. When managers hear they are individually responsible for hazards, their ears perk up, like my dog. That's what the law says. After all, it's not the CEO who will go to jail—it's you, the manager. A CEO might go to jail, depending on the corporation and how big the issue is and what the evidence shows. But the immediate management is much more likely to take it in the neck, and they won't be able to duck. The Eichmann defense, "I was following orders," doesn't work well anymore. People are much more aware of this today than they were just a few years ago. And they should be! It's real! Someone will catch it one of these days.

Physicians also fear that management may deliberately leave judgment calls to physicians in the belief that the physician rather than the employer may be liable if the decision turns out badly.

Prosecutors have pursued companies with criminal charges on behalf of communities, as they did after the Bhopal disaster in India (see Kaplan, Weisberg, and Binder 1996, 997–1032; Bixby 1990; Ferrey 1988, 11; for discussions of the events surrounding the Bhopal disaster, see Melius 1998; Cassels 1993). Professionals perceive a growing threat of criminal charges against individual executives; in the Chicago Magnet Wire case, five corporate officers were charged with aggravated battery and reckless conduct for causing injury to employees by failing to provide necessary safety precautions.[9] A telecommunications company physician said:

The Chicago Magnet Wire case was a totally different kettle of fish because it was intentional. The company was liable, but those company officers were in fact the same as the company when it came to criminal liability. You can't commit murder and say, "The company made me do it."

Physicians may in fact succeed, however, by saying, "The company made me do it. I was afraid of losing my job, and this was a company policy." Prosecutors have focused on finding out who set the policy. In a criminal case, if it is the company president, then that person would ordinarily be held liable. But in civil cases physicians are more likely to be held liable (see Plater et al. 1998, 869–904; Willborn, Schwab, and Burton 1993, 985–97).[10]

Corporate professionals fear jury trials, in which the standard of care for what they should have done is determined in the courtroom. Doctors serve as expert witnesses and medical associations are consulted when juries and judges later identify the appropriate standard of care or interpret statutes. Professionals worry—along with managers—about shifting community standards for what a reasonably prudent doctor would do. The public may increasingly believe that professionals are individually responsible for decisions in their corporations, and public opinion influences the outcome of jury trials, with potentially massive awards. Some physicians say that they try to imagine what a jury might think in five or even twenty years, anticipating the future standard by which they might be judged.

Environmental groups and individuals outside the corporation may sue company physicians over environmental hazards. One oil company physician was named in a citizens' lawsuit over the public health effects of the chemical emissions from his company's refinery fumes that were drifting into the community. He said:

> I have been sued personally for, quote, "environmental crimes" of the company against the community in a "clinical ecology" lawsuit. That's the latest vehicle for suits brought against us personally. Our outside lawyers advise me how to testify. The plaintiff typically sues the company, but an increasing trend for regulatory suits and outside plaintiffs is to name responsible individuals in the company. People seem to want to accept that any chemical exposure, no matter how minor, can cause serious illness. You never know what a jury will believe and these things drag on a long time, so it's distressing.

Physicians who want to be perceived as team players are loath to be associated with trouble and sued from outside the corporation. This can lead them to practice "defensive medicine," which is common outside the corporate context as well. A major oil company physician said:

> Health and medical issues are increasingly high-liability problems. When one is responsible for a large administrative network, as I am, the courts assume that you knew, or should have known, what was going on. But that's not always possible. How do you find out about all the health and environmental practices in a vast organization, with complex administration? You can't, but you're held responsible. It certainly makes our medical practices more defensive. It goes beyond being careful and thorough.

Lawsuits have been filed for breaches of medical confidentiality in cases where physicians gave management data that employees considered private or withheld important medical information.[11] A United Steelworkers official said:

> An airline company doctor who did fitness-for-work exams discovered a pilot had cancer but never told him. It took several months for this to be detected. The pilot sued him, and the jury found no doctor-patient relationship. In cases where we have to go after a company doctor to stop a questionable practice, we tell the doctor, "Look, you may think no doctor-patient relationship exists here, but that's for a jury to decide if it comes to that; and I'm happy to oblige if you want to take your chances with that kind of trial."[12]

Statutes under which individual doctors may be held liable are becoming more common. For example, the California Labor Code specifies a criminal penalty for company retaliation against employees who pursue their rights under workers' compensation. A major computer company physician said: "One of these days a California case on that section 132a statute will send a bigger tremor through the state than the Loma Prieta earthquake."

The California Corporate Criminal Liability Act is sometimes nicknamed the "be a manager, go to jail" act. This act provides for significant fines (up to $1 million for a corporation) and the imprisonment of managers found to be out of compliance with the law. It criminalizes the conduct of managers who know of a serious concealed danger associated with a business practice or product but knowingly fail to notify the state occupational health agency and affected employees within fifteen days (or immediately if an imminent risk of great bodily harm or death exists). Under the act, managers "have knowledge" if they possess facts that would lead a reasonable person in the manager's circumstances to believe a serious concealed danger exists.[13] A government official familiar with companies' occupational health programs and the statute said:

> The Corporate Criminal Liability Act was passed at the same time as the new Injury and Illness Prevention Program regulations, so everybody thinks Cal-OSHA will put you in jail if you don't have an Injury and Illness Prevention Program. It's a big mess, but at the same time it's another in-

centive for behavior. It's more than a regulatory incentive—it's a criminal incentive.

Criminal penalties also apply under the Occupational Safety and Health Act and the Toxic Substances Control Act.[14] Corporations must designate certain corporate officials who are individually responsible for TSCA-related decisions and could be held criminally liable and go to jail if the company does not report.[15] A services company physician said:

> In every corporation you have to say who the person responsible for this [TSCA] area is, and it can't be some low-lying official like a second lieutenant; it has to be like a general, and that person must have that responsibility. The first time I went to the company fifteen years ago and met the medical director's boss, the first thing he said was, "Yes, I'm the guy who goes to jail if you violate the law, and I don't want to go to jail." The fact that you tell a corporation to designate ahead of time who goes to jail if you violate the law makes the designated person a lot more cognizant about what's going on.

The Americans with Disabilities Act supports professional standards and professional judgment by increasing the scrutiny of their decisions regarding who is fit for employment.[16] Before the ADA, a physician's decision about an individual's employability or capacity to do a specific job was a professional opinion; the employer could accept it, seek another physician's opinion, or do something else. Now, under the ADA, any employer who makes a placement or refuses to hire someone for a health reason must be able to defend that decision in a court of law. Employees can sue employers for saying they are not fit to work at a particular job. The government has increased the fines for intentional discrimination with regard to ADA to $300,000 per instance.[17] Insurance for that kind of liability then becomes more expensive or more difficult to obtain.

Physicians trained in occupational medicine are less vulnerable to litigation because they generally know more about what to look for in evaluating an individual's abilities. Companies that realize this are more likely to solicit advice from trained occupational physicians. However, physicians with minimal training in occupational medicine still deliver most medical services to employees. To contain costs, these services are increasingly provided by contract physicians who are technically not co-employees and therefore are liable to suit without that corporate protection. Some of these private physicians are now refusing to do exams for companies because they want to avoid subjecting themselves to this kind of liability. A physician with a major oil corporation said:

> How long will the local doctor call himself the corporate medical director now with the ADA? He won't like that title the minute a lawyer slaps a lawsuit on him, or the minute a company questions him and says we might have trouble with this decision.

Some corporations buy an insurance umbrella that covers not only the full-time but also the part-time physicians and outside consultants who act on behalf of the corporation. More often, corporations pay only in-house physicians' malpractice insurance costs.[18]

The perceived threat of individual legal accountability strengthens physicians' leverage with management. A major oil company physician explained how he has talked to corporate managers:

> I tell them, "I have a specific job to protect this part of the company that's been given to me. I am told to do things that are medically appropriate and to keep the information confidential. If you don't like that, then you have to take it up with the person who set the system up this way. The company gives me this piece of the job to do, and you'll get into a lot of trouble if I don't do my job." I tell them, "If I release this confidential record to you and someone complains, then I'll go to jail and you'll go to jail too and so will your boss. So if you don't want your boss to go to jail, just listen to what I say and you won't keep asking for records because I won't give them to you."

The impact of the law on physicians' decisions can be quite different from what one might expect, even when "the law" is codified, court decisions seem clear, and legislation appears straightforward. A narrow and local but well-publicized legal decision may spread fear through entire industries. For example, in the Chicago Magnet Wire case, where corporate officials were personally charged with the poisoning of workers, the court ruling in fact had limited scope, but the case cast an ominous shadow over corporate practices, resulting in new corporate policies.[19] Conversely, OSHA regulations requiring that lung function tests be performed or records kept on the workdays lost due to occupational disease may have little actual effect unless vigorous government enforcement makes corporate employees believe the regulations are important.

THREATS OF LITIGATION AND REGULATION OF HEALTH HAZARDS

Conservative analysts bemoan the litigiousness in our society, tracing social ills to greedy claimants, zealous lawmakers, and rapacious lawyers. (For discussions of the social effects of litigation, see, for example, Galanter 1994; Huber 1990; Meier 2000; on the overestimation of litigiousness, see Saks 1992.) They argue that these pressures have drained corporate vitality and skewed corporate work away from its proper goals. The business press also condemns what it describes as an epidemic of tort litigation—the many millions of dollars in occupational and environmental health claims that corporations and insurance companies have paid over the past twenty years. Similarly, physicians of all kinds complain that too much time and money is spent on lawyers and others who find fault with the conduct of employers and doctors, as did these physicians from an airline and a computer company:

> Employees often sue the company for job stress if there's an aircraft accident or an occupational injury, or even a non-occupational injury that affects fitness for work. If they sprained an ankle slipping on the water in the kitchen, they come over here, get treated, and the next thing I know they have a lawyer for a seemingly minor problem, especially if they think that they might get terminated for some other reason, like a language or cultural barrier.

> Everything in the law is somebody's fault: it's somebody's fault if I get sick or if I work with asbestos and get lung cancer. But if you smoke cigarettes and work with asbestos, you may be ten times more at risk for lung cancer. A technological society has risks of illness that it continues to be willing to have, by default or by informed decision. All of us deal with what's acceptable risk every day. The law has not necessarily caught up with that.

A physician with a major bank complained about a huge monetary award to an employee with lung cancer after a jury found that another physician in the company had failed to diagnose the man's condition adequately when he came to the medical department complaining of chest pain. He stated:

> The court awarded him $7 million. They accused us of not doing an adequate exam. The court was unreasonable, but there was nothing we could do. The man should feel lucky he's still alive.

Despite doctors' complaints, government regulation and—even more—the threat of litigation have created powerful pressures on employers to reduce health hazards.

Government Regulation

Occupational health changed because of OSHA, along with the ensuing regulations and litigation. Thirty years ago, before OSHA, the occupational medicine field was smaller and much less active. Petitions and lawsuits that labor and public interest groups brought gave rise to OSHA health standards. Legislators who responded to the pressures of the time also changed the widespread perceptions of occupational and environmental problems. In some cases lawyers were the driving force.[20] The effects of OSHA show that laws can empower professionals to do what they want to do. A physician who worked in a large metals company said:

> Those of us who were laboring in the vineyard welcomed OSHA, because it brought recognition to the importance of what we were doing. Some said the OSHA acronym meant "Our Savior Has Arrived." Things have improved immeasurably in the last forty years that I've been involved in occupational medicine. Even though the OSHA program is pilloried and has had difficulties, it has been a major influence in improving workplace health protection and the recognition of hazards. Now there's no place to hide from hazards in company operations. The awareness is way up with the right-to-know OSHA rules and the understanding that working people now get, especially through their unions. With the right to know, people insist on knowing what the hazards are.[21]

A national labor official with the United Steelworkers union said: "Companies had certain responsibilities after OSHA came along, and to that degree their safety and health people came out from underneath the bushel. Employers had to listen to them."[22]

Many companies developed a more lax approach to compliance in the 1980s as deregulation in many ways succeeded and OSHA enforcement declined. The need for doctors, hygienists, and safety engineers declined along with it.[23] When they experienced pressures to downsize, some companies replaced medical departments with contracting services. An aerospace company physician said:

> OSHA enforcement certainly isn't the hot button that it was back when OSHA first came into place. Some companies that in desperation went out and hired staff now feel more comfortable with what the problems are and how to control them.

It costs a great deal more to inspect many small companies, which are thus less threatened by the possibility of enforcement of occupational health and environmental laws and have fewer incentives to invest in safety measures. A newspaper company physician said:

> In some cases legislation was good because companies weren't investing in engineering controls without OSHA and EPA. Somebody had to tell them to do it. Regulators spend more time with big companies, but most people work for small companies, where regulators don't even go unless they get a complaint. Small companies have consultants who probably never visit their premises, or they may not even contract out at all. They hope the regulators won't fine them for their practices, and the employees don't get protected.

OSHA requires regular medical testing of employees who are exposed to one of about twenty-five specific toxic substances or who are involved in emergency response, but company physicians do not always conduct those tests. Although corporations are supposed to have doctors on staff or on contract, many do not. OSHA enforcement varies between regional offices, but in general not enough people and resources are available for inspections, and inspectors often examine only a small part of a given workplace. A high-level OSHA official said:

> OSHA has moved very slowly with health standards over the years. We've never bounded forward in occupational medicine. The agency has had to go the long way around in setting standards in the first place. It's a slow and painful process. Nevertheless, we've done a great deal by osmosis,

because we have a general duty clause, which states that the employer must provide a safe workplace, and companies who appreciate the need to run a safe and healthful workplace are aware of OSHA and the need to employ appropriate qualified physicians. The word has gotten around that OSHA's likely to come in and fine you if you don't do the right thing, and fines have gone up dramatically: what used to be a $7,000 fine can now be a $70,000 fine. Companies have learned that they can be in big financial trouble if they don't do what they are supposed to do. Still, the government's general philosophy largely dictates whether companies think they need the expense of physicians when the laws are so few and far between and will be fewer in the future. Companies say, "Let's just have a contract doctor in an HMO who knows something about occupational medicine and use him when we need his services. We don't need to employ somebody permanently."

Occupational medicine benefits from having the threat of OSHA in a company's backyard. Many doctors have a positive view of OSHA, in part because it helps give them their jobs and preserve their role. Occupational medicine tends to expand when regulation expands.[24] In the textile industry, for example, the cotton dust standard required that companies maintain medical surveillance conducted by a doctor or industrial hygienist, and this requirement increased the number of staff physicians hired to deal with it.[25] Doctors in corporations recognize that new regulations can help them promote company health programs. However, doctors or unions cannot rely on the threat of regulation if it is toothless. A national AFL-CIO official stated:

Requirements of the last decade have greatly expanded resources in the environmental protection area, whereas programs and people are dying in occupational health, with no impetus for putting money or people into these programs. We hope OSHA law and regulations will change to bring about the same kind of developments in safety and health. If we pass OSHA reform and put in place a medical surveillance standard requiring an overall comprehensive safety and health program, companies will need somebody there in-house to figure out what the program is and oversee it.

Despite the limitations of OSHA regulation, many employers give greater attention to occupational health than they did twenty years ago because more OSHA rules now have testing requirements and medical provisions requiring company compliance.

Doctors who once did only a few types of examinations now do many more, partly in response to new regulations.

Effects of Litigation

Although lawsuits do not serve the same function as regulation, liability is a deterrent to unsafe conditions. OSHA regulations, by requiring employers to provide occupational health services to employees, give company doctors a job in medical monitoring. Regulation boosts company medicine in ways that lawsuits do not because companies are shielded almost completely from employee lawsuits for occupational disease, and because employers facing a third-party lawsuit can always hire outside medical experts rather than company doctors to testify in litigation. A computer company physician said:

> Companies do things that they have to do that aren't optional, like regulations. You have to do asbestos or lead testing if you work with asbestos or have lead levels that trigger OSHA requirements. The same is true for people working with a host of other hazardous chemicals. If it costs the company money, that's too bad. It's a cost of doing business. People will regulate their exposure if the government tells them to, or if they must do it to avoid getting sued. A properly designed regulation is more effective and costs less than the threat of lawsuits.

Nonetheless, the threat of litigation has had some of the same effects as regulation. It often is effective, for example, in convincing companies to curtail hazardous conditions. Cutbacks in government occupational health rule-making and enforcement in the 1980s and early 1990s reduced the incentive for companies to do medical monitoring and incur preventive health expenses. In addition, workers' compensation generally has not forced employers to clean up hazards, aside from notorious cases like asbestos, even though preventing illness has been a stated goal of the compensation system. Under these conditions, the threat of third-party lawsuits or lawsuits for intentional misconduct now serves some of the same functions as regulation did in determining what corporations will do to protect their interests. Litigation has restrained excessive short-term profit-seeking at the expense of preventive health programs. The specter of another asbestos debacle and jury

trials in which companies can be held liable for health effects—
with the attendant adverse public opinion—works as a deterrent.
Fear of lawsuits has led corporations to put more money into
health and safety than they otherwise would have—sometimes
they even achieve a standard stricter than OSHA's.[26] These two
doctors, employed by a major computer company and a chemical
company, respectively, had this to say:

> We've been proactive when we have a company product where a large
> number of people might be exposed. We assess the literature and decide
> whether it's reasonable or not. We set up an internal standard that's more
> stringent than OSHA, just because we know OSHA will be a long time
> getting around to it, and we know that we can be faulted down the line
> because following the standards is not a defense. Most people in the com-
> pany and the attorneys certainly recognize that we have to do what we
> know is right if we know the standard is not right.

> I have advised the company on testing various products they are develop-
> ing. One example is a product the company makes that it sold to another
> company that used it to make the silicone material for breast implants. It
> doesn't appear to cause pulmonary or lung damage as much as crystalline
> silicate. Dow and manufacturers who made products for the implants got
> sued, so we've been sued over that. Just the specter of toxic tort has raised
> senior management's concerns: "We want to make some new formula-
> tions. Are we testing these things properly ahead of time? How do we
> know if it's safe?"

Lawsuits for damage from toxic chemicals can be large, multimillion-dollar cases. A physician who has provided occupational
health services for many companies said:

> Environmental and occupational medical litigation is a generally positive
> force toward health and safety. The win rate against companies is pretty
> high in occupational disease. Toxic tort cancer cases resulting from ben-
> zene and other substances can be settled in the millions. Financial incen-
> tives are high. Those lawyers know how to pick their cases. You don't see
> them giving up occupational or environmental law because it's running
> out of money.

Employers are concerned about heavy litigation costs and adverse publicity from major chemical spills or disaster contamination of the sort that Union Carbide had in Bhopal (see Melius
1998; Kurzman 1987). Third-party suits have been filed against

equipment manufacturers whose machines have injured workers. Such suits have made manufacturers more reluctant to rush to market with products before considering their potentially harmful health effects on workers. A physician who directs an occupational medicine clinic and a manufacturing company physician said:

> The toxic tort drives a lot of what goes into occupational and environmental health today. Liability often drives the whole thing. I'm not sure that's helped a lot, but it's been good to have more demonstrations that you need to have careful corporate health responsibility. Personal injury and toxic torts have been extended, and asbestos lawsuits have frightened people. The belief that management can look past health issues and they will just go away just doesn't exist anymore. The threat of lawsuits has led corporations to be more concerned about health in the workplace than they were.
>
> The medical department may cost something to the company, but it is there to protect the employee. It's just like the Pinto that blew up—look how much it eventually cost the company to cut corners.

In-house medical services can save companies money from workers' compensation awards or lawsuits, whereas cutting them back may add to their expenses. Companies that once tried to save money by hiring comparatively untrained contract physicians have sometimes paid heavily for misdiagnosed illnesses and other mistakes. On the other hand, having a medical department within the company also creates fears of litigation among managers, because any health facility makes mistakes. Employers worry about the possibility of a malpractice settlement that exceeds their insurance coverage limits and cuts into corporate profits. A banking company physician and a physician who has provided occupational health services to many companies said:

> The legal element can have an inhibiting influence on occupational medicine. Given the litigiousness of individuals and society in general, an adverse legal experience—even simply a nuisance suit—can easily discourage corporate management from having an occupational medicine entity on premises, especially in a setting like this bank, where it's not mandatory, as it is in a chemical or oil company like Mobil or Exxon.
>
> What little medical activity went on in companies started to decline out of the legal fear of getting too close to health care.

One way employers deal with this fear of suits stemming from their in-house medical staff is by spreading the risk. For example, a corporation may ask occupational medical researchers from a university to join projects and work on tests. The university then shares responsibility for any legal problems that may occur.

The legal structure has been beneficial for occupational medicine in some respects, but lawsuits also have wasted money that could have gone instead to preventive health measures. Asbestos litigation, for example, was beneficial in uncovering hazards and company misconduct in the early cases (see Brodeur 1985). As the litigation spread, it hastened the drastic reduction in the use of asbestos and other toxins. But then the role of the lawyers began to change: less time was spent working methodically to uncover hazards and more time was spent processing claims and making money without unearthing much new information.

Tort litigation has been unsuccessful in preventing the occurrence of occupational disease in general.[27] Part of the dilemma for physicians is that such litigation is strictly reactive. It sends a message—like a ripple effect—to corporate officials: "You'd better watch out to avoid another slew of lawsuits like those against Manville." However, tort litigation does not necessarily send that message effectively, and it is no substitute for prevention through a public health approach.

Public Concern About Occupational and Environmental Health

Public opinion may help create statutes and regulations, but public opinion alone will not necessarily move employers to act. Nonetheless, changing public opinion affects workplace health and the climate in which physicians carry out their work—particularly the prevailing corporate attitudes toward risk, access to medical information, and responsibility for chemical hazards. Information from the media contributes to public concern about health hazards and indirectly to company medical programs.[28] A physician for a major airline said:

> Airline safety made big news in the 1980s in media coverage and in Congress, and some speculated that financial difficulties in the airline industry

were compromising maintenance and the health of pilots and flight atten-
dants was not monitored appropriately. Many corporate officers decided
reestablishing the medical department would be worthwhile so they could
better monitor employees to determine if they were physically fit.

The public's environmental concerns and expectations for safe
conditions generally have intensified since the 1970s, and interest
in environmental issues continues to be strong.[29] Concern is generally greater about environmental hazards than about occupational
hazards, and the environmental movement has had a considerably
greater impact than the occupational health movement. Environmental laws have also had more effect on business than workplace health laws. The EPA, for example, is generally stronger
than OSHA, and its penalties are higher (for discussions of OSHA
and EPA regulation, see Ashford 2000; Wahl and Gunkel 1999). As
a physician in the chemical industry said: "OSHA is still an extremely weak sister to EPA. Occupational medicine is a profession
in search of a law; we don't have an effective law."

Environmental hazards such as water and air pollution affect
large numbers of people, creating a broader base for political action than occupational health can attract. Media coverage of environmental health is also a great deal more extensive, and that is
one reason the public and corporate management are less concerned about workplace health. A physician for a major oil company said:

> Public opinion has done very little because the public doesn't care about
> occupational illness and what goes on in the plant as long as it doesn't get
> out of the plant. They care about environmental stuff. It's very difficult
> to get attention paid to occupational issues. That's a big problem for the
> field.

Nevertheless, public opinion has helped legitimize the role of
occupational physicians within companies and society. It has
helped corporate management understand more clearly what the
issues are—as the public perceives them—and why companies
need a medical staff, including occupational physicians. A physician employed by a large computer corporation said:

> The factory used to be that place remote from the community you didn't
> have to worry about. Today the public views the factory as part of the

community; they realize that the risks extend beyond the factory boundaries. That's engendered a big change in the way the media, courts, and prosecutors look at it. It's sent a message to executives that they have to be responsible.

Corporate physicians and managers are public citizens and professionals as well as employees, and as such they are affected by public attitudes about disease risks and the allocation of responsibility to pay for health damage. A physician for a major chemical company reported:

> There are managers in my chemical company who are absolutely convinced on a personal level that toxic chemicals cause cancer in their families. I talk to people at lunch, and I'm amazed at it all the time. They compartmentalize their lives; they can work for a chemical company, but on a personal level they are very fearful of so-called toxic chemicals for their families, and they run around getting tests done all the time and putting detectors in their homes.

However, it would be easy to overstate corporate concern by quoting a few executives in companies with known risks or recent major litigation. A chemical company physician stated:

> Executives may read the *New York Times,* but they are not interested in health and environmental issues. They are interested in having people in the corporation handle that for them so they can run the business. They might take an interest if it's not being handled well, if it starts to affect their ability to produce and sell chemicals.

Jury trials are an obvious reflection of public opinion. Juries have held manufacturers and their insurers liable for health hazards. Employers have complained that the tort system is out of control and must be reined in through tort reform measures such as restricting third-party liability, suits against product manufacturers for the effects of dangerous products, punitive damages, and other jury awards. Corporations and their insurers have spent many millions of dollars to persuade the public that a lawsuit crisis exists and that jurors should be tougher on plaintiffs. Juries are more likely to give lower and fewer awards to plaintiffs if they think there is a lawsuit crisis. Tort reform contributes to toxic hazards in companies, however, if its success in reducing jury awards and limiting company liability leads employers to take fewer preventive measures.

RESPONSIBILITY FOR HEALTH RISKS AND COSTS

Conceptions of responsibility for health risks have changed in the past four decades, along with trends in personal, professional, public, and corporate liability. Employers and the public have been faced with the steadily growing costs of work-related disease, including many millions of dollars in medical care, lost work time, insurance, and disability payments. Spiraling health costs in the 1980s and 1990s left employers almost desperately seeking solutions that would lower their costs and shield them from liability (see Mintz and Palmer 2000; Gabel et al. 2000).[30] These health costs have been under close scrutiny as part of a larger debate over health-care delivery. Employers argue that health costs have badly hurt the economic well-being of their companies— even causing them to lose half the profitability of American industry in the last ten years. Thus, they argue, they must save on health-care costs either by screening workers better to remove expensive people from the payrolls or by making them pay a higher share of the cost. Employers generally use medical management strategies to try to control costs rather than increasing spending to create a safer work environment. Corporations employ physicians to screen workers and provide health care to them in the belief that having in-house physicians is cheaper than just insuring employees. Even then, few see the advantages of using their physicians not only for providing health care but for helping to create a safe environment through medical surveillance and prevention.

Employers try to characterize the expenses of workplace hazards as a social cost that they need not bear, and they have largely succeeded in doing so. Individual employees, their families, and the public pay most occupational disease costs in the form of Social Security Disability Insurance, Medicaid and Medicare, and out-of-pocket medical payments. And they also bear the burden of disease and death, of course (see Ashford 1998, 1713; Rosenblatt, Law, and Rosenbaum 1997, 129–38; Ashford and Stone 1998). Companies push for more lenient workers' compensation provisions, less restrictive regulatory penalties, and laws that will hold employers less accountable for chemical health hazards—all of which would further shift costs onto workers and the public.

The Difficulty of Measuring and Justifying Prevention

Doctors who believe they provide valuable preventive health services in the corporation bemoan the fact that they have been unable to demonstrate the cost-saving value of their services to corporate management. They try to show that preventing lawsuits and reducing workers' compensation claims and absenteeism save the company money. Their best efforts generally are unconvincing when management asks, "How do you know you did that?" Managers do not see the health benefits and decreased workers' compensation expenses that in-house doctors claim to produce. Thus, companies cut back their in-house staffs in part because managers do not believe that a large in-house staff saves the company money. A telecommunications company physician said:

> No officer of this business would disagree that my objective of healthy, productive people contributing to the success of the business is a desirable objective. Where we part ways is my proposing that the company spend money in order to save money, and other people who compete for those resources say, "While you save money, we won't have any money coming in to upgrade the network." How the corporate leadership prioritizes those competing demands for limited investment capital in allocating resources is tricky.

Justifying preventive programs is difficult, in part because the cost savings of some goals in occupational medicine, such as health education, are hard to quantify. The medical community itself is just now beginning to accept preventive medicine and overcome the belief that curative practices are the only true medicine. As a mining physician explained:

> Nobody bats an eyelash about paying a million dollars to transplant a liver, but it's still hard to get anybody to contribute ten cents to prevent that liver from being damaged. That concept still permeates medicine. The controller immediately can put the value of digging ten tons of coal on the line. You get the same value through health education, preventive programs,

ergonomic factors, and engineering designs, but it shows up in three to five years, not immediately.

The telecommunications company physician articulated another aspect of this difficulty:

> Physicians put successful programs in place after companies say the disease or accident rate is unacceptable. Then a new CEO with none of this knowledge comes in and says, "We haven't had any accidents in five years. Why spend so much on this safety program?" He doesn't know what the rate was without the prevention program. That's the paradox of prevention: you can't count things that don't happen. When you've had a comprehensive program in place for years and a new corporate leadership team looks at your health-care costs, they don't appreciate what the situation was before. Their attitude is, "Get rid of these expensive things, and we'll wait and see. We can always put 'em back in if it goes up, but we've saved a lot of money if it doesn't."

An important reason doctors have had difficulty in clearly demonstrating the benefits of their health services is the challenge of proving a negative. Preventive programs, by their nature, are difficult to justify because it is difficult to point to illness prevented and justify a budget based on prospective savings, to prove that companies get what they pay for. These physicians, from an oil company and a retail sales company, respectively, said:

> You can crank out numbers, but they're not convinced by it, and in some ways they shouldn't be, because how do you know you saved money unless you could do a controlled study, which you could never do. Still, organizations will always get asked, "How much do you think you return to the company, and in what ways?" So you write a report about what you saved. The budget for all medical expenses in the company is about $18 million, including all the staff, services we provide, computer support, rents, and supplies. That doesn't even reach a significant portion of 1 percent of our company's expenditures in a year. The company spent about $5 billion last year to explore and produce and refine oil. Our medical department cost is just a drop in the bucket, but it's an easy figure for them to look at and say, "Do we want to spend $18 million? Can we do it other ways?"

> They can't measure the ineffable benefits *because* they are ineffable. How do you measure somebody waking up in the year 2000 on a Tuesday, fifty-four years old, and saying, "Oh my, I didn't have a heart attack today because in 1970 they persuaded me in my periodic to quit smoking, get

my blood pressure under control, bring down my cholesterol, stick with a diet, do regular exercise." There's no measuring that, but the payoff could be tremendous.

Unfortunately, paying serious attention to occupational disease and prevention may not make good sense purely on economic grounds. Employers compare the frequently high cost of reengineering a work process with potentially increased workers' compensation premiums for diseases that tend not to be recognized anyway. They may conclude that the disease costs are less significant than the engineering costs of reducing hazards. The rise in premium costs for workers' compensation is an insufficient deterrent to poor control practices in a corporation. Hazards that companies ignore may never hurt them. The real risk to employers outside of workers' compensation claims may be negligible unless a company is shown to be willfully negligent. Paying serious attention to occupational disease does make good sense, however, if a company wants to protect a skilled workforce that is difficult to replace, or wants to promote employee goodwill, or has a genuine interest in protecting workers' health.[31]

Keeping people well adds to pension costs. Healthier workers may live longer, use more pension benefits, and then develop disease later. Preventive health measures may thus delay disease so that costs are for seventy-year-olds instead of sixty-five-year-olds. A telecommunications company physician and an aerospace physician spoke about this possibility:

> You can say, "Look, we saved all this money because we prevented so many heart attacks," but if your company insures people from the time they work for you until they die, it doesn't show on your bottom line today, and maybe you just delayed the heart attacks and didn't prevent them.

> Workers live longer if you improve their health; they'll enjoy their pension longer at an increased cost to the company, so you have to be conscious how you present your material in a company totally oriented towards the dollar. You have to show that the overall return will be better than something that might be written off as humanitarian.

Complaints by managers and physicians that people may live longer are truly astonishing. Surely concern over higher pension costs is not a good reason to avoid preventive health programs; having employees live longer and healthier lives should be considered advantageous in itself. A chemical company physician pointed out additional economic justifications:

> When I put in a wellness program corporatewide, the argument of our benefits guy always was, "You'll increase our pension cost." My counter to that was that I hoped he was right; I hoped that we would be so successful that people would live longer. The advantage is that health-care costs are paid out of operating income. Pensions are vested, so we put aside money for a pension whether people use it or not. We pay health care out of our net profits, so it's a whole lot cheaper to have somebody pensioned longer if you can lower their health-care costs. That's the only way to go.[32]

Because top executives typically are judged by their short-term performance, they have little direct incentive to invest in disease prevention. Preventive steps represent a short-term cost and a special burden in times of corporate retrenchment. Many corporations treat their health and environmental staff as easily expendable, overlooking their potential contribution to the company's long-term well-being. In contrast, company managements with a long-term perspective believe that spending for preventive services makes good economic and employee-relations sense; they sustain a level of profitability that can support that longer-term need more easily than the many American corporations suffering from declining profits. (On corporate management's and employees' responses to downsizing, see Bluestone and Bluestone 1992; on corporations' declining concern with historic community ties, see Galston 1996.) American companies lack long-term vision when they pursue quick profits to satisfy stockholders and ensure good bonuses for management—a phenomenon not limited to medical issues. These two physicians, from a chemical company and a conglomerate, stated:

> Management thinks their job is to return money to stockholders, with an extreme emphasis on short-term profitability, which has been a pathology of the American economy. Lawyers are there to let managers do that and reduce liability.
>
> At a meeting the medical benefits people were showing the CEO on a blackboard ways we could save money. He had two choices: on the left, save a little bit now through Band-Aid items, or on the right, go for the big

bundle about three years down the road by implementing the approach that could save us considerably more. The CEO looked at it and said, "I'll take the left," which told me that he's being judged by the present. He probably decided he might not even be around long enough to see the gigantic savings down the road if he doesn't show profit now.

In addition, focusing the attention of executives on reducing occupational disease becomes more difficult when the projected savings are small relative to other company expenses, including health benefits. These two physicians, with a conglomerate and a publishing company, respectively, described unsuccessfully pressing for cost-savings plans in their companies:

> We tried to promote a plan to save the company money and we got an audience with a division president. He paced the floor, and we showed him how we could save $2 million, and his response was, "I appreciate your efforts, but this amount is just too small for me to spend much time and energy on. Right now, I have $20 million issues in savings." Medical departments don't account for much. You're small compared with other departments, and services are expendable.

> Companies are struggling with health care, and paying their medical bills is probably their biggest fear now. Our company [of ten thousand people] paid $20 million for health insurance last year. It's just staggering. That's the big issue. We've shown how we can save them money and provide a great service to our employees by putting an X-ray machine in here, and we can save them $275,000 if we put in an in-house pharmacy, but they haven't done it. They think about too many other big problems—like health insurance and getting a new plant up and running—to put things like that in.

One mining company physician said he saved the company $55 million in benefits by instituting tests showing that people making claims either were not ill or had an illness unrelated to their work. He said:

> When I came here, black lung [or coal workers' pneumoconiosis] cost this company $60 million a year in workers' comp benefits. The fund created to pay these benefits was going bankrupt. When I started reviewing all the cases we were involved with, I found the black-lung awards were granted with no medical evidence if you worked in the mines fifteen years. So we did a study and found that 88 percent of the cases awarded benefits had normal X-rays, blood-gas studies, and pulmonary-function studies. Requiring medical input reduced the company cost to $30 million within eigh-

teen months, and to $5 million in five years. The fund is no longer bank-
rupt; the people who deserve compensation get it and others don't. When
I saved the company $55 million, we showed operating management that
the medical function has a bottom-line value they can see.

But such savings do not necessarily persuade employers that
in-house physicians have continuing value. The employer can still
say, "You served your function. We've brought down costs and
instituted new procedures, but what have you done for us lately?"
Large companies often believe it is cheaper to buy a service than
to pay employees, whether physicians or maintenance workers,
especially in view of the benefits they save.

Workers' Compensation and Contested Claims

Workers' compensation payments to victims of occupational disease historically have been low in most companies, shielding employers from costs as well as lawsuits for disease. But as discussed
earlier, new laws that widen the scope of employers' compensation payments for chronic illness, as well as lawsuits against employers who intentionally inflict harm, have undercut employers'
traditional immunity to financial responsibility for occupational
disease.[33] Also, the minimum requirement for being considered
a compensable injury has recently been lowered throughout the
United States. The number of conditions that are considered work-
related is expanding, as are the incentives to file claims. Even coronary artery disease can be considered a compensable job-related
injury if an employee has a heart attack on the job, despite personal risk factors such as a family history, diabetes, and hypertension. A person with AIDS and job stress could claim that all the
medical care required is compensable because the job stress ac-
celerated or aggravated the AIDS symptomatology (on workers'
compensation costs, see Boden 2000; Willborn, Schwab, and Burton 1993, 715–867).

Rising health-care costs have increased the incentives for employers to reduce disease among employees and to screen workers according to health risks. Employers also have strong incentives to describe workers' illnesses as unrelated to work or to deny
disabled workers a medical impairment rating and force them to

continue working even though they are clearly disabled. A labor health official said:

> Doctors don't provide the sort of services workers need because they aren't trained to understand the work-related claims and they don't diagnose the illnesses as occupational. The employers get away scot-free because those illnesses aren't being properly classified, so they aren't paid out of workers' compensation.

One important reason health costs are shifted onto the workers' compensation system is that many people have no private health insurance.[34] In that situation, both the patient and the provider have an incentive to find a reason why the illness is work-related. Providers of medical services traditionally have sought reimbursement through workers' compensation whenever possible, even when the workplace causation is questionable.[35] At other times they have realized that individuals do not have complete coverage and that workers' compensation limits are less strict than their group health plan on the number of medical visits and treatments allowed.[36]

Doctors describe the workers' compensation system of payments for medical expenses as the last sort of unregulated "cash cow" in the medical field. However, it has come under intense scrutiny and is likely to change over the next decade, especially if any kind of national health insurance integrates medical services. For now, however, it is a unique niche in the economics and practice of medicine, one that has been relatively free of intervention for a long time.

Many employers, insurers, and company doctors maintain that payments for medical care under workers' compensation are in crisis and riddled with fraud and abuse (see Schwartz 1993, 988). They complain that the compensation system favors employees over employers and encourages tremendous waste, especially in the handling of stress claims (particularly in California) and "soft tissue" injuries (such as back pain of unclear etiology) that can be treated with physical therapy.

Overall, litigating workers' compensation cases has been lucrative for attorneys. However, attorneys need to handle many such cases to earn a living because individual disease claims generally yield settlements of only a few thousand dollars. Disease claims also tend to be time-consuming and more difficult than injury claims, unless attorneys can find many people with the same disease or the same employer. Third-party tort cases are potentially larger because there is generally no cap on the size of the awards to plaintiffs. In some jurisdictions, plaintiffs without symptoms of a disease may nevertheless be able to collect because exposure has increased their risk of developing cancer, based on evidence from epidemiological or animal studies that the exposure causes cancer.[37]

Physicians often advise corporate loss-control personnel of ways to control workers' compensation costs, serve as witnesses for the company in contested cases, and heavily influence whether employees are permitted to return to work after illnesses. They also, along with attorneys, absorb money from the compensation system. Although the workers' compensation system was set up to be non-adversarial, it is in fact highly adversarial and litigious. The two sides have developed sets of doctors to serve them, so that over time physicians become claimants' doctors or carriers' doctors, just as different sets of lawyers represent the different interests.[38] Employers require workers to go to doctors who consistently support judgments in the companies' favor. A power company physician explained:

> Good-quality physicians don't want to be a part of the worker comp system because it is so polluted with fraud. It is a legal process, not a medical one. I have difficulty finding good clinicians to evaluate people for workers' comp because they don't like paperwork and the process and how things get polluted. This is one of my ongoing battles with the claims litigation people too. I treat injured employees and refer them to good clinicians who I know will take care of their medical condition. My good clinicians don't always write the legal reports that management would like to see, so they want me to change my referral pattern and send them to *their* little preferred provider network they'd like us to use for worker comp injuries. Those are poor-quality physicians who write magnificent legal reports that the claims people like to see, but don't provide good clinical care. The vast majority of patients would not file claims and litigate if we took good care of them and treated them better. Patients get totally lost in the system; they're utterly confused by evaluators and treaters and who's supposed to be their doctor.

Workers can say they want to change doctors only under certain circumstances, such as the presence of a state law or a collective bargaining agreement that permits a choice of physician. A labor official with extensive experience in health issues said:

> If companies send you down to Doctor Jones, an independent, and don't like what he sends back, they shop for another doctor until they find somebody who gives a prescription they can accept, even in workers' comp cases. You have a right to see your own doctor under workers' compensation in some states or if there's a union, so you might be able to quarrel with them about what your own physician said and present medical evidence in an arbitration, but most people don't have that protection.[39]

Health-care reform has already changed the way employers handle medicine by focusing their attention on the rising cost of providing medical services to employees. Chief financial officers now worry about how they will footnote their potential liability in their annual reports.[40] Increased costs and potentially increased liability have become critically important economic issues to employers and insurance carriers as medical costs continue to mount as a proportion of the total workers' compensation bill. However, the issue of health-care quality for employees, whether companies provide it themselves or contract it out, has not changed substantially. Moreover, the workers' compensation system draws attention only to the care given to workers after they are hurt rather than to the need for preventive practices in the workplace.

Physicians' Evaluation of Health Risks in the Context of Disability Law

Discrimination and disability laws have had a major effect on workplace medicine. Examples are the Americans with Disabilities Act, the Johnson Controls Supreme Court decision barring fetal exclusion policies in employment, and state discrimination laws that restrict workplace medical screening.[41] Recent legal decisions have challenged the ways in which employers and policy advocates think about screening policies. They also have increased the likelihood of further costly litigation related to health risks. However, current laws reinforce the power of managers to define risk and screen out workers, even as new protections for disabled workers restrict the right of employers to hire and fire according to health risk. This area of the law is in great flux, with cities, states, and the federal government actively contending with medical screening issues and the extent of employee rights and employer prerogatives (see Colledge, Johns, and Thomas 1999; Wolkinson and Block 1996).[42]

The Americans with Disabilities Act explicitly prohibits pre-employment medical examinations to detect disabilities (unless the tests offer information about the individual's ability to perform job-related functions), and it prohibits discrimination against the disabled by most private employers.[43] Employers must make some accommodation for disabled individuals, but they may justifiably refuse to hire them if no reasonable accommodation would allow them to do the job. However, an employer cannot eliminate disabled individuals from work as long as they can perform the essential functions of their job without endangering themselves or others.[44] Physicians protest that the ADA compels them not to reject high-risk individuals, as this computer physician explained:

> The ADA essentially says an employer cannot restrict the person from doing a job unless you can prove there's an imminent danger to life involved. Courts ask for real proof, not just, "I think it'll happen." At the same time the corporation has to pay for injuries a worker may suffer if some negligent act occurs. The definition of what's disabled is ludicrous. It's everything, with no limit. You are covered under the ADA if you *believe* someone *perceives* you to be disabled. Maybe someone *believes* you have AIDS and you don't have it—how ludicrous can they get? People who are incapable of working will slip through, and it will create problems. I don't know how you can be competitive today with this kind of stuff. To me, it's just like shooting yourself in the foot and then asking, "How come I'm limping?" It troubles me that the ADA is so unreasonable: we have to give a job offer before examining them. What's the sense in that?

The ADA makes it more difficult for companies to restrict workers from certain activities because of current or future impairments and to use medical guidelines to reject people from employment. It may not result in less testing, however. As an electronics company physician said:

ADA changes the order in which testing and job offers are done, but if anything, more testing will be done. It is still perfectly okay to do a medical evaluation after the job offer, so we'll continue with our evaluations. As soon as people get on board, they can always claim that you put them into a job that aggravated their condition. You still have to make sure you have a good match.

Although employers generally cannot test people or ask medical questions before offering them employment, section 12112 of the ADA stipulates that they can test for high-risk workers and use questionnaires after they have made conditional employment offers (see also Rothstein 1992, 38). Physicians may determine an individual's physical or mental capabilities to do the job once he or she has accepted it. Employers have the opportunity to ask about work history and to link it to future susceptibility, and they can still screen out individuals rather than take risks with people who have prior health claims or potential health problems. An employer can also decide whether a reasonable accommodation to the employee's abilities would enable that person to do the job. A pharmaceutical company physician said:

We can do a placement examination with no restrictions as long as we do it after we've made an employment offer. Then we can do whatever we want, and it doesn't have to have a job relationship.

The ADA permits drug testing and does not require employers to accommodate drug users,[45] but it leaves unclear which other kinds of mental or physical disabilities employers can screen for and which disabilities must be accommodated. Case law will clarify how much an employer must do to accommodate a particular disability. Courts also must determine whether particular conditions qualify as disabilities. How employers should consider biological and psychological differences in employee selection is unclear; what testing and prophylactic restrictions for future harm the ADA permits also remains unsettled.[46] An airline company physician said:

We're asked to discriminate, but we're asked not to discriminate illegally, so I try for what is fair according to my lights. Unfortunately, I don't always guess what other people will decide later was fair. I've come to loathe being in that position; physicians are forced to make decisions about prophylactic restrictions, with no clear guidance available at all. It gets harder and harder, because when I make a decision, I know I'll be reading it to some damn judge in court, so I write everything and make every decision as if I'll have to sit and defend it to judges and lawyers. I've been practicing thirty years, so I say, "This person has a good chance within a year or two of needing back surgery," and I won't let them work. That used to be okay, but now there's some question about whether I can make prophylactic restrictions at all that pertain only to the individual's safety. We know if we restrict people inappropriately, they'll bring a grievance and file an EEOC complaint and then sue us if they exhaust all those options. Government agencies for discrimination against employees investigated us a number of times for our decisions about employees, and we know they come in here loaded for bear. They assume that you intend to discriminate, and they give people back pay and reinstate them.

Employers have access to genetic information from medical records and from claims for medical reimbursement that employees file. According to the EEOC, the medical examinations that employers give after they make a conditional employment offer may include a genetic test. But it would be illegal to withdraw an offer after a genetic test if the test is not job-related.[47] It remains difficult to determine whether the ADA covers people who might be perceived as having a genetic disability (see, for example, Alper 1995, 169).[48] State discrimination statutes and case law restrict workplace medical screening and certain uses of medical information, but few laws that explicitly regulate genetic information in employment have been enacted to date. (For discussions of state laws that restrict the uses of genetic information in employment, see Jeffords and Daschle 2001; Pear 1997b; Rothenberg 1995; Preston 1996; McEwen and Reilly 1992, 638.) Subsequent court cases, congressional amendments to the ADA, or legislation such as the Genetic Privacy Act may well change the circumstances in which medical data can be collected and circulated legally.[49]

The ADA affects workplace medicine in significant ways. It already offers employees more protection in companies that formerly did pre-employment physicals. It also may prove to be a boon for physicians who serve corporations by determining whether individual employees can perform specific jobs. Physicians help companies comply with the ADA in job descriptions, in hiring processes, in the matching of abilities with job requirements, and in deciding what accommodation is necessary for people with potentially limiting medical conditions. They have a major role to play in selecting workers because they make fitness determinations. The prospect of numerous discrimination suits under the ADA makes doctors and managers more careful about screening out employees who may not be fit for a particular job because of possible health risks in the future. That kind of screening requires greater sophistication and is not easily farmed out to a clinic (as employers can do for treating injuries). The ADA may thus strengthen corporate medical programs. A utility company physician said:

> A lot of decisions concerning "Is this person able to do that job?" are medical. Before the ADA, a corporation could just have applicants fill out a sheet with twelve thousand disabilities, asking, "Have you had this?" and if they had, just tell them, "No, thank you," and get them out. You can't do that anymore.

Although the ADA's requirements for medical assessment increase the need for occupational medical services, they do not necessarily require in-house corporate physicians and may promote off-site corporate medical screening instead.

In some industries labor market demands limit the ability of companies to refuse to hire. For example, the textile industry has not stopped hiring smokers, even though corporate officials know that smoking amplifies the effect of exposure to cotton dust and smokers are easy to detect (through simple observation). A national textile union official stated:

> Half the workforce in textile industry areas in North and South Carolina smoke like fiends, yet companies keep hiring them. They talk about moving to a no-smoking policy in plants, but not hiring smokers would make them unable to fill their basic staff needs. These are real labor market problems. They need every dependable worker with qualifications who can do the job.[50]

Employers try to manage costs by identifying employees and applicants as potentially expensive or inexpensive. Companies may save money by putting people on weight reduction programs and helping them to lower their blood pressure, but the incentive to screen arises more from the cost of a few expensive illnesses (see Emmons et al. 1999; Aldana and Pronk 2001; Pelletier 1996). In view of the huge cost of procedures such as liver or heart transplants, employers increasingly direct individual employees to lower-cost health-care providers, thus allowing considerations of cost to prevail over those of quality.

Workers may also be considered high-risk for health-care costs because of their spouses or dependents. As this chemical company physician explained:

> The biggest expenses are from spouses and dependents, and we don't examine them. Here I think I'm employing all these Jack Armstrong wonderful guys, and their teenage kid winds up in a psychiatric hospital for a year and costs us a quarter of a million dollars.[51]

Companies that self-insure have reason to be particularly interested in medical information because they are exempt from state regulation of how they manage their benefits and treat employees.[52] Even if employers do not use medical information as a reason to bar high-risk workers outright, they can still use it to exclude individuals with special risks from medical benefits or to charge them exorbitant insurance premiums. In McGann v. H&H Music Co., a small music company in Texas decreased the lifetime medical benefit for AIDS-related claims from $1,000,000 to $5,000 after it became self-insured, thus effectively denying benefits to John McGann, a man with AIDS.[53] In deciding against McGann, the court ruled that self-insured companies may, in response to an employee's claim or test results, change their benefit plans to provide inferior benefits for a certain condition or raise premiums for workers with a risk of contracting that condition.

The ADA has no effect on the post facto McGann scenario because of the ADA's permissive approach to employer practices after the employment offer. Employers may change their coverage the same day they receive an employee's claim in the mail. They can argue that they never offered permanent benefits, and that providing one high-risk employee with the benefit they initially promised would hurt all the other employees. Companies that self-insure argue that their responsibility is to make a profit for their shareholders.[54]

Despite the tangle of laws, possible jury trials, and conflicting

scientific evidence, employers and physicians continue to differentiate workers by their health risks. They screen for characteristics that appear to make individuals more likely to develop diseases that could cost the company more than their wages. More
testing is available because technologies have improved, but employers perceive that they cannot easily restrict a person, even if
they identify a special risk, because of government regulations
and case law, which limit company testing practices.

Screening employees as a primary control strategy becomes
less economically attractive to employers if they must absorb the
costs of screening and employee lawsuits. A corporation's legal
liability could increase, for example, if workers learned that it
knew specific individuals were susceptible to harm but failed to
modify working conditions. Thus, to reduce their need to defend
against litigation or internalize the costs of screening, employers
may choose to avoid finding out who is high-risk.

CONCLUSION

As we have seen, the perceived threat of legal liability is double-
edged. It diverts resources away from hazard prevention and into
defensive actions against perceived litigation risks, such as hiding
information about hazards. Corporate professionals tend to respond to such a threat by practicing preventive law rather than
preventive medicine. But the perceived threat of liability also provides incentives for managers to invest in engineering controls
and safer practices, to warn workers of health risks proactively,
and to strengthen physicians' leverage with management when
they advocate measures that are more health-protective.

Here and in the previous chapter on toxics, this study reveals
the complex role of lawyers in corporations in relation to health.
On the one hand, lawyers have worked to ensure that information
that is damaging to employers is not revealed. They have worked
to undermine the credibility of critics of corporate practices who
point to health hazards. In addition, they have dampened scientific concerns about the health effects of workplace practices.
However, lawyers have also sometimes been a force for fuller dis-

closure of hazards and other potentially damaging information—
even for the amelioration of hazardous exposures at work.

The legal environment defines company physicians sometimes
principally as corporate employees but at other times as autonomous professionals. Company physicians now know they can be
sued individually, held personally responsible for their actions in a
corporation, and even face criminal charges as individuals.[55] This
perceived threat of individual legal accountability reinforces professional standards and bolsters independent professional judgment in corporations.

Chapter 9

Conclusion: Implications for Society and for Social Policy

M OST THEORETICAL AND empirical studies approach professionalization and corporatization as if they were two very different and conflicting processes. But in fact, the professionalization process has oriented professionals to work in organizations, often large bureaucratic organizations. Professionals no longer identify only with their professional reference group; they also identify strongly with, or acquiesce in, the pursuit of corporate goals. Corporate pressures on physicians have intensified over the past four decades, as lawsuits, publicity about chemical risks, government regulation, and higher insurance and workers' compensation expenses have raised employers' costs. *Professionalization and corporatization are intensifying simultaneously* and in many ways reinforce each other: corporate professionals are becoming more professionalized even as they cede greater control to their employers.

The dilemmas that corporate physicians face concerning loyalty and the treatment of workers are in part ethical problems. However, the conflicting organizational demands from being both a corporate employee and an autonomous professional constitute a social and structural problem rather than a problem of individual ethics. Professionals can be well intentioned and conscientious, but if companies employ them, they usually end up conforming to the corporate culture and advancing the corporation's ends—or losing their jobs unless they can convince the management to alter its practices. Doctors become involved in such activities as deter-

256

mining fitness for work and reducing employer liability, not because they have "bad values," but because they are doing the job they were hired to do. Thus, though white coats' values are different from those of team players, the working conditions generally determine what the person does. The social and legal context of the workplace and the position of individuals within the organization's power structure largely determine that company professionals will be pro-management.

The critical look this book has taken at the corporatization of professional life has implications for how we study and understand society. The conventional approach of medical ethics has been to apply a set of principles (such as autonomy, beneficence, nonmaleficence, and justice) to discrete decisions by physicians (see, for example, Beauchamp and Childress 1994). This book has taken a different approach. By locating physicians in their social and organizational context rather than treating them largely as free-standing decisionmakers, we can better understand how they view their work as well as their obligations to employee-patients, employers, and the public, how they approach ethical concerns, and how they conduct themselves day to day. Where people are located in the organizational structure and in society warrants close attention, since it so strongly shapes their moral beliefs and actions. The decisions and views of individuals are thus best understood in this broader social context.

The focus of much of the literature in the social studies of science has been the effect of intra-lab politics on bench scientists. Here, the focus instead has been on professionals in corporations, where economic and power relations become especially important factors in shaping the ethics and conduct of individual actors. What is at stake is not intra-lab politics but the interests of multibillion-dollar industries. As we have seen, the ethical dilemmas of individuals reflect power and economic conflicts over whose interests, points of view, and definitions of the problem should prevail.

To bring about effective policies to protect the long-term interests of companies, their employees, and society—including the protection of health and the environment—we must increase the power of corporate professionals and employees. Any such empowerment should include facilitating structural change that strengthens safeguards for them when they act to protect such long-term interests.

POLICY IMPLICATIONS

Alternative policies that could encourage the use of medical information in more protective, equitable, and rational ways should have three goals: promoting effective preventive health measures to reduce long-term corporate and social costs, creating organizational incentives for more individual accountability and social responsibility, and separating health services from employer control.

Promoting Effective Preventive Health Measures

Prevention must be institutionalized in society as well as in the workplace through case law and regulations maintaining standards in business. Preventing illness is often far less costly in human and dollar terms than acting after the fact, even though it may not be less costly to a specific employer. Effectively removing the health hazards that employees perceive could also increase job satisfaction, make the workplace less stressful, and promote worker health generally.[1] At the very least, recognizing ways in which adverse working conditions contribute to job dissatisfaction and disease could be a first step toward beneficial alternative policies.

Preventive steps can represent an unwelcome short-term cost for managers, especially in times of corporate retrenchment, when many American corporations are struggling with declining profitability and loss of worldwide market share. Nevertheless, corporations should be given incentives to adopt measures that are cost-effective over the long term as well as incentives to evaluate how managerial job performance meets the needs of corporations and society to prevent illness and death. The goal should be to promote more thorough consideration of the workplace practices that impose costs on employees and the general public. Physicians tend to give little consideration to these social costs when they tailor their decisions to fit their allegiances within and outside the corporation.[2] Social policy and the law could help ensure that employers, rather than individual workers or society as a whole, bear most of the financial burden of dealing with occupational disease.

Individuals identified as high-risk for disease need further safeguards. Companies should rely less on exclusion as a means of protection and take stronger steps to reduce exposure hazards. The ability to introduce new screening practices has outdistanced the dissemination of information about potential consequences. Medical technologies and scientific information about risks are often misapplied to the workplace.

Employers could change specific features of their employment practices related to their medical practices; their privacy protections; and their policies concerning access to health care, job security, and antidiscrimination measures. In the case of drug testing, employers are unlikely to abandon it as long as government agencies such as the Nuclear Regulatory Commission and the Department of Transportation require it. Still, even for government-mandated drug-testing programs, employers could be required to change their surveillance programs, disciplinary policies, and the rehabilitation they offer, as well as their safety and privacy provisions.

Workplace screening should not gain support without careful examination of the evidence for it—especially since genetic and drug screening do not necessarily offer proof of impairment at work. By seeking to identify individuals with specific risk factors, company physicians implicitly argue that all others are safe and so no further substance regulation or change in company policies is needed. It is important to understand how employers use such claims about safety. Their arguments that workplaces are safe for all but a few high-risk individuals who should be screened out resemble the long-standing corporate arguments that low-level nuclear radiation is safe and that smoking does not cause cancer. Employers should take measures to ensure that the scientific evidence for screening is strong and that all tests relate to job performance. In addition, antidiscrimination laws should be extended to cover employees' preexisting health conditions and genetic predispositions, to guard against the labeling and penalizing of individuals as high-risk.[3] The search for high-risk individuals should not limit the use of effective strategies for reducing environmental hazards and disease that are already widely recognized but underfunded (see, for example, Collegium Ramazzini 1999; Aldana and Pronk 2001; Ducatman and McLellan 2000; Cushman 1997; Pelletier 1996). Priorities in health policy should be redirected toward reducing risk and giving sufficient attention to broad health hazards without falsely making it appear that high-risk workers or drug users are the problem or needlessly penalizing individuals perceived to be susceptible. Investing in improved management policies and working conditions could prevent disease more effectively than broad employee screening.

Corporate enthusiasm for screening, though understandable as a business interest, has had a destructive effect on employees and the public and diverted attention from pressing environmental health hazards and problematic management policies. Moreover, companies need to look at the coercive quality of these policies when individuals with few job alternatives and incomplete information on workplace hazards are pressured to take tests and provide medical information, when they are threatened with losing their employment or insurance, and when they find that the truly voluntary and independent counseling recommended for private patients is unavailable to them. (On informed consent in medicine generally, see Appelbaum, Lidz, and Meisel 1987; Kahn, Mastroanni, and Sugarman 1998; Brody 1992; on confidential medical counseling for individuals outside their workplace, see Mehlman et al. 1996.)

If risk is conceptualized in terms of the personal habits or biology of individuals, it naturally appears beneficial to develop screening programs to identify people who take drugs or have genetic characteristics that may present a health hazard on the job. But if risk is conceptualized in terms of workplace hazards that all exposed workers confront, then employers should tighten engineering controls, monitor exposure hazards, replace hazardous products, and collect scientific information on risks to populations. Only such efforts can reveal whether working conditions are indeed safe. Finally, national health coverage and a health-care system of government-financed services could mean that individuals and groups considered high-risk would no longer be denied health coverage or affordable medical care.[4] They thus would have less to fear from screening under such a system.[5]

Legal and Social Policy Protections and Organizational Incentives

The legal environment affects the ways in which company physicians work and think of themselves as professionals and corporate actors. They cast social questions and moral quandaries as legal matters. Whereas forty years ago employees could not sue company doctors because they were considered fellow servants or co-agents, now company physicians are becoming increasingly vulnerable to malpractice and other lawsuits even after they give up the comparative autonomy of private practice. Also, workers' compensation and OSHA regulation are expanding the realm of willful negligence and the possibility that corporations and individual professionals can be held liable for it.

Organizational incentives could encourage professionals and employees to speak up in organizations, government, and in public forums, and those who do so should be protected against retribution for engaging in socially responsible conduct (see Richter, Soskolne, and LaDou 2001; Miethe and Rothschild 1994, 338–40; Willborn, Schawab, and Burton 1993, 79–112).[6] Managers companywide should be held accountable for health and environmental protection. Professional societies and laws can increase both appropriate loyalty and individual accountability among company professionals for hazards and errors. For example, the Corporate Criminal Liability Act of California provides for significant fines (of up to $1 million for a corporation) and the imprisonment of managers who violate the law, such as those found responsible for workers' deaths.[7] Extending medical malpractice to corporate professionals could serve a similar purpose. The threat of lawsuits against physicians and managers could be useful in expanding individual accountability, getting companies to curtail hazardous conditions, and promoting beneficial social policies, even though, as we have seen, lawsuits are a blunt instrument, and fear of them sometimes has adverse consequences, such as information suppression strategies and wasteful defensive medicine.[8]

Physicians generally frame their relations with patients in terms of personal trust and integrity, downplaying any power problems. After having been socialized to believe that they have extraordinary power in society, doctors are beginning to realize how little power they have when they are caught between the tectonic shifts that are occurring between the law, insurance companies, large corporations, powerful medical organizations, and the government payers that largely control medical services.[9] When employees fear getting fired, have no employee organization to appeal to, and see doctors use information against them, it matters little how friendly the company physician is. Good doctor-patient relationships depend on the larger corporate and social structure. In theory, employee demands could actually make it easier for physicians to function in the corporation, because the doctors could advise their employers on how to respond to employee pressure. Most doctors focus on demonstrating their integrity and trustworthiness to employees while maintaining the illusion that they must protect employees' health on their own. Although they often align themselves with management and clash with employees and the public over working conditions, they criticize workers' tendency to mistrust them rather than acknowledge the real conflicting interests and power dynamics of corporate employment. Company physicians find it hard to admit that laws and corporate structures largely govern their relationship with patients, for that would seem to strip them of their own power—an assault on self-image that few people (especially doctors) can willingly tolerate. Still, doctors conceivably could refrain from simply exerting their own power over workers and instead seek workers' empowerment in the recognition that doing so would be in their own professional interest.[10]

Employees could strive to improve their own health by gaining a greater ability to identify health hazards and influence their working conditions. Company medical programs could be made responsible to the workforce as well as to the employer through joint labor-management committees like those set up by General Motors and the United Auto Workers (UAW).[11] Union membership is at its lowest point since the 1930s; with only 9 percent of the private sector unionized, union influence on company policies is certainly limited.[12] Unions also have been constrained by limited information and lack of power under restrictive labor laws. Moreover, basic economic issues take precedence for unions over issues of health and employee participation, especially in periods of layoffs. Nonetheless, organized labor in heavily unionized indus-

tries and workplaces has pressed for specific services, a prohibition on certain tests, more access to information, expanded employee representation, and greater independence of company
doctors (see, for example, Silverstein and Mirer 2000; Bayer 1988;
Dwyer 1991; Judkins 1986). Along with public interest and community groups, they have tried to counteract business's flexibility,
wealth, and power in a globalizing economy.[13] However, gaining
influential transnational resources is overwhelmingly daunting for
citizen groups. It is thus difficult to be optimistic about the prospect of a globalized counterweight to corporate power and control. Much depends on the strength and vigilance of community
and labor organizations in demanding that corporations change
their practices.

Separating Health Services from Employer Control

The rapid expansion of medical information presents many opportunities for its inappropriate or harmful use by company physicians, employers, and insurance companies. Individuals should
have more rights over access to test results than current laws provide. People also ought to be fully informed about risks, the nature of tests, who will get the results, and what impact they may
have. Most employees now have the right to obtain company
medical records if they request them so that they can find out
what tests have been conducted.[14] Since misrepresentations of information can have devastating consequences for employment, insurance, and stigmatization, people should be able to learn of
inaccuracies in or unfair uses of their medical records. They need
information on tests and health hazards collected by agencies independent of their employer so that they can evaluate their employer's warnings or assurances more effectively. And they need
trustworthy information about risks to individuals as well as aggregate data that may reveal patterns of health hazards and which
groups have been screened out.

Physicians' services to employees are likely to improve if control over them is separated from employment. Physicians could
instead work for a third party chosen by both management and
employee representatives.[15] Regulation can serve a critical function in protecting health, but regulatory oversight has been limited

by cutbacks in enforcement and by a slow and cumbersome process of setting standards. (On the competing pressures on government regulation from business and from social groups advocating stricter rules, see, for example, Ashford 2000, 211–36; Wahl and Gunkel 1999; Domhoff 1998; Calavita 1983; Szasz 1986; McCaffrey 1982, 31–69.) Government should strengthen health standards and provide greater support for training occupational medicine physicians, thereby encouraging the growth of a professional base that can advise companies on reducing work hazards. Because most physicians receive little medical school training in occupational health, regional health resource centers staffed by board-certified occupational physicians could support them in many ways: by offering health consulting services, developing surveillance programs, dispensing information about work hazards, offering physical exams, and evaluating individuals who might be at special risk (see Rosenstock et al. 1991; Castorina and Rosenstock 1990).[16] These centers could more credibly study hazards and protect medicine from the constraints imposed by employers whose main concern is maximizing company profits. Companies and the government would jointly pay for the professional services of these centers. Neither of them would employ doctors themselves or retain a legal right to see any of the center's medical data about employees. Such a system would allow doctors to address health risks without worrying that employers could question their allegiance or threaten to fire them; it could make both research and clinical practice more independent of management control. Such independence of physicians' services could help counter the encroachments on the latitude of professionals that we see in company medicine, which prefigures in a more distilled form what is occurring in medicine and corporate professional employment generally.

Social concerns about the control of medical expenses and liability risks are unlikely to disappear anytime soon. Efforts to control these costs, however, have given rise to adverse social effects, including the suppression of information about health hazards, policy shifts further away from preventive medicine, and discrimination. Employees' efforts to control their own costs have sometimes extended disease risks and costs without effectively preventing or treating disease.

Current conflicts over whether individual workers, corporations, or society as a whole should bear the work-related costs of chemical exposure risks and medical care are likely to expand over the next decade. The legal and social policy measures presented here would help protect health and alleviate the adverse social consequences of the distribution of medical information about employees. The initiation of new health and employment policies that could curtail health hazards and the detrimental uses of medical information is likely to involve legal challenges, government regulation, education, and collective bargaining. Problems of health hazards, privacy, and discrimination will not be solved without adequately addressing the power dynamics, laws, and economic interests that affect the work of corporate professionals.

—— Appendix ——

Study Data and Methods

THE PRINCIPAL DATA and methods used in this research are one hundred in-depth interviews and other fieldwork, documents, cases, and an analysis of historical and statistical materials.

INTERVIEWS

Interview Informants

For this study I conducted semistructured, in-person interviews with one hundred people across the country, many of whom are key players in the field of occupational medicine. The informants can be categorized into two groups: sixty company physicians and medical directors working in companies with in-house medical staffs; and forty individuals with particular expertise in corporate medicine.

The latter group can be further broken down into three subgroups. The first subgroup is made up of government officials who are concerned with occupational medicine or charged with employment and health policymaking. They are employed in agencies concerned with occupational health, employment, and medical technology, such as the Occupational Safety and Health Administration, the Department of Labor, the National Institute for Occupational Safety and Health, and state departments of labor and health.

The second subgroup includes labor officials who are knowledgeable about employee health risks and worker selection. Among them are national labor officials from the AFL-CIO; the Oil, Chemical, and Atomic Workers International Union; the United Steelworkers; the Union of Needletrades, Industrial and Textile Employees; the United Mine Workers; the United Auto Workers; state Committee on Occupational Safety and Health (COSH) organizations; and other labor organizations.

The third subgroup includes three types of professionals. The university clinic physicians and scientists in occupational health include directors of occupational medicine residency training programs and other physicians in universities and medical centers (including Massachusetts Institute of Technology, Johns Hopkins, Mount Sinai School of Medicine, University of California, University of Texas, University of Pittsburgh, University of Southern California, Columbia University, University of Oklahoma, and other institutions). The medical and trade association representatives work for the American College of Occupational and Environmental Medicine, the American Public Health Association, the American Medical Association, the American Petroleum Institute, and other organizations. And finally, attorneys, physicians, nurses, and others outside government agencies and corporations who specialize in or are familiar with occupational health come from law firms and legal advocacy organizations, medical centers, and occupational health and public health organizations. Scientists who provide medical research or screening services to employers are of particular interest, as are physicians who direct occupational medical residency programs and attorneys involved in litigation over medical screening.

In complex and controversial areas such as this, relying on survey research as the major source of data certainly seemed out of the question, because in doing so I would have missed important information. I wanted to allow the interviewees to describe their employment practices in detail without being limited to multiple-choice or otherwise brief, easily quantified responses. I also wanted to encourage them to discuss their experiences and perspectives in ways that would go beyond what they might say in a public forum. Thus, this study committed me to the labor-intensive enterprise of interviewing a broad range of people in person with flexible interview guides, as well as to studying documents and observing people as they functioned in their daily work in order to capture the complex reality of their social world. (For discussions of intensive interview data and analysis and the constructed social world they can illuminate, see Strauss and Corbin 1998; Mishler 1991; Lofland and Lofland 1995.) This approach allowed me to assess the significance and meaning that social actors gave to corporate professional work and the relationship between their perceptions and actual workplace practices.

Large manufacturing corporations that confront significant medical hazards in their line of work typically retain occupational physicians on staff. Corporate informants were primarily from large firms in the chemical, oil, automobile, metals and mining, pharmaceutical, airline, telecommunications, aerospace, transportation, utilities, computers, and electronics industries. These companies generally have substantial medical programs, more sophisticated technologies, and extensive experience with health hazards. They also are heavily involved in the medical selection of workers. The health effects from hazardous chemicals and the identification of high-risk groups have also been salient issues at these work sites. Further, the toxic exposure problems in these industries are often "upstream" and therefore magnified versions of exposure in the industries they supply.

For the sake of comparison, I also investigated physicians in smaller firms and other types of corporations and government organizations that use medical information, including textiles, banking, publishing and broadcasting, consumer products, conglomerates, retail sales, financial services, and other manufacturing and service corporations. As explained earlier, my principal theoretical interest, and the research focus of this study, is in large nonmedical corporations that employ medical professionals, not in corporations such as hospitals that revolve around physicians' professional activities.

Physicians who are corporate medical directors offered a special perspective stemming from their management of other company physicians, their relationship with other high-level corporate managers, and their heightened visibility, which they had typically attained by participating in medical associations and testifying at government hearings. Corporate medical directors usually have considerable direct contact with the legal, personnel, environmental affairs, and other corporate departments that contribute to medical decisions. They have usually worked as lower-ranking company doctors, and most of them come in contact with many other company physicians.

I interviewed former in-house physicians who now do consulting for companies as well as in-house physicians who had worked as consultants or contractors in occupational medicine. I also talked with physicians with experience in the military and HMOs for comparison to gain insight into their work structures and processes.

The interview informants who were not company doctors were knowledgeable about the occupational medicine practiced in corporations and well acquainted with the work of corporate physicians, if from a different vantage point.

Medical and trade association data on company physicians (such as from ACOEM) provided overall information and facilitated the selection of physicians to be interviewed. The selection method for this study yielded a broader and more informative and truly representative group of informants than could have been obtained by drawing a random sample from existing data sources. No national sampling frame adequate for this study existed for drawing a random sample of informants. For example, medical associations do have data on their physician members, but these data omit too many of the types of physicians in large companies who are the focus of this study. Further, medical association data do not offer information on the variables (such as training and circumstances of corporate employment) that this study uses and that informed the selection of informants.

I selected the individuals to be interviewed from a national population, to allow for regional variation and to ensure that I interviewed federal officials and informants located in many states. Approximately half of the company physicians and other informants are from the eastern half of the country, and approximately half are from the western half of the country, with the South and Midwest represented along with the East and West Coasts. I selected informants so as to achieve a broad regional and industrial distribution across the country, as the research design required for analyzing the data. The age range of physician informants both inside and outside corporations also is wide, reflecting the populations they represent. I interviewed people fresh out of residency programs along with physicians who have practiced in corporate medicine for ten to twenty years and people close to retirement. The sexual and racial composition of physician respondents is heavily white and male, reflecting the population of occupational physicians that corporations employ.[1] Overall, I chose informants so as to ensure breadth in type of organization, company position, and perspective. I chose nonphysician informants in such a way as to attain diversity within the categories of informants, including variation by region and organization represented.

I interviewed people in a broad range of industries. Approximately two-thirds of the physician respondents and nonphysician corporate personnel are employed at Fortune 500 companies in the chemical, oil, metals and mining, automobile, pharmaceutical, aerospace, telecommunications, airline, transportation, utilities, computers, and electronics industries. In addition, approximately two-thirds of the labor officials are from these industries. The remaining third of the physician and labor individuals are from smaller companies in those industries and from other employing organizations.

Typically I selected one physician from each company, but occasionally I selected more than one, especially if the physicians were from different geographical regions of the country in a large company and widely separated by length of employment in the firm and in occupational medicine. As with government, union, and university informants, I interviewed more than one individual from organizations that were important cases.

I identified individuals to be interviewed by consulting the professional literature and by using methods of key informant referral to achieve the demographic, industry, and regional distribution that the study sample and research design defined. I obtained the names of most interviewees from publications and documents such as articles, legislative hearings, professional publications, and conference proceedings. Although I obtained the names of most interviewees from documentary sources, other names came from contacts familiar with the field of occupational medicine.

Names of corporate medical directors were readily available through medical and trade association publications. Other physicians provided the names of specific physicians in the firms I selected for study. Referring physicians were from professional societies, corporate medical departments, and occupational medical clinics. I initially contacted the individuals I interviewed directly by phone or letter.

The majority of the corporate, labor, academic, legal, and government personnel I selected for interviewing are leaders rather than lower-ranking members of their organizations. These informants are prominent in their fields and known for their expertise in occupational medicine. For example, those interviewed include the directors of occupational health agencies and programs, labor officials responsible for health and safety in international unions, directors of university occupational medical clinics, legal scholars specializing in corporate medical liability and workplace health issues, the president of a national occupational medical association, and the environmental affairs director of a major chemical company. My research design decision to interview more leaders than lower-ranking members of organizations reflected a desire to find particularly well-informed respondents—individuals who are not only highly knowledgeable about occupational medicine and the conditions affecting it but also aware of the range of perspectives on it in their own and other organizations.

The comparative design of this research ensured that interview informants were acquainted with the concerns of this study from a range of important vantage points. For example, they offered varying perspectives on medical information as it is used in large corporations.

The research design identified individuals to be interviewed because of their structural location in specific positions and organizations. That is, they were chosen to be typical of those in the same types of positions and organizations. I chose the interviewees for sound methodological and sociological reasons, not because they fell into arbitrary categories that seemed plausible or because they offered to be interviewed owing to their strong views about occupational medicine.

Interview Questioning

Most of the initial and follow-up interviews were conducted between 1992 and 2000, with some initial and exploratory interviews conducted between 1980 and 1992. Interviews generally lasted from one to three hours, and some of them extended over more than one session. They were conducted in an office, home, or other location, as the interviewee preferred.

Confidentiality of informants' identities was maintained in that their names were not used in the analysis and presentation of the findings, except for those individuals who wished not to be interviewed anonymously and formally allowed their names to be revealed. Although all those interviewed were willing to talk with me at length, company physicians predictably were more reluctant to be quoted by name than union officials. Still, several company physicians formally permitted me to attribute their statements to them. The position or affiliation of individuals who are quoted by name or cited anonymously is generally the one they held at the time of the statement.

When physicians who have worked within and outside companies discussed their work as corporate physicians, I often identified them as a physician working for the company they described in the interviews. Because of job mobility and movement between companies, government, and universities, I ended up interviewing more than sixty physicians in depth who had been employed by a company.

I had no significant problems in gaining access to corporate officials and professionals. Through previous research, I was familiar with the field settings and network of physicians, corporate officials, and other contacts who facilitated access to a broad range of informants. As in earlier research projects using interviews, the individuals interviewed for this study were generally cooperative and willing to talk at length. I had discovered in prior interviews with occupational physicians—as well as with corporate, government, and labor officials—that they generally speak knowledgeably, often eloquently, about the changing conditions affecting their work and about their own views and decisions.

The interviews were focused and semistructured. To prepare for the interviews, I examined documents and publications for relevant data and leads. I developed and revised interview guides with detailed questions after exploratory discussions with informants. I questioned the individuals in areas such as: their background and experience in occupational medicine and corporate employment; their knowledge of the ways in which medical information has been applied and employees with health risks have been identified; their views on the broader topic of health and employment practices as a context for corporate medical professional work; cases of workplace medical screening; and the legal and political dimensions of health risks and workplace practices. Individuals described their general perspective and their own experience. Actual cases that physicians discussed yielded more valuable data on decisionmaking than a discussion of hypothetical cases and imagined consequences would have. I analyzed the major cases of corporate medical practices that emerged from the research.

I asked the same questions of nonphysician informants, but from the perspective of their own area of expertise. In addition to asking questions similar to those asked of physicians, I questioned union officials about union pressures on medical professionals and the experience of the union with company physicians. In the same vein, I asked medical association personnel about professional influences on company physicians and the experience of their association with company physicians, and I asked nonphysician corporate personnel about corporate influences on company physicians and their experience with company physicians.

Interviews with directors of occupational medicine residency training programs around the country provided insight into the skills, training, and goals of physicians who join corporations. They also illuminated the perspective of doctors who join consulting companies, government, and universities. In addition to the program directors, I interviewed many doctors who teach or otherwise contribute to the residency programs.

Most of the interviews were taped and transcribed. Interview transcripts provided the crucial detail and direct quotes that were important to this research. The data could be analyzed repeatedly to discover previously unnoticed phenomena and to verify patterns suggested by the ongoing analysis. Thus, analysis did not depend entirely on what I had thought was interesting or significant before analyzing the data. Transcripts also enabled me to analyze the interviews in detail.

In addition to the one hundred interviews, I observed and talked informally with many people at conferences and hearings on occupational risk, at meetings of the doctors' professional organizations, in medical departments within corporations, and in a wide range of other workplaces that employ occupational physicians. This field research was a valuable supplement to the data obtained in interviews, surveys, and documents. It offered insight into the people being studied and provided telling details from their daily work environment and interaction with others at meetings.

This study drew from existing survey data on company policies, medical screening, and risk perspectives. National opinion polls and surveys from medical and trade associations offered valuable data. Medical associations collect data from their members, just as trade associations collect extensive data from their member company officials and corporations. For example, the American College of Occupational and Environmental Medicine conducts surveys of the member physicians, occupational medicine, and screening programs related to this study. Much of this information is summarized in the *Journal of Occupational and Environmental Medicine* and other publications, and detailed survey data often are available beyond those that are published. I asked officials from medical and trade associations, government agencies, public interest organizations, and labor unions for survey data on members and other groups. Legal analysts, medical researchers, and academic scholars also had survey data relevant to this study. The literature review, document collection, and interviews unearthed new survey data sources and facilitated access to them.

DOCUMENTARY, STATISTICAL, AND HISTORICAL RESEARCH

In addition to the interviews, I drew on numerous other sources of data on company physicians, including government documents, conference proceedings, hearing transcripts, employment records and health data, scientific publications, trade and medical association data, and unpublished documents. I also reviewed historical and sociological materials on the history of corporations, medicine, the professions, occupational health practices, and employment trends; literature on specific professions such as lawyers and engineers; and legal cases, regulations, statutes, and proposed bills.

Documents provided valuable evidence regarding occupational medicine and corporate professional work. I examined evidence of company practices, positions taken by various parties, and social contexts through documentary, statistical, and historical data sources that included: historical and sociological materials on medical professionals, occupational health, employment policies, and regulatory developments; government documents, including health and employment data, regulatory standards, laws, and proposed bills; transcripts of testimony at legislative, regulatory, and judicial hearings on the rights and responsibilities of medical professionals, liability for disease, employment discrimination, and other data on important legal cases; scientific, medical, legal, ethical, and policy sources on physicians in corporations; conference proceedings on major occupational health issues; policy position papers and other written material that gives evidence of the various perspectives on medical professionals in corporate organizations; statistical data, particularly health and employment data; corporate documents, including employment records, policy statements, health information, trade association reports, public relations material, research reports, internal corporate memoranda, and press releases; labor union documents, including position papers, employment and health information, and research reports; and general news periodicals, particularly the *New York Times,* the *Washington Post,* and the *Los Angeles Times,* and periodicals, including the *Journal of Occupational and Environmental Medicine, Environmental Health Perspectives, Business Week,* and *Chemical and Engineering News.*

Informants wrote or were quoted in many of these data sources. Some of these documents are readily available to the public. I obtained other documents through the people I interviewed, medical and trade association representatives, government officials, attorneys, corporate employees, and other resources. My previous research experience and familiarity with many organizational representatives facilitated access to these documents. As with the interview component of the research, my emphasis in the documentary, statistical, and historical research was on large corporations as employing organizations.

INTEGRATION OF DATA SOURCES

A major advantage of the research design was that it generated a large volume of comparative data from several types of people. The diverse data sources also allowed me to collect crucial contextual information pertaining to each interview. This included data on the litigation and regulatory history of the company, the economic conditions affecting it, the location of company medicine in the changing corporate structure, and the work and publications background of the person interviewed. I examined the data sources on a particular organization and informant before carrying out the interview, thereby enabling the questioning to be more specific and informed. Linking these other types of information with interview data also provided a deeper understanding of the legal, professional, corporate, and public pressures on decisionmaking than could be obtained from the interviews alone.

I used the field research methods of data collection and analysis that I have developed in several previous research projects and fine-tuned in advanced graduate field research methods courses I have taught. I conducted the interviews, took primary responsibility for analyzing them, and developed theoretical conceptualizations and analyses of the study data. Research assistants carried out specific delimited tasks of data collection and organization.

The systematic field research methods used in this research offer an understanding of the social context of corporate professional work that abstract investigations, literature reviews, or social surveys alone cannot adequately provide. In-depth personal interviews combined with documents and field observation provide crucial missing information and allow corporate professional work to be analyzed from a range of perspectives.

—— Notes ——

INTRODUCTION

1. A few studies have considered the work of physicians in large organizations. Investigators have paid some attention to physicians on
the staffs of large hospitals and health maintenance organizations
rather than manufacturing companies (see Starr 1982; Freidson
1986). Field (1957, 1966) has examined the work of Soviet physicians; Lifton (1986) has analyzed Nazi doctors; Daniels (1969) and
Howe (1986) have discussed military physicians; Walters (1984) has
analyzed Canadian occupational physicians; and Walsh (1987) has
examined physicians who manage corporate medical departments.
Yet the number of studies that attend to the conditions of corporate
employment remains small.

2. For a discussion of the role of physicians in Manville Corporation
and firms that have used large amounts of asbestos, see Castleman
(1996) and Brodeur (1985).

3. Employer concern about the ways in which their practices may
clash with the values of their employees and of the public waxes
and wanes; it has led at various times to more values training for
MBAs, heightened interest in corporate responsibility, and greater
attention to the linkages between work, family values, and religious
beliefs.

4. On conflicts of interest of doctors engaged in clinical practice and
research, see, for example, Korn (2000), Speece, Shimm, and Buchanan (1996), and Lo, Wolf, and Berkeley (2000).

5. Professions are concrete forms of organization developed by particular occupations historically. The category of professionals should
be disaggregated, because each group has its own history and differs in its approach to problems of independence, autonomy, and
professional control. On the history of professions, see Brint (1994),
Abbott (1988), Freidson (1984), Burrage and Torstendahl (1990),
and Halpern (1992).

6. This model in the literature reflects not only analysts' neglect of certain issues but also the changing locus of professional work as corporations employ growing numbers of professionals. On the rise of professionals, see Hughes (1958), Merton (1940), Scott (1966), Parsons (1939), Freidson (1986), and Vollmer and Mills (1966).

7. On scientists, see Sassower (1993), Gilbert and Mulkay (1984), Kornhauser (1962), Latour and Woolgar (1979), Marcson (1960), and Glaser (1964). On lawyers, see Abel (1997), Heinz et al. (1998), Nelson and Nielson (2000), Heinz and Laumann (1994), Suchman (1998), Nelson and Trubek (1992), Devlin (1994), Spangler (1986), Kagan and Rosen (1985), Smigel (1964), Auerbach (1984), and Granfield and Koenig (1992). On engineers, see Meiksins and Smith (1996), Kunda (1992), Zussman (1985), Whalley (1986), Meiksins (1982), Noble (1977), Miller (1967), and Ritti (1971). See also Thomas (1994), who examines the social and ideological distance between design engineers in their labs and manufacturing engineers on the shop floor.

8. A major concern in the large literature on professionals is whether professionals are a powerful new class or whether they are instead becoming proletarianized or deprofessionalized. One set of analysts argues for the growing strength of professionals relative to other workers and corporate managers. Bell's (1973) postindustrial theory maintains that salaried professionals, rather than becoming subordinate to their new employers, manage to gain control in their employing institutions and wield considerable influence within them. Moreover, professionals in the new postindustrial order wrest power from the previously dominant group: those who control capital. The growing influence of professionals stems from their valuable specialized knowledge. Other related theorists also argue that professionals have ascended in relation to corporate owners and managers. These include Galbraith (1967), who portrays professionals as part of the powerful technocracy; Steinfels (1979), who sees growing social control by a "new class" of professionals; and Illich et al. (1987), who describe the rise of professional authority in a process of "professional imperialism." Freidson (1970) argues that although professionals have undergone increased bureaucratization of their work, they have not experienced the "deskilling" to which nineteenth-century industrial workers were subject, instead often retaining high levels of both skill and autonomy. In contrast to these theories of professional ascendance, theories of professional decline emphasize the shift from professional self-employment to salaried employment and the resulting similarities be-

tween professionals and other workers as power and control over work is transferred from professionals to employers. Theorists of professional decline and proletarianization include Larson (1977, 1980), who shows the tendency of professionals to be increasingly subject to the constraints of corporate- or state-dominated markets. Derber, Schwartz, and Magrass (1990) argue that a new system of labor process control—"ideological proletarianization"—shifts power from professionals to managers. Oppenheimer (1970, 1973) explains processes of rationalization and routinization that professionals experience in bureaucratic organizations.

CHAPTER 1

1. The 1981 film *Outland* (written and directed by Peter Hyams) is set in a remote location where over two thousand workers are mining titanium ore. The workers take amphetamines that initially increase their productivity but later make them psychotic. The corrupt general manager sends assassins after the security officer (Connery) after he, along with the company doctor (Sternhagen), discover the cause of several workers' deaths. The film portrays the company's workers as unwilling to risk their jobs to oppose the general manager and stop the drug promotion that is threatening their health and lives. My thanks to Eric Frumin and anonymous others for interesting discussions of the portrayal of company doctors in film and literature.
2. In the 1945 film *Brief Encounter* (directed by David Lean), the occupational physician (played by Trevor Howard, here not a company doctor), speaking to the woman with whom he has fallen in love (played by Celia Johnson), describes his specialty of pneumoconiosis as "a slow process of fibrosis of the lung due to the inhalation of small particles of dust" (such as dust from coal mines, metal dusts from steelworks, or stone dust from gold mines, which cause silicosis). He is an occupational physician leaving England to join the staff of a new hospital in Johannesburg, South Africa. In explaining his enthusiasm for preventive medicine, the doctor says: "Most good doctors, especially when they're young, have private dreams. That's the best part of them. Sometimes, though, those get overprofessionalized or strangulated."
3. The 1954 movie *Salt of the Earth* (directed by Herbert T. Biberman) is a quasi-documentary drama about a thirteen-month strike at a zinc mine in New Mexico, featuring many of the actual striking

mineworkers as nonprofessional actors (along with the actors Juan Chacon, Rosaura Revueltas, and Will Geer). The film describes how the strikers' wives took up the cause of their miner husbands and portrays anti-Hispanic racism.

4. The environmental doctor who discovers that the medicinal baths are contaminated is fairly contemptuous of the townspeople and unwilling to deal with their concerns. He never fully understands the community's failure to support environmental concerns or the insecurity that prompts their response. He takes for granted that the people will think he has acted heroically and is stunned when they attack him. He reacts defensively against them and sees them as essentially the same as the bath owners, the mayor, and the town fathers, who have more money than the people who might lose their livelihoods.

5. Illinois Central Hospital in Chicago, for example, was founded to deal with traumatic injuries, such as the mangled legs and arms of railroad workers in need of amputation. Park City, Utah, had a special hospital for railroad miners, predominantly Chinese, who were afflicted with silicone tuberculosis. The railroad hospitals at the turn of the century functioned as little more than places to hold workers until they died and could be buried.

6. Before 1911, when nine states enacted the first state workers' compensation laws, employers could terminate injured employees without compensating them. By 1920 most states had passed workers' compensation legislation. Nevertheless, employees still tried to avoid reporting injuries or accidents so as not to be fired or otherwise have their employment records blemished. For discussions of workers' compensation, see Ashford (1998) and Berman (1978).

7. Coal mining is a fairly isolated industry, and only in the last twenty years, as major corporations have bought mining companies, have mineworkers negotiated contracts that require employers to provide health plans similar to those that employers in other industries provide and to contract out health care. Companies in rural areas generally no longer hire doctors to provide day-to-day acute or chronic care. Fifty years ago, if a company like Exxon wanted to explore for oil in Argentina or Venezuela, there would be little medical infrastructure for its two hundred employees setting up a camp in the tropics, so the company would have to import its own doctors, hospitals, and equipment. Now, with some exceptions, an indigenous health-care system of doctors and hospitals exists locally when companies go to Argentina or Venezuela. For discussion

of the history of health and safety in coal mining, see Krajcinovic (1997), Donovan (1988), and Seltzer (1988).

8. The AMA's hostility to corporate medicine is one reason company physicians have a separate medical association. The AMA objected to the code of ethics of the American College of Occupational and Environmental Medicine (ACOEM) and retained a more stringent code of its own. Medical societies had concerns about the quality of company doctors and the competitive threat they posed to physicians in private practice. See Starr (1982, 200–4) for a discussion of the tensions between the medical profession and company doctors.

9. Jesse Lang, physician at Hughes Corporation, personal interview. He added: "Paying for medical care was foisted on employers by pressure from unions, legislation, and the development of the occupational medicine specialty, not because they wanted to spend the money and were great humanitarians."

10. Kaiser never had a large in-house medical staff to provide medical services for its employees, as did General Motors and AT&T. But at its height during World War II the company medical programs covered about two hundred thousand people (Starr 1982, 322). In 1945 Kaiser opened its health plans to the public. Kaiser Permanente continued to expand and make money even after Kaiser Industries went out of business.

11. Hallett Lewis, a physician who formerly worked at Kaiser Steel and Kaiser Industries, personal interview. Lewis described the hostility toward Kaiser Industries doctors from doctors in private practice in the community: "I was blackballed when I applied for membership to the San Bernardino County Medical Society. Two of the four original Kaiser physicians joined the County Medical Society before the fence between the doctors practicing privately and the Kaiser physicians got put up. So when a Kaiser Permanente doctor—or in this case, I—applied, they would have two of these four guys recommend the individual, which was the clue to the membership to vote against him." Nonetheless, large steel companies sent their staff who dealt with health insurance to study health-care delivery and costs in the Kaiser health plans to learn how Kaiser could generate financing internally to build hospitals.

12. Current company physicians sometimes commend the characteristics of company medicine that Kaiser's critics once condemned as socialized medicine. A major airline physician said: "We practice a kind of socialized medicine: the patients don't pay us for our ser-

vices; a corporation pays us, whether we work forty or one hundred hours a week, and the pay is the same if we see twenty or two hundred patients in one day. Patients get any tests they need—an X-ray or blood work—free, and the corporation pays for physical therapy through its insurance company as a workers' compensation claim for occupational illness. Private practice has an RVS code with a certain price tag for all those things, and we don't."

13. For brief discussions of the origins of occupational medicine, see Starr (1982), Walsh (1987), and Berman (1978). New technologies for measuring contaminants also facilitated the growth of the field, as did computer technology that enabled researchers to link disease and exposures, using large data banks. Some state health departments, such as New York's, became active in occupational medicine beginning in the 1950s.

14. OSHA standards appear in 29 *Code of Federal Regulations,* sections 1910.1000–.1450 (2002), and the Toxic Substances Control Act is at 15 *United States Code,* sections 2601–2692 (2000).

15. Whereas plant physicians may supervise some employees but also do hands-on medicine, medical directors are administrators who worry about liability, regulations, quality assurance, and companywide policies. They hire local contractor doctors, deal with company policy and regulators, and do the medical part of reviewing product safety. Setting policies at a higher level involves consulting the other parts of the organization that deal with health regulations and insurance. Promotion within the company usually means moving away from the exercise of clinical skills into the exercise of management skills. In-house physicians need administrative ability to advance within the company or to become a medical director in another company.

16. A metals company recently had sixty in-house doctors plus many more contractors. In 1992 the utility company Southern California Edison had 227 people in its medical department, including forty-five in-house doctors, eight regional clinics, and a network of doctors under contract for in-house doctors to refer people to. The nonphysicians were nurses, claims people, preventive health personnel, and budget officers. The company in the mid-1990s dismantled much of its extensive in-house health-care apparatus. On the structure and components of oil company medical departments in the 1980s, see Gibson (1988).

17. In 2000 two-thirds (67 percent) of all small firms (those with between 3 and 1,999 employees) reported offering health coverage to their workers, and nearly all firms with fifty or more employees

offered coverage (Gabel et al. 2000, 149). These figures are based on an annual survey of employer-based health plans (the Kaiser Family Foundation/Health Research and Educational Trust Survey of Employer-Sponsored Health Benefits), which in 2000 surveyed employee benefits managers from 1,887 private and public employers.

18. For example, DuPont had a full-time physician in a facility with about six hundred employees that made tetraethyl lead because it was highly toxic and had posed major problems for predecessor companies, whereas another kind of company with only six hundred employees would not have a full-time physician.

19. The industrial and mining sectors have disproportionately employed physicians, although public employers and utilities also have maintained large medical departments. Some newer industries, such as high-tech and semiconductor companies, have opened clinics or become interested in developing occupational health services.

20. Similarly, researchers tend to wind up doing the kinds of research for which grants are available rather than those for which money is unavailable.

21. As with dry cleaners and spray paint shops, construction firms are typically small and usually do not hire company doctors. Workers in stationary work environments report to the same employer daily at the same place, whereas construction and maintenance employees are sent out to different contractors as the need arises for constructing, demolishing, or renovating buildings and roads. A worker might go to ten employers during a month or a year. Lead and asbestos abatement, along with hazardous and nuclear waste, require examinations for workers to be deemed fit for duty. Building and construction companies contract with clinics and mobile vans to test employees. They rarely send this workforce to company doctors.

22. In 1917 occupational physicians belonged to the American Association of Industrial Physicians and Surgeons, which in 1951 changed its name to the American Industrial Medical Association, then to the American Occupational Medicine Association, and in 1992, to the American College of Occupational and Environmental Medicine.

23. For discussions of training in occupational medicine, see Rom (1998b), ACOEM (1998), Burstein and Levy (1994), Institute of Medicine (1991), and Pransky (1990). The University of Cincinnati created a pioneering residency training program in occupational medicine in 1947. Researchers there investigated the diseases resulting

from wartime radiation exposures and from beryllium and other dust exposures during World War II munitions manufacture. Several medical directors of major corporations (DuPont, Eastman-Kodak, and Ethyl Corporation) taught at the few university residency programs that existed in the 1950s and 1960s.

24. Several medical research reports published over the last three decades pointed to the need for specialists in the field and bolstered efforts to improve training in occupational medicine (see, for example, Institute of Medicine 1988). These studies showed a critical need for physicians in occupational medicine and preventive medicine as well as for industrial hygienists, nurses, and environmental health specialists. They focused on needed improvements in quality as well as quantity. For example, a 1988 National Academy of Sciences Institute of Medicine study of occupational medicine identified a great need for improved training and greater specialization of occupational physicians. Castorina and Rosenstock (1990) estimated that 4,600 to 6,700 board-certified physicians in occupational medicine are needed, so that every major corporation, large group practice, medical school, and public health department would have a specialist; whereas only 1,200 to 1,500 of these board-certified specialists are available. To expand primary-care practitioners' training in occupational medicine, Rosenstock et al. (1991) recommend that the American Board of Family Practice and the American Board of Internal Medicine provide certificates of added qualifications to diplomates in family practice and internal medicine who have advanced training or experience in occupational medicine. They recommend an extra year of clinical training in the specialty and streamlined dual board certification in family practice or internal medicine. Company physicians such as former medical directors of Exxon and Ford also pressed for upgrading the field of occupational medicine. Earlier reports—such as the Flexner Report (1910)—had pointed to poor-quality medical training in general. See also Dinman (2000), who argues for improving the training of occupational physicians, and Rudolph (1996), who argues for improved quality in occupational health care.

25. The NIOSH-funded educational resource centers include occupational medicine residencies and graduate programs in industrial hygiene and safety. By 2001 about forty medical schools in the United States had approved residency training programs in occupational medicine (American Medical Association 2000a). Money for training more occupational physicians is not growing, however. Federal NIOSH funding (the major federal funding source) has been level

in year-to-year dollars over the past twenty years—or has even gone down, once inflation is factored in. (NIOSH funding for training grants in occupational medicine, occupational safety, industrial hygiene, and occupational health nursing was $12.9 million in 1980 and a high of $14.2 million in 2000, with a low of $5.8 million in 1982 and 1983, according to John Talte of the National Institute for Occupational Safety and Health (personal communication, March 7, 2001; see also Frumkin 1994, 676). The limited availability of research money is a major obstacle to the further growth of the field. Some new training programs support residents through means not dependent on the federal government, such as through income generated from hospital services and other types of services, or through having residents work for sponsors such as corporations or managed care organizations that sell occupational medical services. See also Frazier et al. (1999), who discuss NIOSH's efforts to train faculty in family practice and internal medicine residencies in occupational and environmental medicine.

26. There are about 721,000 professionally active physicians in the United States (American Medical Association 2000b; U.S. Department of Commerce, Bureau of the Census 2001, table 153), so ACOEM physician members practicing occupational medicine represent about 1 percent of U.S. practicing doctors. However, the actual proportion of physicians who practice occupational medicine is much larger, since most physicians who practice occupational medicine do not belong to ACOEM. Instead, they are primary-care physicians who do workers' compensation and other work-related cases on the side, or they have contracts with companies to do their occupational medicine, or they are emergency room or family practice doctors who treat work-related illnesses and injuries. A far larger proportion of physicians work in circumstances similar to those of company doctors, that is, in nonmedical corporations and large organizations. In addition to physicians, about 3 percent of U.S. physician's assistants work in occupational and environmental health services (Deitchman 2000, 298).

27. Specialty groups for specific industries (mining, auto, aircraft and aerospace) hold independent meetings at the time of the national ACOEM meeting.

28. In February 2001, 1,836 (26 percent) of the 6,930 ACOEM members were board-certified in occupational medicine (Mike Thompson, membership director, and Jeri Garcia, information systems support associate, ACOEM, personal communication, February 9, 2001; see also Deitchman 2000, 297). The distribution of in-house and con-

tract doctors varies considerably by region. Northern California, for example, has had fewer medical directors than in the East but for forty years has had a tradition of occupational medical consultants who were strong competitors to the in-house company doctors. Most companies in the region's newer industries, such as electronics, have not invested in company doctors at all.

29. Connie Highland, administrator, American Board of Preventive Medicine, personal communication, January 12, 2001; Patricia Socha, database manager, American Board of Medical Specialties, personal communication, February 9, 2001; see also Levy and Wegman (2000, 8).

30. ACOEM appoints a representative to the residency review committee of the ACGME, the accrediting agency.

31. The physicians who train those residents state that only 10 to 20 percent of the residents in NIOSH-sponsored training centers (educational resource centers, or ERCs) go into corporate employment, though the percentage is higher in some training programs. Of 151 current occupational and environmental medicine residency trainees in the United States and Canada surveyed in 1994 (84 percent of the 180 occupational and environmental medicine residents at that time), 32 percent said corporate or industry practice was their short-term career goal (34 percent stated that it was their long-term goal), 29 percent cited hospital-based or university-based clinical practice as a short-term goal (27 percent long-term), 22 percent said their short-term goal was academia (28 percent long-term), 22 percent said it was the government or military (10 percent long-term), and 18 percent said it was consulting (39 percent long-term). Fewer than the 32 percent who seek corporate employment are likely to find corporate jobs (Schwartz, Pransky, and Lashley 1995, 743).

32. Few worker clinics exist, state agencies mostly do research, and physicians in corporations are often high-level administrators who need years of prior experience. The fact that most graduates of occupational medicine residency programs now do not go to work full-time for corporations or have corporate employment as a career goal is partly due to physicians' preferences but also to the fact that corporations are not hiring many. Aside from what physicians ideally want to do, the job market largely dictates what they will finally do.

33. Residency training programs in occupational medicine with a pro-management reputation include Johns Hopkins, the University of California at Irvine, and George Washington University; those with a pro-worker or public health reputation include Mount Sinai, the

University of Illinois, the University of Washington, and the University of California at San Francisco. In addition, people with different values, interests, and priorities may be drawn to different training programs and to different jobs when they complete residency programs. In their 1994 survey (see note 31), Schwartz and his colleagues (1995, 741) found that residents stated that they selected their residency training program because of geographical considerations (64 percent), impressions from interviews and visiting the program (49 percent), and the "reputation" of the program director or faculty (44 percent) or of the program (44 percent). Physicians with business interests who seek bigger salaries traditionally have gone into corporations rather than government or university research and teaching, and as a government physician said, "More conservative people tend to gravitate toward corporate positions." Those who traditionally were attracted to corporate jobs have increasingly sought employment in private clinics and consulting firms as these positions have become more numerous.

34. Broadening the training of occupational physicians to encompass skills in industrial hygiene, safety, toxic exposures, and company operations has been a core goal of training programs for the past twenty years.

35. Bruce Karrh, physician at E. I. du Pont de Nemours and Company, personal interview.

36. James Hughes, physician who worked for Kaiser Aluminum and Kaiser Industries at the time of personal interview.

37. Richard Alexander, physician at Lockheed Missiles and Space Company at the time of personal interview.

38. Albert Ackroyd, physician at Northrup, personal interview.

39. Serving as an expert in lawsuits is especially lucrative. Consultants who go into chemical company litigation can make over $1,000 an hour.

40. Lloyd Tepper, physician at Air Products and Chemicals Corporation, personal interview.

41. The priority that the military places on medical care waxes and wanes. Military commanders have an acute awareness of its importance when they go into the heat of battle and see casualties coming out or cannot get units ready because they have not done what is necessary to prevent disease. The priority that the military puts on medical care lingers for a time after a war until current circumstances compel them to forget. Then more events and even military training maneuvers can remind the military that medical care is important. For a discussion of military medicine, see Stanley and Blair (1993).

42. Naval doctors historically have had the authority to order a captain to make a vessel go into port for medical reasons or, more recently, to insist on medical evacuations by helicopter; they report to their superiors in Washington, not to the captain.

43. However, some early occupational physicians were trained in the specialty and became leaders in the field.

44. The survey conducted by Schwartz and his colleagues (1995, 739–41) found that the most commonly cited reasons residents were attracted to occupational and environmental medicine were the prevention focus of the field (64 percent), the lifestyle (56 percent), opportunities to work on worker protection, worker training and education, and labor issues (53 percent), environmental health (44 percent), opportunities for consulting practice (44 percent), and interaction with the business world (43 percent). Physicians changing course in midcareer and those who entered the field over thirty years before do not necessarily lack training or competence. Some occupational physicians were highly trained and committed to the field beginning in the 1950s and 1960s. Within occupational medicine now, some prominent internists and occupational physicians in the field—most of them in academia—are trying to move the field into what they are calling clinical preventive medicine and to certify occupational medicine as a subspecialty of internal medicine.

45. The three subspecialties under the American Board of Preventive Medicine are occupational medicine, public health and general preventive medicine, and aerospace medicine. Some company physicians who entered the field with a public health orientation drew their early inspiration from pioneer Alice Hamilton, who came from a prosperous family and rejected a privileged life of leisure to go to work for better working conditions and the welfare of immigrant families (see Hamilton 1943).

46. However, physician researchers in universities, as well as university administrators and corporate donors, may view research into health hazards as politically unwise or as threatening to large corporate donors. They are also likely to encounter barriers to gaining access to records and employees in corporations.

47. The image and reputation of being an HMO doctor have also changed dramatically. Doctors who formerly derided the standard of care and working conditions in HMOs now view working in doctor-directed HMOs such as Kaiser Permanente as a good job. Those positions come with more freedom and fewer hassles than

private practice, and some even view them as the last bastion of private practice left in the country.

48. Within three years in the early 1990s, for example, four companies in the oil and chemical industries eliminated their corporate medical director (Unocal, Sun Petroleum, Tenneco, and Dow Chemical, which also eliminated its entire epidemiology department). Arco Petroleum lost its corporate medical director through attrition but replaced him, then later eliminated its medical department. Private groups of multi-clinics—such as HMOs and groups of one hundred physicians together providing multiple clinical services—now add occupational medicine services. Occupational services have grown recently in hospital-umbrellaed programs in stand-alone clinics, the hospital itself, or a multi-clinic setting of that hospital. These clinics usually have a financial arrangement with the hospitals that house them or helped finance setting them up, and they see occupational medicine as a draw to help fill the beds. Although occupational medicine clinics seek to fill their hospital beds, occupational medicine ideally should reduce the number of hospitalized people if it does its job. Some contracting or consulting firms are set up by medical directors or other experienced company physicians who are laid off and need work. For example, five corporate physicians from competing companies who anticipated that their companies' medical departments were likely to be severely cut got together to lay the groundwork for a new group medical practice. One of them worked for years setting up the new firm and targeting clients while still employed as a corporate medical director.

49. IBM, for example, had a huge medical structure of sixty to seventy physicians worldwide and a large hierarchy with a medical director, area and division medical directors, managing physicians, physician specialists, and staff physicians. Management had advocated full employment in the company—employees would always remain with the company if they did a good job—but then later concluded that too many medical services were offered on the inside and started contracting out more of those services. Other companies have moved from a medical model to a nurse-directed model with interdisciplinary health teams of employee assistants, counselors, nurse managers, sickness-absence disability managers, and health promotion managers. They tailor their services to the specific needs of particular business groups.

50. Bruce Karrh, physician at E. I. du Pont de Nemours and Company at the time of personal interview. As of March 2001, DuPont in the

United States employed full-time eight doctors, four physician's assistants, and eighty nurses. A physician in another company that
lost 90 percent of its full-time doctors in seven years—and was one
of only three full-time doctors remaining—said: "The company
supported broad health promotion when I got here. We are now
on the down side, cutting programs and saying, 'It was all well and
good then, but now we can't afford it anymore.'"

51. See Bluestone and Bluestone (1992) and Reissman et al. (1999) on
corporate management's and employees' responses to downsizing.
See also Galston (1996) on corporations' declining concern with
historic community ties.

52. Kaiser Permanente, for example, developed this specialty extensively. It collects employer reimbursement for work-related illness
in addition to its regular fees.

53. For example, between 1981 and 1984, after deregulation of the airline industry, most U.S.-based airlines either replaced their medical
departments with vendors or reduced their departments to one or
two physicians at a corporate level; then, from 1984 on, airlines
started to rebuild their medical departments.

CHAPTER 2

1. Divided loyalties for physicians serving their profession, workers,
and employers remain an active issue. The individual's role as a
doctor may in fact conflict with his or her position as a corporate
employee and manager. In addition, the ideal care of patients
clashes with legal and economic pressures, such as cost constraints,
new regulations, the threat of lawsuits, and corporate restructuring.
On the influence of nonmedical parties on doctors and health services more generally, see Mechanic (1976, 2000), Mintz and Palmer
(2000), Bergthold (1990), Rubin and Zoloth (2000), Sharpe and
Faden (1998), Mechanic and Schlesinger (1996), Stone (1986), Bosk
(1979), Katz (1999), Fuchs (1974), Zola (1983), Shrader-Frechette
(1991), and Reiser (1978).

2. For the ACOEM ethical code, see ACOEM (1994). ACOEM circulates
the ethics code and publishes it in its professional journal (*Journal
of Occupational and Environmental Medicine*) and elsewhere. The
ACOEM "Code of Ethical Conduct" states that each ACOEM member is expected to comply with it. It states that physicians should:
(1) accord the highest priority to the health and safety of individ-

uals in both the workplace and the environment; (2) practice on a scientific basis with integrity and strive to acquire and maintain adequate knowledge and expertise upon which to render professional service; (3) relate honestly and ethically in all professional relationships; (4) strive to expand and disseminate medical knowledge and participate in ethical research efforts as appropriate; (5) keep confidential all individual medical information, releasing such information only when required by law or overriding public health considerations, or to other physicians according to accepted medical practice, or to others at the request of the individual; (6) recognize that employers may be entitled to counsel about an individual's medical work fitness, but not to diagnoses or specific details, except in compliance with laws and regulations; (7) communicate to individuals and/or groups any significant observations and recommendations concerning their health or safety; and (8) recognize those medical impairments in oneself and others, including chemical dependency and abusive personal practices that interfere with one's ability to follow the above principles, and take appropriate measures (ACOEM 1994, 28).

3. As noted in note 2, doctors are to keep medical information confidential except as allowed by the law, overriding public health considerations, accepted medical practice, or individuals' permission to release information (ACOEM 1994, 28). The ethical code of occupational physicians, like that of many other professional groups, points us toward some of the important problems in the field. It also serves to remind physicians of the important ethical questions that remain unresolved. However, the ACOEM ethical code does not tell us much about the actual behavior of this professional group in view of the competing demands on occupational physicians that stem from management policies and laws affecting medical practice. Some occupational physicians and others have criticized the current 1993 ACOEM code of ethics as weaker than the 1976 version it replaced. For example, the Association of Occupational and Environmental Clinics board of directors, along with six physicians and scientists, criticized the 1993 ACOEM code for, among other things, failing to address avoidance of conflict of interest, the need for familiarity with workplace hazards, and the obligation to contact the scientific community and government agencies when workers' health is threatened, and for not actively opposing unethical conduct (Brodkin et al. 1998). Rothstein (1997b) proposed changing the ACOEM code to reintroduce elements of the 1976

code, arguing that the revised code demands too little of physicians in such areas as conflicts of interest, reporting unethical or incompetent colleagues, and confidentiality of medical information.

4. Although doctors can use the ethics code to justify their resistance to managers' demands for medical information, they do not routinely oppose management or use the code to articulate their reasons for doing so.

5. The *Journal of Occupational and Environmental Medicine* and other professional journals from time to time discuss the problem of conflicting loyalties for physicians who serve patients but also work for large corporations. They include periodic reminders to company doctors that their responsibility is to their patients and that general medical ethics principles of informed consent and confidentiality apply in corporations.

6. James Weeks, United Mine Workers of America, personal interview.

7. Dean Belk, physician at Aluminum Company of America at the time of personal interview.

8. Eric Frumin, Health and Safety Director, Union of Needletrades, Industrial and Textile Employees, personal interview.

9. OSHA standards are at 29 *Code of Federal Regulations,* sections 1910.1000–.1450 (2002); ADA rules are at 42 *United States Code,* sections 12101–12213 (2000); the ERISA rules that apply to employer-provided benefits, including health insurance and pensions, are at 29 *United States Code,* sections 1001–1461 (2000); and COBRA, which provides continuation of health insurance coverage to individuals who have left their job and would otherwise lose their employer-sponsored health benefits, appears at 29 *United States Code,* sections 1161–1168 (2000) and 42 *United States Code,* sections 300bb-1 to 300bb-8 (2000).

10. Women who favor the team player approach wear more standard business attire, with a white coat nowhere to be found.

11. MPH training also can be principally in administrative health services.

12. Bruce Karrh, vice president, Integrated Health Care, DuPont, at the time of personal interview. Karrh was indeed replaced by a non-physician when he retired, but as of 2001 DuPont's chief medical officer is a physician.

13. To a great extent, "networks" have replaced community and loyalty to an organization for professionals. Networks of professionals and managers—such as Reich's (1991) "symbolic analysts" and Lasch's (1979, 1994) upper-middle class—involve cross-cutting linkages that transcend geographical communities. These networks serve

elites well. They facilitate their influence while also increasing social polarization and contributing to the decline of community and
civic culture in the broader society. See also Osterman (1996), on
diminished expectations of security among managers, and Heckscher's (1995) account of the responses that middle managers and
human resources personnel have to restructuring and downsizing.

14. Similarly, the public commonly discounts the statements of company physicians who evaluate risks in the media—by appearing on
television, for instance. Although company managers may successfully affect the public perception of hazards by using company
doctors this way, companies may be shortsighted in using less credible spokespersons.

15. Bruce Karrh, physician at E. I. du Pont de Nemours and Company,
personal interview.

16. Comprehensive Environmental Response, Compensation, and Liability Act of 1980 (CERCLA), 42 *United States Code,* sections 9601–
9675 (2000).

17. The pharmaceutical company physician also said, "We use outside
consultants when we don't want to appear to be bought. We use
them to come in for problems, because then it doesn't look as
though it's all in-house and we're hiding anything."

18. Dean Belk, physician at Aluminum Company of America at the
time of personal interview.

19. The doctor went on to say: "Physicians are revered in this society
socially; that's what every mother's son is supposed to be, a doctor.
Suddenly you have this doctor who now just can't wait to become
one of us, which managers don't consider that wonderful—business isn't like a *physician,* with their high ideals and all that. So
they don't trust you anymore because you've abandoned what they
consider sacred ideals."

20. Lloyd Tepper, physician at Air Products and Chemicals Corporation, personal interview.

21. Although professionals blame themselves for their failure to market
themselves within the company, they also assist the company with
locating blame in employees, in part by screening workers and
eliminating those they deem "high-risk," as we shall see in chapters
5 and 6. Corporate professionals increasingly have become team
players who focus on employees' inappropriate lifestyles and individual risks rather than on workplace hazards such as asbestos.

22. Comparable to company physicians are engineers who have worked
on mainframe technology for years; if that is all they know, they
find themselves in trouble when they are laid off. Their engineering

skills have withered, and some find it impossible to change as networks come along.

23. Empowerment and participative management programs do not exist at most corporations.

24. Budrys (1997) examines the exceptions—physicians who join unions.

25. See ACOEM (1994) for ACOEM's code of ethics. ACOEM's ethics committee is charged with evaluating possible breaches of professional ethics. ACOEM physicians investigating charges of ethics violations sometimes cannot find anything specific in the code to address the violation, since the code is general. Still, they use the code as justification and usually identify specific sections to apply in evaluating a suspected violation.

26. The doctor on the committee went on to say: "I always feel you are known by the company you keep. It's easy for people to get into this organization to begin with, but once they are in and you tell them the rules you play by, then you're stuck if you can't get rid of the person who you find out didn't play by your rules. It's like being associated with criminals; I don't want to be known for associating with criminals. We should strive to have a purpose to this organization higher than a social function or providing a little education, such as it is."

27. Hallett Lewis, formerly physician at Kaiser Steel Corporation and Kaiser Industries Corporation, personal interview.

28. The physician went on to say: "I went to a private-practice session of ACOEM and was stunned by the breadth and depth of what I consider unethical practice. A vivid example I heard there was a doctor who could have told a company that wanted low-back X-rays for all employees coming in, 'The evidence is pretty clear now that giving X-rays does not help and probably harms patients because of the radiation dose.' But he went along with it and didn't say anything because he got money to do it and might have lost the client altogether if he had said no. He was willing to do something medically harmful to keep the client. That's pretty shocking, but he saw nothing wrong with it." Similarly, a chemical company physician who has also worked as a contract physician for corporations said: "The implication to the outside world of being employed by a corporation is that you are in somebody's back pocket. But I have *more* ethical challenges as a doctor doing occupational medicine for small businesses in an outside clinic than in corporate work. You want a little business and management pressures you at the clinic to do back X-rays to predict back injuries, and you tell them

that back films can't do that. They want lobotomies too. Where do you draw the line?"

29. Roy de Hart, director of occupational medicine at the University of Oklahoma, personal interview.

30. As with company doctors, U.S. corporations have reduced the number of middle managers, at times with little regard for an individual's services to the company.

31. Similarly, a metals company physician said, "One day a high-level manager said to me, 'We didn't have any problems until you came around.' I was regarded as the guy who went around and found problems." James Hughes, physician who worked for Kaiser Aluminum Corporation and Kaiser Industries, personal interview.

32. For example, occupational medical journals and professional societies have grown substantially since the 1950s, with greater professional participation by company doctors.

CHAPTER 3

1. Dean Belk, physician at Aluminum Company of America, personal interview.

2. James Weeks, United Mine Workers of America, personal interview.

3. For discussion of multiple chemical sensitivity (MCS) and psychological explanations of symptoms, see Cullen and Kreiss (2000), Ducatman (1998), and Sparks et al. (1994). In 1999 ACOEM characterized MCS as a controversial designation that should not be defined as a distinct entity because evidence does not exist to support it. The American Medical Association's 1992 council report on MCS stated that no well-controlled studies establishing a clear causal mechanism exist and that the efficacy of the diagnostic and therapeutic modalities have not been confirmed (AMA Council on Scientific Affairs 1992). For a parallel argument on musculoskeletal disorders, see Hadler (2000), who maintains that psychosocial factors such as low job satisfaction and inability to cope with pain are more important than workplace biomechanical hazards in producing reports of prolonged musculoskeletal symptoms. He uses these arguments to oppose tighter OSHA ergonomics regulations. See Punnett (2000) for a contrasting view that work-related musculoskeletal disorders that are causally related to preventable, physical ergonomic stressors in the work environment occur with high frequency. Punnett concludes that the epidemiologic evidence linking physical ergonomic workplace exposures with musculoskeletal dis-

orders is extensive and methodologically adequate to inform primary prevention and justify stricter OSHA ergonomic regulation.

4. Robert Larson, physician who evaluates employees for employers, personal interview.

5. Eric Frumin, Health and Safety Director, Union of Needletrades, Industrial and Textile Employees, personal interview.

6. Lloyd Tepper, physician at Air Products and Chemicals Corporation, personal interview.

7. Michael Wright, United Steelworkers of America, personal interview. He added: "It happens more often in unorganized workplaces than in organized workplaces, but it's not rare." Another labor official, a former smelter worker, described a company doctor's role in providing a health justification for removing him for reasons unrelated to his health: "I worked as a smelter worker on staff with the union, and I had open-heart surgery while I was on leave of absence from the plant. That company would have poisoned me with arsenic if they could have. The company canceled my leave of absence and said that the only way they could sustain my medical benefits was if I retired immediately. They decided that I had to see their company physician, who just signed the forms without examining me, without even asking what the blood values were, without asking *anything,* and they officially retired me from that company. They just didn't want me back on their property for any reason. Their getting rid of me entirely had to do with my political activities and had nothing to do with my health." Paul Falkowski, United Steelworkers of America, personal interview.

8. Michael Wright, United Steelworkers of America, personal interview.

9. Albert Ackroyd, physician at Northrop, personal interview.

10. The doctor went on to say: "Doctors are supposed to take responsibility. If you give somebody a medication and let him jump in his car and drive home, you must be confident he can do it. We say, 'Put it down for all to see.'"

11. The physician went on to say: "I help executives get through the health-care system and choose specialists for them or their families, serving as their advocate in getting what they want done in the medical arena as efficiently and expertly as possible. I'd like to get it up on the table with my management; I'd say, 'Look, it's 20 or 30 percent of my time, so if you want me to take care of all the health needs of our senior executives, their spouses, and their children, let's talk about it honestly.' They can't talk about it honestly, because some benefits laws prohibit giving excessive benefit perks to

executives. They're nervous about formalizing that as a function even though we all know that executives in this country get all sorts of benefits and perks, including health benefits."

CHAPTER 4

1. Difficult economic conditions, increased competition, and a more conservative political climate tend to diminish attention to toxics. Cost containment in occupational medicine gets more attention in such times. Workplace health hazards have become a major problem, with about 500,000 new cases of occupational disease and 100,000 deaths in the United States each year. In 1995 employers reported 495,000 new cases of occupational disease and 6.6 million work injuries (U.S. Department of Labor 1997). Toxic exposures are not limited to large corporations, but less scientific and public attention goes to hazards in smaller firms. Medium-size and small companies typically do not have in-house doctors to deal with hazards, and many believe that they cannot afford to hire outside doctors.

2. Hallett Lewis, physician at Kaiser Steel Corporation and Kaiser Industries Corporation, personal interview.

3. Only a fraction of occupational disease is diagnosed as work-related. Primary-care physicians fail to identify illnesses as work-related partly because they do not ask about workplace exposures and are not trained to link disease to work. (On history-taking by primary-care physicians, see Thompson et al. 2000.) Company physicians may uncover hazards through blood tests and other physical examinations, while safety and industrial hygiene units routinely monitor hazards, but they fail to identify many cases of occupational disease as such (Boden 2000).

4. The physician added, "Some of it is perhaps out of laziness, because raising an issue tends to make more work. That's perhaps the biggest reason that some people say that." The organizational, political, and economic pressures on physicians not to focus on workplace exposure hazards are more important, however, than personality characteristics such as laziness in explaining why physicians do not draw attention to such hazards.

5. The physician went on to say: "You have to go to management as not a joker or a panicking person but as somebody who knows what you're talking about. They have to know you're a solid citizen

who means business and isn't just agitating a scarecrow, if you tell them, 'Listen, you're heading for big trouble.'"

6. For example, a company's infection control program under OSHA's blood-borne pathogens standard is not properly constructed if physicians are not responsible for it. 29 *Code of Federal Regulations,* section 1910.1030 (2002).

7. Cigarette smoke is an easy explanation if employees have chronic bronchitis or emphysema, for example, but chemicals can also cause those diseases, and physicians will not recognize chemical hazards as the cause unless they investigate them. Some sophisticated large chemical companies understand the work environment better because they have a staff of physicians, toxicologists, and industrial hygienists, along with greater scientific capabilities. However, most companies hire doctors who know little about the production process and plant environment. For example, small clinics that contract to provide health services often have little or no training in how to interpret job descriptions or determine the value of health-surveillance programs. They look for pathology in laboratory results or physical examinations, whereas surveillance programs could reveal disease trends rather than simply pathology.

8. Eric Frumin, Health and Safety Director, Union of Needletrades, Industrial and Textile Employees, personal interview. Another labor official stated: "Physicians in this country are ignorant about occupational medicine. I am concerned about the lack of knowledge, caring, and interest of many physicians who end up working for corporations. It's a fifty-year-old mentality of dealing with accidents and not diseases. I typically send workers to see about one hundred board-certified occupational health physicians and another one hundred physicians from various specialties because I believe they are competent and give workers a fair shake and speak in English and give them information."

9. Similarly, an OSHA doctor said: "Sometimes a physician is an auxiliary called in from a local university or some place close by to come sign papers, and that of course is not adequate. Too many physicians still are just not qualified to do this kind of work, and they don't get involved in fieldwork, even in their own companies."

10. Melena Barkman, an occupational health nurse with the United Steelworkers of America and assistant director of the union's Health, Safety, and Environment Department, said: "Typically smaller companies get a local doctor to come into their dispensary for workers' comp and emergency first-aid one or two days every week or every month, or just send their workers to his office; 95

percent of the time, in our experience, that doctor has never toured that plant and doesn't understand the circumstances they work under. Companies typically prefer to deny that health issues even exist because they don't want to get into compensation. It's a bad setup, but it's even worse from a contractor, who is less likely to be able to deal with any occupational health problems." Primary-care physicians are untrained in occupational medicine and do not practice medicine in the work environment, yet they deliver most of the health care provided to U.S. workers and do so without any real knowledge of the work environment. Based on their analysis of 4,261 industrial facilities in NIOSH's National Occupational Exposure Survey, Pedersen, Venable, and Sieber (1990) found that off-site physicians providing occupational medicine services to companies under contract conduct far fewer screening tests and medical exams and engage in less extensive and continuous record keeping than physicians in on-site occupational medicine programs. For example, off-site physicians are considerably less likely than on-site physicians to conduct blood, urine, and pulmonary tests, radiography exams, and post-illness exams. (Pedersen and his colleagues define as "on-site physicians" both corporate employees and contract physicians who conduct their practices at the work site; "off-site physicians" have a contractual relationship with management and provide their services at off-site locations or travel to the facility intermittently on an on-call basis, only upon specific request.)

11. Former medical directors with experience designing and monitoring occupational health programs also provide contract services. Contract services are bifurcated. Services by laid-off in-house doctors with expertise in occupational medicine and by board-certified or otherwise highly trained new occupational medicine professionals differ from those of contractors with little knowledge of workplace health. Contract services provided from outside the corporation may give superior care and more professional services in some arenas in that they may be connected with hospitals and less under the control of plant managers.

12. When companies cut back on in-house doctors, they usually retain nurses to conduct tests and supervise first aid.

13. He added: "The happiest corporate physicians I've ever met simply defer everything to their nurses. Nurses who don't know their limitations go until they make mistakes that others must straighten out."

14. For example, ACOEM coordinates the educational efforts of the organization's physicians with those of occupational health nurses,

holds its annual spring meeting in conjunction with that of the American Association of Occupational Health Nurses, and holds training seminars jointly with that organization.

15. He went on to say: "We had an ACOEM president who wanted to have the doctors meet alone, but the nurses were furious with his proposal, and the ACOEM president got no support from his physician colleagues in ACOEM for it. It's a sensitive topic."

16. On nurses, see Chambliss (1996), who describes nurses working in hospitals who occasionally advocate strongly for patients or come into conflict with doctors or administrators over patients. Often they say they know what should be done but do not have the power to do it when others object. Nurses routinely juggle patient needs with the demands of doctors, families, administrators, and the law. Anspach (1993) and Zussman (1992) find in their studies of intensive-care nurseries that the nurses caring for chronically ill infants—who spend more time with these infants than the physicians do—are more willing to withdraw treatment than are the doctors.

17. For cancer incidence, estimates of the proportion due to work exposures range from less than 1 percent to 40 percent (see Garte 1998; Ducatman 1993; Draper 1993b). Estimates of cancer causation are an example of the effect of social location on people's perspective toward medical information concerns. The epidemiological and other evidence linking disease to work exposure is complex and equivocal. Methods for establishing occupational causality vary widely. In the current climate of scientific uncertainty, social actors believe different estimates. In general, corporate officials maintain that chemical risks are less extensive and dangerous than does the public, and company physicians generally find work-related disease to be a less significant concern than do university research scientists. See Engelhardt and Caplan (1987), Beryllium Industry Scientific Advisory Committee (1997), Lynn (1986), and Epstein (1979), who discusses corporate efforts to show that a small proportion of cancer cases are due to toxic chemicals found in the workplace. See Frumkin and Thun (2000) for a discussion of animal testing in the study of carcinogenesis.

18. Robert Larson, physician who performs examinations and evaluations of employees for corporate employers and other clients, personal interview. See Ducatman (1998) for a discussion of the literature on multiple chemical sensitivity.

19. Private practitioners who treat employees also report fewer company health hazards when they see the minimal compensation in-

volved with reporting symptoms as work-related and billing workers' compensation as not worth the time and aggravation involved.

20. About another company, this physician said: "This preposterous safety record of [the chemical company] that no one can believe, including every professional in the world, can only be explained by fudging the numbers."

21. Doctors frequently complain that they do not get the ear of the top executives or gain access to information about the planned production of new products. Whether management consults them generally depends on employers' relationship with their professionals and employers' experience with doctors handling previous problems. In the case of Rockwell, the Environmental Protection Agency found the company guilty in courts of law and imposed on them the largest corporate fine in history for environmental damages: $19 million for their role in the Rocky Flats land and groundwater pollution in Colorado. Physicians obviously were unable to prevent this environmental and occupational health catastrophe. High rates of chronic beryllium disease have been identified among the more than 7,500 current and former workers screened at the Rocky Flats Environmental Technology site, which had been a nuclear weapons production facility. For a discussion of community responses to the pollution and health hazards, see Lodwick (1993).

22. Various laws and penalties make trying to hide information potentially costly. Examples are OSHA rules covering hazard communication and access to employee exposure and medical records (29 *Code of Federal Regulations,* sections 1910.1200 and 1910.1020 [2002]). Under the Toxic Substances Control Act (15 *United States Code,* sections 2601–2692 [2000]), employers must put new information that is reportable as a significant adverse effect on their material safety data sheets within sixty days. Significant penalties attach to missing those deadlines. Managers are generally aware of these disclosure obligations, whether or not they agree with them. In addition, failure to warn is a common tort claim that propels employers at times to share adverse information with their employees and send letters about risks to their customers and suppliers. On government regulation and tort claims, see Howard (1998), Ashford (2000), and Rothstein (1994).

23. Lloyd Tepper, physician at Air Products and Chemicals Corporation, personal interview.

24. Lloyd Tepper, physician at Air Products and Chemicals Corporation, personal interview.

25. Exceptions are medical directors of Monsanto Chemical and Du-Pont, among others, who have spoken to the public extensively.

26. The threat of lawsuits in the area of asbestos certainly has done much to change attitudes about what kinds of medical services and preventive measures are necessary. Other areas of litigation with similar effects as asbestos are benzene and leukemia, lead-based paint and central nervous system damage, and polychlorinated biphenyls (PCBs). The Johnson Controls Supreme Court decision also effected change in the area of reproductive hazards (International Union, UAW v. Johnson Controls, 499 U.S. 187 [1991]).

27. For a discussion of the Santa Barbara oil spills and related social and legal developments, see Freudenburg and Gramling (1994) and Molotch (1970). The "Superfund" act is the Comprehensive Environmental Response, Compensation, and Liability Act of 1980 (42 *United States Code*, sections 9601–9675 [2000]). It is broadly concerned with the cleanup of hazardous substances in the environment; its main focus is on removing hazardous waste and remediating waste sites. When Congress passed the Superfund Amendments and Reauthorization Act in 1986, it replenished the original $1.6 billion fund with $8.5 billion and generally tightened regulations directed toward cleaning up waste sites. For a discussion of the initial Superfund and subsequent legal developments, see Boston and Madden (1994, 475–526). On issues of race and social inequality concerning environmental hazards, see Bullard (2000), Stretesky and Hogan (1998), Kamieniecki and Steckenrider (1997), and Bryant and Mohai (1992). The National Environmental Policy Act appears at 42 *United States Code*, sections 4321–4370 (2000). See Melius (1998) for a discussion of the Bhopal catastrophe, in which the release from a chemical plant of over thirty tons of methyl isocyanate and other chemicals into the air killed thousands and injured hundreds of thousands of others.

28. High disease risks from asbestos exposure confront employees working in asbestos manufacture as well as in jobs cleaning asbestos brake linings or restructuring buildings with asbestos in them. See Rom (1998a) and Collegium Ramazzini (1999) for a discussion of asbestos-related disease.

29. For example, Brodeur (1985) discusses Raybestos Manhattan's and Manville's early knowledge of asbestos hazards in the 1930s and 1940s. Castleman (1996) also discusses the asbestos controversy, legal and scientific disputes, and efforts by employers and company physicians to withhold risk information from employees and the public beginning in the 1930s.

30. Irving Selikoff was a pulmonary physician who found his first cases of asbestos diseases among his patients in Paterson, New Jersey. He identified many cases of lung disease among asbestos-insulation workers from a factory near the community clinic he operated and established a pattern of disease. His study began, not when he drew associations after coming across them individually, as doctors would usually do with patients in their sixties, but when a cohort of workers approached him, suspecting that asbestos was making them sick. In 1963 he gave pulmonary function tests, blood tests, and X-ray exams to 1,117 asbestos-insulation workers in two union locals and asked them about their working conditions. He found evidence of asbestosis in half of them, and he found that the extent of damage was strongly correlated with the duration of exposure.

31. Eric Frumin, Health and Safety Director, Union of Needletrades, Industrial and Textile Employees, personal interview.

32. Anthony Mazzocchi, Oil, Chemical, and Atomic Workers International Union, personal interview. Similarly, a university occupational physician said: "Manville, which had a plant in New Hampshire, hired a physician to work for them whose main job was to talk widows out of autopsies. The physicians were supposed to tell the widows how mutilating autopsies were and that they shouldn't let their husbands go through this process—presumably to keep the lungs from being looked at to find out the real cause of death."

33. The physician went on to say: "Employers and the EPA will walk away from its sites requiring cleanups because risk analysis makes hazards look trivial. On the other hand, you can make risk analysis sell things. If you want to sell incinerators to neighborhoods, risk analysis can lessen the objection to the incinerator by showing that the smoke is one one-millionth as dangerous as not wearing your seat belt."

34. An example comes from the industry making vinyl chloride, whose management told employees it would cause manufacturers to go out of business and cost workers thousands of jobs if exposure standards were tightened. After prolonged controversy over standard setting, OSHA reduced the workplace maximum exposure level dramatically (to one part per million [ppm] parts air, averaged over an eight-hour period, falling from 250 ppm in 1971). Nevertheless, the industry continued to do well and even profited from adhering to a tighter standard and capturing emissions that previously had escaped into the atmosphere. Companies that do not wait to clean up until too much damage is done—that do not resign themselves to remedial action after substantial health effects

occur—could have similar outcomes. On vinyl chloride effects as well as company and government responses, see Brown (1992). The vinyl chloride OSHA standard is at 29 *Code of Federal Regulations,* section 1910.1017 (2002).

35.   On the social and political factors contributing to health-related scientific controversies, see Caplan (1995), Dembe (1996), Shrader-Frechette (1995), Short (1994), Sheehan and Wedeen (1993), Cook-Deegan (1994), Epstein (1996), Gusterson (1996), Bayer (1993), Slovic, Flynn, and Layman (1991), Salter (1988), and Tesh (1988). A university occupational physician described corporate physicians' concern with the potential costs to management of a physician's findings: "We had just finished doing a study showing acute, measurable effects on pulmonary function at fairly low exposure levels, and I presented the results at a meeting on the health effects of isocyanates, sponsored by the federal government. A medical director from a big chemical company came up after my presentation and seemed very angry. He said, 'Do you realize that what you're doing could cost American industry millions of dollars? This could be very expensive if you're right.' That surprised me, because I thought I had presented some interesting findings and everybody would do what they could to pursue it. The corporate medical people did not react that way. That experience certainly woke me up to the way the world works."

36.   The physician and *Journal* editor went on to say: "I might feel I have to do the author a favor if it's a friend or somebody I know, so I could just pick two reviewers whose opinion I know and get the answer I want. I've done test runs. I'll take a paper on one side of a controversy and send a copy to each side. One side says, 'Oh, this stinks and should never be published—all these methodological flaws and the data don't warrant the conclusions,' and the person from the other side says, 'This is the best thing that's ever been done.'"

37.   One such organization is the International Agency for Research on Cancer (IARC) of the World Health Organization (WHO), which publishes the *IARC Monographs on the Evaluation of Carcinogenic Risks to Humans.* For each volume of the *Monographs,* an international and interdisciplinary working group of about twenty individuals with expertise relevant to the topic under consideration meets in Lyon, France, to finalize the text and evaluation of the agent or process under consideration. Another organization that publishes documents on the carcinogenicity of substances is the American Conference of Governmental Industrial Hygienists (ACGIH). Physi-

cians are on the ACGIH threshold limit values (TLV) committees—some from corporations. Critics of the TLV process and standards maintain that the heavy influence of corporate participants in the process undermines the credibility of the resulting standards. Watterson (1993) reports that the manufacturers ICI, DuPont, and Hoechst wrote the first drafts of the International Program on Chemical Safety (IPCS) reports on chlorofluorocarbon refrigerants and the fungicide benomyl. (The IPCS in Geneva is jointly sponsored by the World Health Organization, the International Labor Office [ILO], and the United Nations Environmental Program.) Watterson identifies the conflicts of interest of the corporate consultants on expert task groups assigned to write IPCS documents. He states that industry representatives at IPCS task meetings rarely were balanced by representatives from organizations outside industry or government. Castleman and Lemen (1998) describe the substantial influence of corporate representatives on ILO and WHO bodies that write reports about toxic substances. They describe efforts by corporate interests to influence ILO reports on asbestos and argue that such efforts undermine the technical quality and scientific objectivity of the resulting international reports. LaDou (1998) describes the ties between the asbestos industry and the International Commission on Occupational Health (ICOH), an organization that plays an important role in developing scientific documents and policy recommendations on asbestos and other materials.

38. For insightful discussion of scientific controversies and the social context of knowledge construction, see Kuhn (1964), Berger and Luckmann (1966), Merton (1973), Mannheim (1952), Cozzens and Gieryn (1990), Clarke and Fujimura (1992), Knorr-Cetina and Mulkay (1983), and Nelkin (1992).

39. ACOEM is growing, largely because of new members from private clinics outside of corporations rather than from in-house programs. ACOEM's business, legal, and basic science concerns have changed along with its membership, taking the organization even further from its earlier days as the American Association of Physicians and Surgeons in Industry, and then the Industrial Medicine Association, an era when physician members more often focused on treating industrial accidents.

40. Bruce Karrh, physician at E. I. du Pont de Nemours and Company at the time of personal interview.

41. The physician added: "Our profession said, 'If public health people won't pick up on this big field of environmental medicine because they are still too busy immunizing people and checking people for

tuberculosis and AIDS, all of which are extremely important, then maybe our field is the logical profession to jump into that.' I worry that workers will get the short end of the stick as we chase all these chemicals in the environment, some of which are probably important."

CHAPTER 5

1. Sheldon Samuels, director of health, safety, and environment at the AFL-CIO Industrial Union Department at the time of personal interview (currently director of the Ramazzini Institute for Occupational and Environmental Health Research).

2. Company employee assistance programs started dealing with drug dependency and alcoholism in the 1970s, then broadened to encompass other factors affecting worker health and productivity, such as depression and family problems. Many companies offered incentive plans for wellness, such as additional benefits if employees stopped smoking or lowered their cholesterol levels. Other companies established fitness facilities and no-smoking policies. See Ducatman and McLellan (2000), Aldana and Pronk (2001), and Erfurt, Foote, and Heirich (1991).

3. The Drug-Free Workplace Act of 1988 requires any company with a federal contract or grant of $100,000 or more to agree to provide a drug-free workplace (41 *United States Code,* sections 701–707 (2000). It requires contractors and grantees to have a written substance abuse policy, but it does not require drug testing. Transportation companies do extensive random drug testing of workers covered by DOT rules. Most large companies I examined in my research on workplace medicine test all new employees who are provisionally offered a job, pending the drug test results. The American Management Association (2001, 4) found that 79.7 percent of the 1,627 corporations it surveyed conduct the same tests on all job applicants.

4. Sixty-one percent of the surveyed companies test all new hires for drugs in preplacement exams. The AMA analyzed surveys from 19 percent (1,627) of its 8,500 U.S. corporate members, which are relatively large firms that together employ one-quarter of the U.S. workforce. (The AMA sent the survey to human resources managers in AMA member and client companies, which are half in manufacturing and half in services.) The proportion of companies conducting drug testing rose in its annual surveys from 21.5 percent

in 1987 to 81.1 percent in 1996, then fell gradually to 66 percent in 2000. Companies reported a positive test rate in 1995 of 4.0 percent among new hires and 1.9 percent among current employees. The AMA (1996, 7) stated: "Drug testing, where utilized, ought to be part of a comprehensive policy on workplace drug abuse that includes education, supervisory training, and opportunities for counselling and treatment."

5. See, for example, Loder v. City of Glendale, 14 Cal. 4th 846 (1997). See also Willborn, Schwab, and Burton (1993, 175–98).

6. Federal agencies have established regulations for antidrug programs, including the Nuclear Regulatory Commission, the National Aeronautics and Space Administration (NASA), and the Departments of Defense, Energy, and Transportation. The California constitution does not permit random testing beyond what is required by federal law or by a compelling employer interest, but random testing programs outside of California typically apply either to everybody in the company or to people in safety-sensitive jobs, as defined by the DOD and DOT. See Wolkinson and Block (1996, 287–307); see also Loder v. City of Glendale, 14 Cal. 4th 846 (1997).

7. From 1989 to 1995 the positive test rate of companies that routinely test job applicants and use for-cause testing fell from 8.1 percent to 1.9 percent (American Management Association 1996, 2–3). I discuss reasons for the decline later in the chapter.

8. See, for example, "Drug Testing: Cost and Effect: Cornell/Smithers Report on Workplace Substance Abuse Policy (1992)," in Willborn, Schwab, and Burton (1993, 195–99) and Marshman (1994, 143–60).

9. The physician went on to say: "I figured out last year it cost us $5,000 to discover each positive. I brought it to their attention, and they said, 'Oh, still, it's better that we don't have them in the workforce.' Okay, I did my job."

10. Lloyd Tepper, physician at Air Products and Chemicals Corporation, personal interview.

11. Aside from their concern about deterring drug users from applying for jobs at their own company, some employers are on the moral bandwagon of using workplace testing to stop drug abuse in the country. For a related discussion of the molecular biological bandwagon in cancer research, see Fujimura (1996).

12. The medical division must be involved in drug testing that the DOT and NRC require because regulations specify that the medical review officer who judges positive test results must be a physician. For example, the NRC's fitness-for-duty rule requires that an MRO be a "licensed physician . . . who has knowledge of substance

abuse disorders and has appropriate medical training to interpret and evaluate an individual's positive test result together with his or her medical history and any other relevant biomedical information." 10 *Code of Federal Regulations,* section 26.3 (2002).

13. See, for example, ACOEM's (then ACOM) ethical guidelines on workplace drug screening, which recommend that MROs be licensed physicians (ACOM 1991, 652); see also Swotinsky and Chase (1990). ACOEM has also promoted drug-testing courses for its member physicians.

14. Under California law, for example, employee intoxication is an affirmative defense in workers' compensation cases, thus creating an incentive for employers to perform tests whenever a worker is injured. See California's workers' compensation statute, which specifies that the employer is not liable for compensation when the employee's injury is caused by the employee's intoxication "by alcohol or the unlawful use of a controlled substance." *California Labor Code,* section 3600(a)(4) (West, 2002).

15. Some employers also use psychological testing to detect drug abuse, reduce theft and absenteeism, or dismiss workers' complaints of medical symptoms of chemical exposures as merely "psychogenic illness," even though psychological test results are of uncertain value for identifying accident-prone or expensive employees. Employers who want to avoid workers with schizophrenia, depression, or other mental and emotional disorders are subject to the restrictions of the Americans with Disabilities Act. The employer must reasonably accommodate disabled workers. However, the ADA generally permits preplacement drug screening. 42 *United States Code,* section 12210 (2000).

16. The next chapter considers a parallel process by which company physicians and employers create company programs to target employee stress but pay insufficient attention to the working conditions that contribute to employee stress.

17. Durbin and Grant (1996, ch. 3:23) conclude from their review of the technical findings and survey data on drug and alcohol use: "Despite the popular attention paid to illegal drugs, alcohol clearly remains the most commonly used, and abused, mind-altering drug in America. This is true for both the general population and employed workers. Survey findings show that while illegal drug use has declined among the general population over the past decade, heavy alcohol use has remained stable."

18. Analyses of workplace fatalities find a minor contribution of non-alcoholic drugs to accidents and fatalities. Alcohol is associated with a significant minority. See Martin, Kraft, and Roman (1994, 6–

7), Durbin and Grant (1996, 3.1–3.29), and Macdonald and Wells (1994, 139), who conclude that "too few empirical studies on the effectiveness of drug screening programs exist at this time to prove that programs are effective in reducing drug use among employees, accidents, and performance problems in the workplace, or drug problems in society as a whole."

19. Eric Frumin, Health and Safety Director, Union of Needletrades, Industrial and Textile Employees, personal interview.

20. Michael Wright, United Steelworkers of America, personal interview.

21. For example, if employees took a drug during their vacation, the drug might show up in tests yet may not affect performance on the job. The surveillance period for workplace drug testing using hair analysis is typically the most recent ninety days (four centimeters of hair growth), so hair testing can identify about seven times more drug users than urinalysis and drug users are far less likely to evade a positive test result by temporarily abstaining.

22. In contrast, HIV testing in private practice is both a diagnostic and a *preventive* tool that educates those who do not know they are infected so they will not pass AIDS on to others.

23. Many companies offer an employee assistance program for employees with drug problems. See Shain (1994, 260–68) and Normand, Lempert, and O'Brien (1994, 241–68). Chapters 6 and 7 discuss EAP programs further.

24. The company has since initiated a random drug-testing program. This physician reported that "there's been very little negative comment regarding it. I don't interpret that for a minute to mean that people love it or accept it or think it's great, but they just realize that this is the way things are, and very few people challenge it."

25. For example, see Gilliam (1994), who found that two-thirds of the union-member respondents to a mail survey opposed random drug testing; see also Alvi (1994), OCAW (1991), and United Steelworkers of America (1991). Unions have been more favorable toward drug testing for cause and for dangerous jobs than toward random drug testing.

26. Anthony Mazzocchi, Oil, Chemical, and Atomic Workers International Union, personal interview.

27. For discussion of the law applying to employer drug testing, see Wolkinson and Block (1996, 287–307) and Lieberwitz (1994, 185–203); see also Loder v. City of Glendale, 14 Cal. 4th 846 (1997).

28. The American Management Association (1996, 7), then representing 9,500 U.S. corporations, stated that data "support, most emphatically, the deterrent effect of drug education and awareness pro-

grams, supervisory training, and employee assistance programs. . . . Testing cannot and should not be expected to take the place of good supervision and management practices."

29. See, for example, Pelletier et al. (1999), Shain (1994, 257–74), Blum (1994, 279–300), and Macdonald and Roman (1994).

CHAPTER 6

1. The American Management Association (2001, 1) reported recently that 68 percent of major U.S. firms—and 82 percent of U.S. manufacturing firms—require medical exams for new hires, current employees, or both. Of the firms surveyed by the AMA (69.3 percent of manufacturing firms), 51.7 percent require medical tests for all newly hired personnel and an additional 13.6 percent (9.6 percent of manufacturing firms) test new hires in selected job categories. For current employees, 5.7 percent of firms (7.1 percent in manufacturing firms) report that all employees are subject to periodic medical exams, and another 28.5 percent (31.2 percent in manufacturing firms) require periodic exams of employees in selected job categories. Testing is most common among manufacturers and least common among providers of business, professional, and financial services. In addition to these regularly scheduled exams for employees, 45 percent of firms require unscheduled exams when the employer maintains that job performance suggests a medical problem, and 18 percent conduct random exams, usually as part of a workplace drug-testing program.

2. Americans with Disabilities Act of 1990, 42 *United States Code,* sections 12101–12213 (2000); International Union, UAW v. Johnson Controls, Inc., 499 U.S. 187 (1991). Fetal exclusion policies are discussed later in this chapter, in the section on Reproductive Risk.

3. Employers have used the ability to screen workers as a justification for potentially harmful exposures. An example of a problematic screening approach concerns the risks of cotton dust, which is regulated as a hazardous substance (29 *Code of Federal Regulations,* section 1910.1043 [2002]). Company officials have stated that only a small proportion of the workforce is vulnerable to cotton dust and should therefore be screened out of jobs in which they would be exposed to it. This claim that almost all workers are safe when exposed to cotton dust, and that therefore no real need to monitor the substance exists, contributes to companies' interest in screening out certain workers as high-risk.

4. Genetic monitoring involves periodic employee testing to detect possible genetic damage over time from exposure to toxic substances. It works the opposite way from genetic screening and therefore tends to be more useful to employees than to applicants. Monitoring can benefit incumbent employees by detecting genetic abnormalities that may indicate exposure hazards to employed populations, whereas job applicants and new hires have a minimal interest in such tests, except for gathering baseline data to compare with later alterations in their genes. Genetic monitoring thus undermines the notion that employee testing is more pernicious than applicant testing and that employees therefore need greater protection. Monitoring information generally is used as evidence of chemical damage to groups of workers rather than as the basis for excluding individuals based on their genetic makeup and presumed predisposition to disease. An example of the screening and monitoring approaches is the contrast between types of genetic testing. Employers have supported genetic screening in which individuals are screened—usually once—to see whether they have a genetic susceptibility to disease. In contrast, workers and union representatives tend to favor ongoing genetic monitoring, which involves periodically testing groups of people to detect damage over time from workplace exposures. Monitoring tends to support reducing exposure levels rather than removing individuals from the environment; see Andrews, Mehlman, and Rothstein (1994) and Draper (1991). The occupational medicine core disciplines that have dominated the field over the past twenty years deal with toxic chemicals and focus on monitoring rather than screening: toxicology, industrial hygiene, and epidemiology.
5. For example, physicians, scientists, and workers who have opposed companies' screening programs have tended to favor testing used to detect chemical damage to workers rather than to exclude individuals or locate risk in workers' own susceptibility to disease.
6. Doctors and managers claim that a low proportion of workers' illness, reproductive failure, and cancer is occupationally related; see, for example, U.S. Congress, Office of Technology Assessment (1990a) and Draper (1991). Unions that have taken positions on genetic testing have generally opposed it, although this is not universally true. Unions have favored genetic monitoring to detect environmental hazards in specific workplaces, while opposing genetic screening for predisposing inherited traits. On competing conceptions of risk more generally, see Vaughan (1996), Clarke (1989, 1999), Perrow (1984), Douglas (1992), Cutter (1994), Freudenburg

(1993), Stallings (1995), Dunlap, Kraft, and Rosa (1993), Dietz and Rycroft (1987), Fischhoff et al. (1981), Kroll-Smith and Couch (1990), Edelstein (1988), and Roberts (1993).

7. Self-insured employers have a particularly strong incentive to reduce their financial risk by identifying high-risk employees. They thus can save medical expenses while (under the Employee Retirement Income Security Act of 1974) avoiding state laws designed to ensure adequate health insurance for employees (for ERISA rules, see 29 *United States Code,* sections 1001–1461 [2002]). See also Ostrer et al. (1993) and Rosenblatt, Law, and Rosenbaum (1997, 159–292, 1001–37).

8. Chapter 8 and the section here on "Social Stratification and Discrimination" discuss legal constraints on screening.

9. Employers and occupational physicians have recommended that employees be tested for a CBD genetic susceptibility marker (Glu-69). Beryllium was also used in making fluorescent lights until the 1950s, when recognition of the health hazards led to discontinuation of its use for that purpose. See also the debate in the *Journal of Occupational and Environmental Medicine* over whether beryllium causes lung cancer: the *JOEM* editorial by Vainio and Rice (1997) defends the International Agency for Research on Cancer report (IARC 1993) classifying beryllium and beryllium compounds as a human carcinogen, and the beryllium industry article (Beryllium Industry Scientific Advisory Committee 1997) criticizes the IARC report and argues that confounding factors of smoking and sulfuric acid exposure undermine the epidemiologic evidence linking workplace beryllium exposure to lung cancer.

10. Of the 1,627 corporations the American Management Association surveyed (2001, 2): (1) 14.3 percent test for "*susceptibility to workplace hazards*" (11.9 percent test new hires and 9.8 percent test employees), 8.7 percent use the test results for hiring job applicants, 8.2 percent use the results to assign or reassign employees, and 2.8 percent use them to dismiss or retain employees; (2) 2.9 percent test for *breast or colon cancer* (0.8 percent test new hires and 2.7 percent test employees), 0.4 percent use the test results for hiring job applicants, 0.6 percent use the results to assign or reassign employees, and 0.2 percent use them to dismiss or retain employees; (3) 1.3 percent test for *sickle cell anemia* (1.0 percent test new hires and 0.8 percent test employees), 0.6 percent use the test results for hiring job applicants, 0.4 percent use the results to assign or reassign employees, and 0.1 percent use them to dismiss or retain employees; (4) 0.4 percent test for *Huntington's disease* (0.2 percent test new hires and 0.4 percent test employees), 0.3 percent use the

test results for hiring job applicants, 0.5 percent use the results to assign or reassign employees, and 0.1 percent use them to dismiss or retain employees; and (5) 20.1 percent collect *family medical histories* (16.8 percent test new hires and 9.7 percent test employees), 4.6 percent use the test results for hiring job applicants, 1.4 percent use the results to assign or reassign employees, and 0.6 percent use them to dismiss or retain employees. In addition, 2.2 percent of the corporations test for HIV infection ("AIDS" testing), 1.5 percent test for sexually transmitted disease, and 0.8 percent test for pregnancy. In its 2001 survey, the AMA was told by two large corporations that they practiced genetic testing (compared with seven in 2000), according to the definition the AMA provided. ("The analysis of human DNA, RNA, chromosomes, proteins, and certain metabolites in order to detect heritable disease related genotypes, mutations, phenotypes, or karyotypes for clinical purposes. Such purposes include predicting risk of disease, identifying carriers, and establishing prenatal and clinical diagnosis or prognosis.") In its 1998 questionnaire, fifty-two corporations (5.7 percent of the companies responding) reported that they conducted genetic testing. The 1998 survey did not include the 2001 survey's restrictive definition of genetic testing, and the AMA stated that some of these employers included in the category of genetic testing their tests for the *presence* of a disease rather than for *genetic susceptibility* to that disease, and that nine of the employers had genetic testing programs under the more restrictive 2000 survey definition (AMA 2001, 3).

11. However, small companies are less likely to screen to determine their employees' health risks.

12. Susceptibility refers not just to the individual with esoteric genes but also to the individual who has worked in the hazardous work sites of the textile industry for fifteen years and is more likely to become sick than somebody who has worked in an office job for the same amount of time but without hazardous exposures. As with drug testing, company doctors have initiated programs that are unjustified on scientific grounds out of concern about disease risks, health costs, and liability. See U.S. Congress, Office of Technology Assessment (1990a), Draper (1999), and Andrews et al. (1994).

13. The beryllium lymphocyte proliferation test of peripheral blood or bronchoalveolar lavage (BAL) cells is used for detecting beryllium sensitization and chronic beryllium disease. On testing for beryllium disease, see Maier and Newman (1998).

14. Sheldon Samuels, director of health, safety, and environment of the AFL-CIO Industrial Union Department, personal interview.

15. As president, Bill Clinton signed into law a medical surveillance bill for former DOE workers that provides for lifelong medical surveillance (Public Law 102–484, as an amendment to the National Defense Authorization Act for Fiscal Year 1993) and directs the Secretary of Energy, in consultation with the Secretary of Health and Human Services, to develop a program of medical evaluation for current and former DOE workers at significant risks for health problems owing to exposures during employment (5 *U.S. Code Congressional and Administrative News* [102d Congress, 2d Session 1992], 2315–2770).

16. The use of genetic information is likely to become even more pervasive as the Human Genome Project uncovers more genetic markers for disease that can be used to screen out large segments of the population from employment. See Buchanan et al. (2000), Pennisi (2001), Murray, Rothstein, and Murray (1996), and Cook-Deegan (1994), on the fifteen-year, $3 billion Human Genome Project, begun in 1991. Designed to map and sequence the human genome, the project could make a major contribution to public health. It will identify a growing proportion of the population who may be presymptomatic for late-onset single-gene disorders, those who may be at increased risk for multifactorial disorders, and those who carry recessive and X-linked traits. See also the January 1995 *Journal of Occupational and Environmental Medicine,* which is devoted to articles about the current use of biomarkers in occupational and environmental health research and proposed uses in the workplace.

17. On genetic discrimination in employment and insurance, see Capron (2000a, 2000b), Schafer (2001), American Management Association (2001), Stone (1997), and Mehlman and Botkin (1998). In a case involving federal and state governments as employers, plaintiff employees filed suit in the state of California against their employer, Lawrence Berkeley Laboratory (LBL; now Lawrence Berkeley National Laboratory) and others, on behalf of past and present LBL employees (Norman-Bloodsaw v. Lawrence Berkeley Laboratory, 135 *Federal Reporter 3d* 1260 [Ninth Circuit 1998]). The plaintiffs alleged that LBL for thirty years tested its employees for medical conditions and genetic characteristics without notice or consent. The plaintiffs claimed that: the conditions LBL tested for were not reasonably related to the administrative and clerical jobs the employees had been hired to perform; LBL used race and gender classifications to decide which employees should be given which tests, in that LBL tested all employees for syphilis (and tested blacks and Latinos more frequently), screened all women for pregnancy, and

screened all blacks for sickle cell trait and disease; LBL's policies and practices violated the Americans with Disabilities Act of 1990 because the medical testing and inquiries served no legitimate employer purpose; and LBL's testing and inquiries violated Title VII of the Civil Rights Act of 1964 because of LBL's discriminatory selection process. The employees contended that they did not give informed consent because they were given no information regarding the specific tests to be performed and the testing was required as a condition of employment. After the defendants prevailed at the trial court level, the Ninth Circuit reversed and remanded the action. The court found that knowledge and consent were material issues of fact. The court held that employers can perform health- and occupation-related medical testing if the testing is based on the reasonable probability of substantial harm to the tested employees or others. See Holmes-Farley (1997, 1, 4), Hawkins (1997, 26), and Cowley (1996, 49).

18.   Genetic screening generally evaluates people according to stereotypes of future ability to function and the probability that disease will occur, rather than on evidence of actual ability or disease (Geller et al. 1996; Brown and Marshall 1993). In addition, employees are exposed to hazardous substances in various combinations, and most new chemicals are not tested. An EPA analysis found that of the approximately 3,000 chemicals ever produced in the United States at an annual volume of at least 1 million pounds, only 7 percent have been fully evaluated for toxicity, and a much smaller percentage have been tested with long-term carcinogenicity bioassays (Frumkin and Thun 2000, 339). Genetic screening as applied has been ineffective preventive medicine. The best the tests can do is show that certain individuals *may* be somewhat at greater risk for one type of ailment when exposed to a specific substance or group of chemicals. But they may be less at risk for another. They may be at lower risk of developing emphysema, but they may develop bladder cancer from the same substance or from other chemicals.

19.   For example, spina bifida is prevalent in highly polluted industrial areas, such as South Wales, and sickle cell trait protects individuals from the environmental threat of malaria (Duster 1990, 53–54). Similarly, phenylketonuria (PKU) is called genetic despite the fact that a specific and careful diet can control the symptoms (U.S. Congress, Office of Technology Assessment 1990a, 10).

20.   California legislation bars genetic discrimination against policyholders by health insurance companies based on genetic disorders that are currently asymptomatic (1994 *California Statutes,* chapter 761, *California Health and Safety Code,* section 1374.7

[West, 2000, and 2002 supplement], and *California Insurance Code,*
section 10123.3 [West, 2002]). Health plans may not offer reduced
benefits based on one's genetic traits (1995 *California Statutes,*
chapter 695). No California statute specifically prohibits employers
from conducting genetic screening in the workplace, but in 1998
California amended the Fair Employment and Housing Act (FEHA)
to prohibit employment discrimination based on asymptomatic genetic characteristics (1998 *California Statutes,* chapter 99 amended
FEHA; *California Government Code,* section 12926 [1992 and West
supplement 2002]). Although existing law already prohibited discrimination in employment-related matters on the basis of medical
condition, physical disability, or mental disability, the new legislation provides that "medical condition" includes genetic characteristics and clarifies the legislative intent to prohibit genetic discrimination in companies with five or more employees. This statutory
protection is particularly important because of the federal law's
gaps in protection. The ADA to some extent protects genetically at-
risk employees under federal law, but it applies only to employers
with fifteen or more employees (42 *United States Code,* sections
12111[5][A] [2000]), thus excluding from ADA coverage the many
California employees who work for smaller companies.

21. Few cases have been decided under the ADA that deal with discrimination resulting from the belief that an individual who is diagnosed with a condition that is currently asymptomatic will become
disabled in the future. See Andrews, Mehlman, and Rothstein
(2002) and Alper (1995).

22. For examples of state genetic discrimination laws, see *Oregon Revised Statutes,* section 659A.303 (West, 2001); 10 *New Hampshire
Revised Statutes Annotated,* chapter 141-H:1–141-H:6 (1996 and
2001 supplement); *New Jersey Statutes,* 17B: 30–12 (1996 and 2001
supplement). New Jersey bars employers and health insurers from
discriminating against individuals based on genetic information, defined broadly as "information about genes, gene products or inherited characteristics that may derive from an individual or family
member." Legislation with a broad definition of genetic information, like the one in New Jersey's law, is desirable because it would
protect genetic information obtained from direct testing as well as
from medical records, physical examinations, and family histories.
New Jersey's law is also advantageous because although life and
disability insurers may use genetic information to set premiums or
deny coverage, they are barred from "unfair discrimination" or discrimination not based on "anticipated claims experience."

23. A major federal bill that would effectively address the genetic discrimination problems described here is the Genetic Information Nondiscrimination in Health Insurance Act of 1995, introduced by Representative Louise Slaughter (HR 2748, 104th Cong., 1995). HR 2748 would prohibit insurance providers from: using genetic information, or an individual's request for genetic services, to deny or limit any coverage or to establish eligibility, continuation, enrollment, or contribution requirements; establishing differential rates or premium payments based on genetic information or an individual's request for genetic services; requesting or requiring collection or disclosure of genetic information; and releasing genetic information without the individual's prior written authorization for each disclosure, which must include to whom the disclosure would be made. See Rothenberg (1995) on HR 2748. Senator Tom Daschle and Representative Slaughter introduced similar bills in 2000 and 2001 (see Pear 2000; Genetic Nondiscrimination in Health Insurance and Employment Act, 107th Cong., S318, January 22, 2001, and HR602, February 13, 2001; see also the Genetic Information Nondiscrimination in Health Insurance Act of 2001, sponsored by Senators Olympia Snowe, Susan Collins, Michael Enzi, James Jeffords, and William Frist, introduced in the Senate S382, February 15, 2001). By executive order in 2000, President Clinton restricted the use of genetic information about federal employees (Executive Order 13145, of February 8, 2000 [3 *Code of Federal Regulations*, 235–239 (2001)]). Federal agencies may not dismiss, refuse to hire, or discriminate against federal workers because of genetic tests conducted on them or their relatives, and they cannot discriminate against workers in job-related decisions because they request or receive genetic counseling or tests. The order contains exceptions: for instance, federal agencies may use genetic information if workers already have medical conditions that affect their ability to perform their jobs, and they may periodically conduct genetic monitoring of employees for chromosomal damage or genetic alterations because of workplace exposures. The order covers about 2.8 million civilian employees, but not federal contract workers or military personnel. See also Pear (2000).

24. The government requires certain kinds of drug testing, as in DOT- and NRC-mandated tests. See, for example, Normand, Lempert, and O'Brien (1994, 284–301).

25. Corporate officials reported that they believed OSHA required them to conduct genetic tests, such as those for sickle cell trait and G-6-PD deficiency (Severo, February 6, 1980). The director of OSHA,

Eula Bingham, responded to the news coverage by issuing a public statement insisting that OSHA regulations should not be interpreted as a mandate to screen (Bingham 1980).

26. An employer must accommodate a disabled individual if the individual's impairments are known to the covered entity and if the accommodations would not impose an undue hardship on the entity's business operation (42 *United States Code,* sections 12112[a], 12112[b][5][A] [2000]). Under the ADA, disability means: a physical or mental impairment that substantially limits one or more of the individual's major life activities; a record of such an impairment; or being regarded as having such an impairment (section 12102[2]).

27. The ADA excludes persons currently using illegal drugs from the term "individual with a disability" as long as the employer took its action against the person owing to the drug use (42 *United States Code,* section 12210 [1994 and supplement IV 1998]).

28. 42 *United States Code,* section 12112(d)(3) (2000). Genetic tests are not specifically mentioned but presumably could be included as part of medical exams and inquiries.

29. In genetic monitoring, periodic genetic tests may detect adverse health effects that reflect managerial choices rather than immutable characteristics of workers.

30. Title VII of the Civil Rights Act of 1964, 42 *United States Code,* section 2000e (2000). If the genetic trait targeted by the employer is found disproportionately among one of these protected classes, the employer may be held liable whether or not the employer intended to discriminate on that basis (42 *United States Code,* section 2000e–2[a][2000], intentional violations; 42 *United States Code,* section 2000e–2[k][1][A][2000], disparate impact violations). In addition to Title VII, Title VI of the Civil Rights Act of 1964 (42 *United States Code,* section 2000d [2000]) prohibits recipients of federal funds from discriminating based on race.

31. Title VII of the Civil Rights Act of 1964, 42 *United States Code,* sections 2000e, 2000k (2000). If an employer policy explicitly discriminates against a protected class, the employer must show that the exclusion based on genetic predisposition is a bona fide occupational qualification reasonably necessary to the normal operation of the business (42 *United States Code,* section 2000–2[e][1][2000]). If an employer is found to have a policy that unintentionally discriminates on the basis of protected status, the employer can escape liability by showing that the classification is related to the position in question and consistent with a business necessity (42 *United States Code,* section 2000e–2[k][1][A][2000]). It is difficult for an em-

ployer to justify a discriminatory policy, as shown by the history of fetal exclusion policies, which barred all women from working in particular positions because of the risk of fetal injury. In 1991 the Supreme Court held in Johnson Controls that such policies violated Title VII (see International Union, UAW v. Johnson Controls, Inc., 499 U.S. 187, 209 [1991]). The Court found that fetal exclusion policies were facially and intentionally discriminatory and therefore required the defendant corporation to show that maleness was a bona fide occupational qualification. The defendant offered a general safety justification, but the Court rejected it because the employer had failed to show that a woman's potential fertility had any effect on her ability to perform her job. The defendant's "fear of prenatal injury, no matter how sincere, [did] not begin to show that substantially all of its fertile women [were] incapable of doing their jobs" (Johnson Controls, at 207). Johnson Controls applies to genetic testing and the exclusion of workers on the basis of genetic predispositions that do not actually affect a person's work performance. However, it may have only limited practical effect on employer practices. Even after Johnson Controls, some employers maintain fetal exclusion policies because they fear tort liability more than Title VII liability.

32. See Johnson Controls, 499 U.S., at 198 ("The business necessity defense is more lenient for the employer than the statutory BFOQ [bona fide occupational qualification] defense.")

33. 42 *United States Code,* section 12113(a)(2000).

34. See Andrews, Mehlman, and Rothstein (2002); Lieberwitz (1994, 192–203); Americans with Disabilities Act, 42 *United States Code,* sections 12101–12213 (2000); and Loder, 14 Cal. 4th, at 877–900.

35. See Title VII of the Civil Rights Act of 1964, 42 *United States Code,* section 2000e (2000); Americans with Disabilities Act, 42 *United States Code,* section 12112 (2000).

36. Chapter 7 discusses data banks and search companies in more detail.

37. Unlike employment policies, tax and transfer programs often address class stratification.

38. See, for example, Wright v. Olin Corp., 697 *Federal Reporter 2d* 1172, 1189–1190 (Fourth Circuit 1982), in which the court held that employers may use a business necessity defense when they restrict women's job access to protect the health of their unborn children through policies such as Olin's, which excluded women from jobs with exposure to known or suspected teratogenic or abortifacient chemicals; and Grant v. General Motors Corp., 908 *Federal Reporter*

2d 1310, 1304 (Sixth Circuit 1990), in which the court found that General Motors' fetal exclusion policy, which excluded all fertile women from foundry jobs involving airborne lead exposure, was discriminatory and that the employer could justify the policy only by using a bona fide occupational qualification (BFOQ) defense.

39. International Union, UAW v. Johnson Controls, Inc., 499 U.S. 187, 204 (1991). The Johnson Controls Company, a battery manufacturer, had a policy of excluding fertile women from jobs with exposure to lead, in the belief that the exposure of working women to lead might damage fetuses and the company could be sued for fetal damage. Johnson Controls held the employer's exclusion of all women except those who showed proof of surgical sterilization to be unlawful discrimination under Title VII of the Civil Rights Act of 1964 (42 *United States Code,* section 2000e [2000]); Johnson Controls, 499 U.S., at 204–206). Before Johnson Controls, American Cyanamid had barred women of childbearing capacity from production jobs that involved exposure to lead beginning in 1978. Five women underwent sterilization procedures as a result of this exclusionary policy.

40. In Johnson Controls, the Court rejected Johnson Controls' argument that potential tort liability for damage to a fetus from workplace exposure made policies excluding fertile women permissible under Title VII. The majority noted that tort liability is unlikely without a finding that the employer was negligent. In addition, the Court held that Title VII's antidiscrimination provisions would preempt state tort liability if states were to impose tort liability for conduct that Title VII requires and thereby create a conflict between state and federal law. Allowing state tort law to excuse or further discriminatory hiring would thwart the goals of Congress in enacting Title VII. The Court concluded that employers cannot implement policies excluding women out of concern for fetal safety without potentially ruinous tort liability. Higher costs from employing women are generally not a defense to discrimination, but costs that are "so prohibitive as to threaten the survival of the employer's business" could constitute a defense to discrimination (Johnson Controls, 499 U.S., at 210–211). Johnson Controls, however, had failed to show that tort liability raised its costs at all. In Johnson Controls, the Supreme Court left unresolved how far state tort law would extend, in view of Title VII's mandates, and whether employers with potentially vast tort liability from employing fertile women could use the BFOQ defense to charges of sex discrimination—that is, that sex is a bona fide occupational qualification for the job in question that is

reasonably necessary to the normal operation of the business (42 *United States Code,* section 2000e–2[e][1][2000]). The Court left open the possibility that employers could show that tort liability raised their costs so much as to threaten the survival of their business. (The Court stated that "ruinous" tort liability could be the basis for a BFOQ defense [499 U.S., at 210–211].) Employers could successfully defend against a discrimination charge with this argument. Moreover, concurring opinions by four justices concluded that higher tort liability costs from hazards to third parties could establish a BFOQ defense to discrimination, even if the increased costs to employers were not ruinous (499 U.S., 212–213 and 223–224).

41. For example, Bruce Karrh, as corporate medical director of DuPont, has said, "When we remove a woman [from a job] it's to protect her fetus" (Bayer 1982, 17). Johnson Controls officials maintained that "the issue is protecting the health of unborn children" (quoted in Kilborn 1990, 1). Earlier, in 1979, American Cyanamid officials had claimed that when they excluded women from jobs, they were protecting fetuses, which they referred to as "the most helpless member[s] of society" (quoted in Sheridan 1983, 73). See also Taub (1996), Vogel (1993), Otten (1985, 27), and Johnson Controls, 499 U.S. 187 (1991).

42. In fact, the application of fetal exclusion policies has been determined in large part by the gendered stratification of the workforce and the related ideologies that reinforce it. See Gatson (1997) and Reskin and Roos (1990).

43. For example, lead can cause birth defects through maternal exposure, but men are vulnerable as well because lead can also damage the heart, kidneys, and nervous system in both men and women (Landrigan 1994, 745–49). In some cases, risks from paternal exposure to hazards are greater than those from maternal exposure (Paul and Frazier 2000). For instance, male exposure to ionizing radiation presents a higher risk for genetic mutations and chromosome aberrations than reproductive risk through female workers, at the same radiation dose. See Draper (1993a, 92–103) and Samuels (1995) for discussions of the selective application of fetal exclusion policies.

44. In fact, the evidence shows that occupational hazards that affect fetuses through maternal exposure alone are rare. Many of the same substances from which women are excluded can harm children through male workers by way of sperm damage or mutagenic effects (Paul and Frazier 2000). For example, the children of men

working with the pesticide dibromochloropropane (DBCP) at an Occidental Chemical plant in California have had high rates of birth defects, and many of the men have become sterile. DBCP and chlordecone (Kepone) can cause male sterility and other health damage; see Whorton (1998, 1245–50); Lemasters (1998, 227). Carbon disulfide also may damage the children of men who have been exposed to it. For evidence of reproductive damage through the exposure of male workers, see Mattison and Cullen (1994) and Blakeslee (1991). In addition, men who regularly bring home lead dust, asbestos, or other substances on their clothes can produce an accumulation of these substances in women and others outside the work environment; see Paul and Frazier (2000), Kreiss (1994, 735), McConnell (1994, 854), and Stellman and Henefin (1982).

45. Lead affects fetal development at low levels of exposure. While some would argue that this fact supports even greater differential treatment of men and women, it supports the opposite point. If low-level dust exposure can cause that problem, then men who come home with dust on their clothes can expose their wives at levels heretofore thought to be safe. So the children of both men and women are at risk from low exposure levels (Landrigan 1994; Bellinger et al. 1987).

46. The pro-choice arguments, which center on the *employer's* choice, appear in hearings on fetal exclusion policies and in the thousands of pages of briefs and transcripts related to the Johnson Controls cases heard by the Seventh Circuit and the U.S. Supreme Court; see Supreme Court of the United States (1990) and Draper (1993a) for further discussion of pro-choice arguments. As with genetic information, the rhetoric of choice concerning reproductive hazards gets used in powerful ways; it is a telling case of the language constructions people use to justify what is in their interests. Employers recognize the power of pro-choice rhetoric and use it themselves. They have argued that they must be allowed to protect fetuses from hazardous mothers and protect women from their own bad decisions.

47. Jaspan maintained that "it would violate common sense and the overriding interest in occupational health and safety to require an employer to damage unborn children" (Supreme Court 1990, 48). After Johnson Controls, a Johnson Controls company spokesperson stated that in light of the Court's decision, the company would consider returning to its previous practice of warning women of job-related fetal risks and allowing each woman to decide what was in her best interest (Kilborn 1991, B12).

48. According to the economist Kip Viscusi (1983, 107), workers are paid $900 more on average for hazardous work and therefore deliberately take hazardous work for specific benefits. Although economic decisionmaking models maintain that people freely choose risk to advance their own interests and preferences, workers are restricted in their ability to pursue their own interests. The assumption of risk requires that the risk be known and the assumption voluntary. However, given the economic necessity of working, limited job alternatives (especially in manufacturing industries that experience layoffs and plant shutdowns), managerial control, and incomplete employee information on hazards, the available choices are limited. See Lester (1998), Wilson (1996), Bianco (1996, A5), and du Rivage (1992) on declining employment opportunities for low-skill workers. See also Ashford and Stone (1998) for a discussion of the externalities and imperfect information problems that economic models of risk often inadequately address. Another major problem with economic decisionmaking models in the arena of occupational health is that company doctors and managers are shielded from the medical, monetary, and moral consequences of their actions. Managers constantly take risks that they do not define as risks because the consequences fall on workers or the public. They correctly perceive that others bear the risks and costs of their decisions.

49. Richard Alexander, physician at Lockheed Missiles and Space Company, personal interview.

50. Getting permission from the parent does not adequately protect the company in terms of the unborn child or shield the company from liability, because the employer does not have permission from the unborn child to expose it. Employees have limited legal ability to waive their own rights or the rights of third parties—such as their damaged offspring—to sue the employer. See, for example, Taub (1996, 454–55), Samuels (1997), Clauss, Berzon, and Bertin (1993), Stern and Tierney (1993), Murray (1993), Kirp (1992), and Johnson Controls, 499 U.S. 187 (1991). As a physician with a major chemical company stated, "Women sign a waiver, but it does not protect the company from having a toxic tort." In addition, parents cannot sign away their workers' compensation rights granted by state law, so a company is responsible at least for workers' compensation. For example, workers can sign an informed consent paper saying they realize they have a higher risk of getting carpal tunnel syndrome or another cumulative trauma disorder because they pack one million widgets in boxes every day. But as soon as they get carpal tunnel

syndrome, the employer is still expected to pay part of the bill for that injury under workers' compensation, whether or not the person knew about the risk. See Boden (2000), 82 *American Jurisprudence* workers' compensation, sections 1 and 62 (1992 and 2001 supplement), and Spieler (1994, 161–73).

51. Proponents of fetal exclusion policies often claim that the fetus is most vulnerable to toxic chemicals early in pregnancy, when the woman may be unaware that she is pregnant, but this is not necessarily true. For example, in the case of lead, the fetus may not be at highest risk during the first trimester. OSHA findings regarding fetal risk and lead exposure appear in the lead standard: 29 *Code of Federal Regulations,* 1910.1025 (2002), and in 43 *Federal Register* 2959 (1978).

52. Employers persist in focusing on the risks of employing women because of reproductive hazards even though male reproductive damage from workplace exposures has already led to lawsuits. Suits for reproductive damage have arisen from men's exposure to DBCP, Agent Orange, and atomic weapons testing. These suits generally have been for military or agricultural exposures, however, rather than for more typical workplace exposures. The suits that male veterans have brought for damage from exposure to the herbicide Agent Orange cite birth defects in their children, miscarriages, and serious illnesses in the men themselves. For discussions of Agent Orange and DBCP suits, see Whorton (1998), Weinstein (1995), and Schuck (1986). In addition, companies that exclude women can still be held liable for damage to consumers or to the community from hazardous conditions. In the Love Canal case, both men and women brought many suits against Hooker Chemical for reproductive and other health damage to the residents of the Love Canal neighborhood near Niagara Falls, New York. The Bunker Hill Company, which has barred women from working with lead, has been sued for exposing children to lead in the area surrounding company facilities. See Levine (1982) and Randall and Short (1983). In their concern over the legal risks, employers typically overstate the special liability that employing fertile female workers may represent, while understating the potential liability of male reproductive damage. They allow their fear of tort liability from employing women in hazardous jobs to outweigh their concern with avoiding Title VII liability.

53. Between 3 and 5 percent of all live births are recognized as having a congenital malformation or a chromosomal disorder; see Mattison and Cullen (1994, 449). In addition, approximately 7 percent of U.S.

newborns are of low birthweight (less than 2,500 grams), and 10 to 20 percent of pregnancies end in clinically recognized spontaneous abortion, with even higher rates of early loss before clinical pregnancy diagnosis (Paul and Frazier 2000, 589).

54. Bruce Karrh, physician at E. I. du Pont de Nemours and Company at the time of personal interview.

55. In other cases, company physicians simply inform women's private physicians of the hazard. For example, one physician in a company whose employees were exposed to lead from the lubricants used in forging operations and PCBs said: "We handle each case individually, and we don't have a formal written policy. We have an informal policy of counseling individuals. We advise women the job might be dangerous, and we make her personal physician aware of this problem." Dean Belk, physician at Alcoa Corporation at the time of personal interview.

56. However, if the treating physician says the job is safe, the employer rather than the outside physician might still be ultimately liable. Doctors in corporations tend to discount private doctors' judgments and medical evaluations except in the case of private physician waivers, when these opinions may limit the company physician's and employer's liability.

57. Private physicians sometimes resist signing these statements, since signing them might make them at least partially liable for any adverse health effects from women's continued employment.

58. Similarly, doctors and employers have given people they consider high-risk because of nonreproductive risk factors the choice of taking on hazardous work if they will sign a waiver of the right to sue. Further, some have required private doctors to sign statements confirming that they believe environmental exposures are safe before employers will permit employees to work in specific jobs.

59. James Weeks, United Mine Workers of America, personal interview.

60. The Americans with Disabilities Act presents problems for employers who want to avoid workers with schizophrenia, depression, or other mental and emotional disorders. The employer must make reasonable accommodation to disabled workers. However, the ADA generally permits employers to do preplacement drug screening and to fire or refuse to hire drug users. 42 *United States Code,* section 12210 (2000); see also Wolkinson and Block (1996) and U.S. Congress, Office of Technology Assessment (1990b).

61. For discussions of the associations between job satisfaction, control over work, and health outcomes, see Reissman et al. (1999) and Karasek and Theorell (1990). Low levels of control over work pro-

cesses, along with performance demands that exceed individual and social resources for accomplishing the required tasks, increase job stress and are associated with a higher risk of cardiovascular and other forms of chronic disease. Martin and his colleagues (1994, 11) report that marijuana and cocaine use is high in lower-status service and blue-collar occupations.

62. Wellness programs include health screening programs such as for breast cancer and hypertension, and health promotion such as smoking cessation, exercise, and stress management programs. See Aldana and Pronk (2001), Emmons et al. (1999), and Peterson and Dunnagan (1998).

63. Nevertheless, the fact that labor organizations generally give more attention to the rights of employees than of applicants in their policies and practices does not mean that applicants need protection less than employees.

CHAPTER 7

1. Anthony Mazzocchi, Oil, Chemical, and Atomic Workers International Union, personal interview.

2. Of the firms that the American Management Association (2001, 1–2) surveys each year, 48 percent report that they conduct complete medical exams; the leading rationale for these exams is "fitness for duty"—establishing the applicant's or employee's ability to perform assigned job tasks. The AMA found that 40.7 percent of the U.S. firms it surveyed conduct fitness-for-duty testing of new hires, and 32.9 percent conduct such testing of employees. As expected, employers use the test results in employment decisions: 42.8 percent use fitness-for-duty test results to hire job applicants; 24.8 percent use these test results to assign or reassign employees; and 17.5 percent use them in dismissing or retaining employees. The AMA reports that new-hire testing generally includes job applicants who qualify in other areas and may have received job offers pending the results of a pre-employment physical. (The AMA definition of job applicants includes current employees applying for new jobs within their organization.)

3. ACOEM's code of ethical conduct states that physicians should "keep confidential all individual medical information, releasing such information only when required by law or overriding public health considerations, or to other physicians according to accepted medical practice, or to others at the request of the individual"

(American College of Occupational and Environmental Medicine 1994, 28).

4. Lloyd Tepper, physician at Air Products and Chemicals Corporation, personal interview.

5. James Weeks, United Mine Workers of America, personal interview.

6. See Norman-Bloodsaw v. Lawrence Berkeley Laboratory 135 *Federal Reporter 3d* 1260 (Ninth Circuit 1998), Hawkins (1997), and chapter 6, note 17, for further details on this case. See also Orentlicher (1997) and Draper (1992).

7. In addition to federal laws, state laws govern the confidentiality of medical records, such as California's Confidentiality of Medical Information Act (*California Civil Code,* sections 56.05, 56.10, and 56.20 [West, 2000]), which applies to the use of health records by in-house medical professionals as well as by those in private practice and HMOs.

8. Doctors who resist management's demands for medical information or records find that it hurts them when they press for medical resources, because managers resent doctors' withholding records that managers feel they need.

9. The doctor went on to say, "But that's bad business; it prevents people from having good care and good relationships with their own medical people." Similarly, a chemical company physician said, "Management pressuring doctors for information on employees is part of the economic stress we're under, and it's going in the wrong direction now. Doctors are modifying their ethics because of their own economic realities. But I would be perceived as losing my credibility if I shared information with management."

10. Bruce Karrh, physician at E. I. du Pont de Nemours and Company at the time of personal interview. He continued by emphasizing the role of a medical director in assisting local physicians who are being pressured by plant managers: "How do you share that information with their management to try to get special consideration for the employee? We are available to assist our site physicians with doing what we think they need to do from an ethical and medical standpoint. We can intervene and help physicians if a plant manager is needlessly ruthless with them."

11. Similarly, as one metals company physician said, "a nurse ran our medical department in many locations. She usually had an office next door to the safety director or labor relations guy. Giving the managers records or medical information became a problem." Another metals company physician said: "Often the safety person would come in and demand of the nurse access to employee medi-

cal records. I had a hell of a time with that. That was a serious bone of contention nurses complained about." For an insightful account of nurses, see Chambliss (1996), who examines the sometimes conflicting interests of nurses, doctors, patients, administrators, and insurers.

12. See Kass (1997, 301–3), Lyon and Zureik (1996), Geller et al. (1996), McEwen (1997), and Annas (1993) for discussions of the possible misuse and misinterpretation of the health information kept by data banks and credit companies. Hundreds of health insurers in the United States share their computerized data on health-care costs and risks. See also Nelkin and Tancredi (1989, 37–50) and National Institutes of Health/Department of Energy (1993, 794, 802–4) for a discussion of the problems of accuracy, reliability, and validity associated with diagnostic testing. Although legal restrictions limit the activities of search companies, these companies describe their activities as credit reporting, which is protected under the federal Fair Credit Reporting Act (15 *United States Code,* section 1681 [2000]).

13. The ACOEM code of ethical conduct states that physicians should "recognize that employers may be entitled to counsel about an individual's medical work fitness, but not to diagnoses or specific details, except in compliance with laws and regulations" (American College of Occupational and Environmental Medicine 1994, 28). See also the position paper on workplace medical confidentiality by the ACOEM Committee on Ethical Practice in Occupational Medicine (American College of Occupational and Environmental Medicine 1995).

14. Roy de Hart, director of occupational medicine at the University of Oklahoma, personal interview.

15. Albert Ackroyd, physician at Northrup, personal interview.

16. An important privacy concern is that managers have access to employees' answers to intrusive questions about their health, which company personnel may ask in anticipation of litigation or workers' compensation claims. Employers still require employees to fill out questionnaires even though under the ADA they may be unable to fire or refuse to hire the person because of their answers.

17. Michael Wright, United Steelworkers of America, personal interview. He went on to describe one company's questionnaire: "One company with a big medical department that used a long, fairly invasive questionnaire said, 'We want to make sure that these people are basically healthy. We have a duty to help them if they have any health problems and to do more than just look at their fitness

to work.' We hoped they would also say that they are in a doctor-patient relationship, to provide people individual medical services. Then we would say, 'Fine! Now that ought to be a voluntary relationship, so you should say that the questionnaire is entirely voluntary when you administer it, and we expect that you will give people good advice on their state of health and provide medical services as well, along with this questionnaire.' Then we could make the case to an arbitrator that somebody should not have to submit to this forcibly. We've had many battles with companies over that problem."

18. Albert Ackroyd, physician at Northrup, personal interview. Similarly, a chemical company physician said, "I have never had to tell management what a medical problem was, except when an employee applies for consideration for medical pension, files a workers' comp claim, or files any type of litigation, because they have put their medical condition into evidence. Once the person files some type of action, then that record is in the case and available to management." Bruce Karrh, physician at E. I. du Pont de Nemours and Company at the time of personal interview.

19. For example, if attorneys request information about a foot while subpoenaing records for a back injury, that immediately alerts the plaintiff's attorney that the company might focus on a different way of litigating the case.

20. In contrast, one physician opposes lawyers who demand employees' medical records without a subpoena: "I try to explain to the legal department, 'You need to go through the same procedure as outside lawyers would with private practitioners, because the medical department deserves the same respect as if these records sat in an outside physician's office. You can't just dip in here.'"

21. In large firms, outside counsel under contract usually handles cases that go to litigation.

22. Robert Larsen, physician who performs examinations and evaluations for corporate employers and other clients, personal interview.

23. James Weeks, United Mine Workers of America, personal interview. In workers' compensation claims, employees could lose their claims for not giving information about their health problems or cooperating with company doctors. In addition, the records from employees' private physicians can be subpoenaed through a court of law. On workers' compensation, see Boden (2000).

24. Doctors often guess the person's medical condition or illness, as when they know that the doctor who signed their paperwork is in psychiatric practice.

25. Robert Larsen, physician who performs examinations and evaluations for corporations, personal interview. He went on to describe
employees' concerns after learning company personnel will review
the doctor's report: "Some patients who come in are very uncomfortable with this; they want to know who specifically will get this
report. Usually it allays some of their concerns if you explain that it
won't go directly to their boss, but rather to the insurance company
that makes the administrative decisions or to the company's EAP
program or medical department. If the report goes to *anybody* at
the company, just the idea that we would explain our findings to
the referral source over the phone without even a written report is
sufficient for them to say they don't want to go through this."

26. Similarly, an auto company physician said: "Ideally you always
want to have doctors report to a medical supervisor—a corporate
medical director or a vice president who's an MD. When I first
came to the company, I had a furious conflict with the personnel
director, who tried to manage the medical department and wanted
to go through the charts. I said, 'No, you're not allowed to do that,'
and yet he signed my checks. You can be intimidated in some companies, where if the doctor is going to stand up for his convictions,
he'll have to leave." A physician from a consumer products company said: "Money speaks. The man who signs the performance
appraisals gets first attention."

27. The doctor added, "I tell plant managers, 'If you don't like the way
it's set up, you can go talk to the CEO, because he set it up this
way, but I was given this job to do, and I can't give you that information.' They can get pissed off at me and talk to my boss, but if I
do my job right they won't, because I make them understand what
I'm doing. You lose when your boss—the manager across the
street who gives you raises—says, 'I want it done this way,' and
you can't do much about it. We are a fairly autonomous unit here,
so when managers tell us what to do, it's difficult for this department to get squashed." This physician later did go to work for a
company with a decentralized medical structure, however. As he
mentioned, most companies are structured that way. A physician in
a conglomerate who reports centrally described the advantages of
more centralized control over medical information: "We've had
problems with plant managers pressuring doctors and nurses to
turn medical records over to management, to give them more detailed information about individuals' health and absentee problems,
and to get somebody back to work just in order to maintain a good-
looking safety record. Having all physicians and nurses throughout

the corporation on the medical department payroll was a big help because we had the budget and a lot more control, without local plant managers trying to save a dime. It is just natural for local managers to want total responsibility for all the people working for them."

28. See Americans with Disabilities Act of 1990, 42 *United States Code,* section 12112 (2000). ACOEM's code of ethical conduct states that physicians should "recognize that employers may be entitled to counsel about an individual's medical work fitness, but not to diagnoses or specific details, except in compliance with laws and regulations" (American College of Occupational and Environmental Medicine 1994).

29. He went on to say: "That makes the union patients uncomfortable, and they'd feel better if the claims were outside. Not a lot of union patients will come to the clinic because management and union leadership have had a bad relationship for years, and ultimately they just want everything totally external. They have no trust in having it here. There's no trust problem as long as you preserve the doctor-patient relationship with management and employees, but what should I put in the chart?"

30. Anthony Mazzocchi, Oil, Chemical, and Atomic Workers International Union, personal interview.

31. The Employee Retirement Income Security Act of 1974 (29 *United States Code,* sections 1001–1461 [2000]) exempts self-insured employers from state laws covering health, pension, and other benefit plans that employers provide. Corporations that become self-insured become like a small insurance company. They live closer to their risk and have great incentives to reduce their risk.

32. In self-insured companies, the workers' compensation personnel are the doctor's co-employees and their departments are co-departments; the lines of confidentiality are weaker than in a doctor's office, where the workers' compensation carrier is another insurer who must write letters and follow additional procedures to gain access to medical records.

33. Contract professionals may be subject to corporate directives and managerial control even more than the in-house doctors they replace. They may generally be more malleable in what they will do, owing in part to highly competitive contractor markets and employers' expectations of access to contractors' information.

34. The physician described his effort to persuade the VP not to fire contract physicians who were reluctant to give managers employee medical information: "I talked to the VP and explained to him that

he was treading on very thin ice, that if the press ever learned that a doctor was fired for doing the right thing and refusing to disseminate medical information beyond stated ethical practices, he might as well just close up his operation, because the occupational health program would be sunk and subject to litigation and a lot of problems for everybody. I said, 'If you want the records, just tell the workers when they come in for their placement exam that everything they write on this form will be transmitted to Joe Smith at ABC Company. You can have the records if you want them, but I'll guarantee that only a fool—the person you won't want to hire—will write all their medical problems knowing they are released to human resources.' "

35. Employers must keep employee medical records for thirty years after employees' separation from the company (29 *Code of Federal Regulations*, section 1910.1020[d] [2002]). The company can write a contract with physicians to say that the contract physicians are the custodians of the records and that the records go with the employer if the employer changes doctors. Employers then can keep the records in a separate, specific place so that they can produce the records if OSHA ever demands them. Physicians must follow the rules about permitting access to the records, but legal requirements do not prohibit employers from entering into a contract with providers. The contract could clearly state that the records are the employer's and that the provider is the temporary custodian. If physician contractors want to keep copies for malpractice purposes or other reasons, then they can arrange for copies to be made at the employer's expense if the employer changes doctors and demands the records. Managers and in-house physicians could explain to contract doctors—if they do not already understand—what should be held as confidential and how they should handle medical records.

36. Laws limit management's and lawyers' access to medical records, and information about health hazards such as lead or asbestos is the focus of regulation and extensive litigation. For discussions of the laws affecting the distribution of employee medical information, see, for example, Snyder and Klees (1996), Rothstein (1994, 1997b), Rischitelli (1995), and Parliman and Edwards (1992). See also OSHA's "Access to Employee Exposure and Medical Records" rule (29 *Code of Federal Regulations*, section 1910.1020 [2002]).

37. The ADA eliminates virtually all pre-employment examinations and has stronger confidentiality protections than OSHA. It affects the information that contracting and in-house physicians give com-

panies. It also requires that medical records be filed separate from personnel records. Permitting unauthorized access to files with diagnoses in them—such as being hypothyroid or having diabetes or having had Hodgkin's disease ten years before—can make the doctor and company liable for improper circulation of medical information. That kind of information must be handled confidentially under ADA, and companies that do not handle it confidentially may be liable; 42 *United States Code,* section 12112(d)(3) (2000). The ADA also made more debatable employers' right to ask questions that do not directly relate to an individual's ability to work or to have employees fill out long questionnaires and in-depth medical histories (section 12112[d][2]). One interpretation is that they cannot ask such questions; another is that they cannot compel an answer; and a third is that they may require answers to non-job-related preplacement questions as long as they use only job-related medical criteria to screen out qualified individuals with disabilities. Any of these interpretations protects employees more than did preexisting law. For a discussion of ADA and workplace medical information, see Rothstein (1994).

38. The OSHA "Access to Employee Exposure and Medical Records" rule gives employees access to their own medical records and to certain exposure information. Current or former employees assigned or transferred to jobs with exposure to toxic substances or harmful physical agents have the right of access to environmental and biological monitoring results, material safety data sheets, and other records disclosing the identity of a toxic substance or harmful physical agent at that work site. Employers must provide the identity of substances and exposure levels, but they may delete trade secret data that disclose the percentage of a chemical in a mixture, as long as the employees or their designated representatives are notified of the deletion. Employee rights of access to medical information are circumscribed, however. For example, employees do not have access to certain physical specimens or to certain records concerning health insurance claims or voluntary employee medical assistance programs because the access rule excludes these from the definition of "employee medical records." According to the American Management Association's (2001, 4) recent survey, 16.9 percent of companies did not notify job applicants who had any sort of medical test performed on them of the test results, and 11.8 percent of companies did not notify employees who underwent medical tests of the test results. The 1,627 U.S. companies surveyed were disproportionately large firms, half in manufacturing and half

in services. The figures could be even higher if companies that gave no answer or said they didn't know are included: in that event, 26.6 percent of companies did not notify job applicants of test results, and 29.6 percent of companies did not notify employees of test results. Aside from individual access to medical and exposure information, government agencies, unions, and doctors outside companies have tried, with mixed results, to get information about employees for research purposes from corporations, as discussed in chapter 5.

39. Toxic Substances Control Act, 15 *United States Code,* sections 2601–2692 (2000).

40. More generally, evidence supporting the economic necessity of layoffs and plant closings has often been contested. On downsizing, plant closures, and their effects, see Dudley (1994) and Bluestone and Harrison (1982).

41. Michael Wright, United Steelworkers of America, personal interview. He added: "The OSHA standard that gives workers access to their medical records helps enormously. In cases where companies haven't wanted to share information with people, we've said, 'Fine. Here's this guy's medical release. Send it all to our doctor for the union,' and they have to oblige." A telecommunications company physician referred to the company policy of consulting the legal department and sending employee records to physicians: "Usually we like doctors to give records only to other doctors. People have a difficult time getting their own records or the union getting them, but we'll be glad to send it to their doctor. We have a whole corporate procedure to go through to get your records, and the legal department determines whether we can give out the record or some medical information."

42. The OSHA hazard communication standard requires employers to give employees information on hazardous chemicals through labeling, providing material safety data sheets and training, and granting access to written records; 29 *Code of Federal Regulations,* section 1910.1200 (2002). Employees have used information from the material safety data sheets that OSHA requires companies to keep to research exposure hazards themselves, such as by analyzing studies that others have conducted or having samples from the company analyzed.

43. Anthony Mazzocchi, Oil, Chemical, and Atomic Workers International Union, personal interview. He emphasized the role of unions in building company medical programs: "We've made jobs for company doctors and nurses and industrial hygienists because of our

aggressive stance on occupational medicine. It changed the nature of company medical departments." In another example, Mazzocchi said: "In the bladder-cancer episodes we had at J. S. Young in Baltimore, the doctor at Johns Hopkins under contract with the company discovered bladder cancer when he examined the workers. He knew they worked with benzidine, a bladder-cancer inducer, but never told the workers the cause and effect. His position was, 'Look, I'm under contract to the company. I told *them*.' That's how they see their responsibility."

44. Melena Barkman, assistant director of Health, Safety, and Environment Department, United Steelworkers of America, personal interview.

45. See "Labor Union Membership by Sector: 1983 to 2000" (U.S. Department of Commerce, Bureau of the Census 2001, table 637). A few unions have been particularly active on health issues in workplaces they have organized, including the Oil, Chemical, and Atomic Workers International Union, the International Chemical Workers Union, the American Federation of Federal, County, and Municipal Employees (AFSCME), and the United Steelworkers.

CHAPTER 8

1. The interviews and field research for this book add perspective to a doctrinal analysis of the law. The words of corporate professionals infrequently appear in the scholarly literature, but field research nonetheless is valuable for illuminating the significance of the legal environment from the perspectives of the social actors themselves and for shedding light on the organizational and cultural context in which the laws have effect.

2. Sheldon Samuels, director of health, safety, and environment for the AFL-CIO Industrial Union Department at the time of personal interview.

3. Attorneys trying to protect the company may scrutinize the records of in-house doctors as they would scrutinize the records of a physician outside the company who supports an employee suing the company.

4. Lloyd Tepper, physician at Air Products and Chemicals Corporation, personal interview.

5. Three occupational physicians, for example, point to the legal protections of corporate employment. "We are protected by the corporate umbrella when it comes to the question of our own liability,"

said an oil company physician. "The limits on liability," according to an airline physician, constitute "the primary advantage of corporate practice." A physician who works in a university occupational clinic has found that, "for the most part, manufacturers are well protected against suits from their own workforce, and they behave accordingly. That devil's bargain was made a long time ago where workers can't sue their own employers, except for the most wanton and willful neglect of their health and safety, and that's a tough one to prove."

6. The doctor went on to say, "We evaluate people in workers' comp cases, and it could always flip from normal workers' comp into something where the person gets a lawyer and sues the company and sues me." Similarly, a physician from a retail sales company said: "The company has a general liability policy. Every doctor knows you can always be sued because you can't stop lawyers from suing whomever they wish. It's just that doctors know the company will defend you—one hopes (laughs)—as long as you aren't grossly negligent in performing your duties for the company."

7. Most states permit employers' intentional torts to fall outside the workers' compensation system's coverage, through statutes and case law. Standards for satisfying the intentional tort exception vary among the states; see Boden (2000), Larson (1999), and 6 Larson's Workers' Compensation Law, sections 68.00 and 68.13 (1997). See also Millison v. E. I. du Pont de Nemours & Co., 501 A.2d 505 (N.J., 1985), in which the court held that although the defendants could not be held liable for the first injuries their products caused, they could be held liable for fraudulently concealing knowledge of these initial diseases. The court found for the employee plaintiff in a tort action concerning workplace asbestos hazards. The company physician had fraudulently concealed important health information and thereby contributed to employees' aggravated disease by failing to warn of the evidence of disease and the further risks that the employees faced. The court stated that fraud is not within the ordinary risks of employment. The court held that the New Jersey Workers' Compensation Act's exclusive-remedy provision (New Jersey Statutes Annotated, 34:15–8 [West, 2000]) did not bar plaintiff's cause of action for aggravation of the diseases resulting from defendant's fraudulent concealment of already discovered disabilities. (The court also held that the employees were limited to workers' compensation benefits for any initial occupational disease disabilities related to the hazards of their employment.)

8. Physicians worry about being held personally liable for their decisions in corporations even though their chance of such a suit is small. Professionals in large companies with occupational health programs are particularly concerned because they generally know more about potential liability than managers in smaller companies, who have few, if any, lawyers to advise them; moreover, plaintiffs' lawyers consider their employers to be especially attractive as defendants in lawsuits because the awards are likely to be larger from major corporations.

9. In People v. Chicago Magnet Wire Corp., 534 *N.E.2d* 962 (Illinois, 1989), five company officers were charged with aggravated battery and reckless conduct for causing injury to forty-two employees by failing to provide necessary safety precautions. The court held that OSHA did not preempt the state of Illinois from prosecuting the corporation and five of its officers (despite the approval of OSHA officials) for conduct that OSHA standards regulate.

10. In United States v. Northeastern Pharmaceutical & Chemical Co. (Nepacco), 810 *F.2d* 726 (Eighth Circuit, 1986), the court held that any corporate officer or employee who personally participates in conduct that violates the Comprehensive Environmental Response, Compensation, and Liability Act (CERCLA) or contributes to a substantial endangerment to the environment in violation of the Resource Conservation and Recovery Act of 1976 (RCRA) may be held individually liable for that violation. The court held that a corporate vice president was strictly liable for arranging for the disposal of hazardous substances under CERCLA (42 *United States Code,* section 107[a][3][2000]) and that the company president was individually liable for contributing to an imminent and substantial endangerment to health and the environment in violation of RCRA. A plant supervisor for Nepacco had dumped drums of toxic chemicals into a trench on a farm near the plant, with the permission of the vice president. The court rejected the defendant vice president's argument that he acted on behalf of the corporation and therefore could not be held individually liable without piercing the corporate veil.

11. See, for example, Millison v. E. I. duPont de Nemours & Co., 501 *A.2d* 505 (New Jersey, 1985). See also Rothstein (1994).

12. Michael Wright, United Steelworkers of America, personal interview.

13. *California Penal Code,* section 387 (West, 2002).

14. Toxic Substances Control Act, 15 *United States Code,* sections 2601–2692 (2000). Criminal penalties apply under the Occupational

Safety and Health Act (29 *United States Code,* section 666[e] [2000]), which states that any employer who willfully violates any standard, rule, or order promulgated pursuant to OSHA (or any regulations prescribed pursuant to that act), shall be imprisoned, if that violation caused death to any employee, for not more than six months or be fined—the amount of which was raised to $500,000 for an organization and $250,000 for an individual after passage of the Comprehensive Crime Control Act in 1984 (or both a fine and imprisonment). See also *California Code of Regulations,* title 8, sections 10447 and 10406, and Howard (1998, 1675).

15. Toxic Substances Control Act, 15 *United States Code,* section 2615 (2000). For a conviction of knowingly or willfully violating TSCA, the statute calls for a fine of not more than $25,000 for each day of the violation, or imprisonment for one year, or both.

16. Americans with Disabilities Act of 1990, 42 *United States Code,* sections 12101–12213 (2000), and regulations.

17. Besides ADA, see also the Civil Rights Act of 1991 (42 *United States Code,* section 1981a [2000]), according to which companies can be forced to pay punitive and compensatory damages of up to $300,000 for each count of unlawful, intentional discrimination. See also section 1981a(b)(3), which sets a cap on compensatory and punitive damages. Under the statute, damages are capped depending on the number of people a company employs. For example, damages are capped at $300,000 for a company employing five hundred or more individuals; damages are capped at $50,000 for a company employing only fifteen to one hundred individuals.

18. The fact that corporations usually pay malpractice insurance costs only for in-house doctors is one reason management may favor using contract physicians rather than physician employees.

19. Similarly, the early rulings on possible corporate liability for fetal damage due to employee exposure to dioxin and lead were circumscribed but nevertheless have had a definite, broad impact: corporate policies excluding fertile women from jobs with exposure to toxic chemicals later became widespread. See International Union, UAW v. Johnson Controls, Inc., 499 U.S. 187 (1991).

20. On the history of OSHA and its regulation, see Ashford (1976, 2000), Wahl and Gunkel (1999), and McCaffrey (1982). Not all workers are covered by OSHA. For example, the Mine Safety and Health Administration (MSHA) in the U.S. Department of Labor, not OSHA, is responsible for issuing and enforcing health and safety regulations for American miners, and longshore workers come un-

der a federally administered program called the Jones Act (46 Appendix *United States Code,* sections 1–1904 (2000).

21. James Hughes, who worked as a physician at Kaiser Aluminum and Kaiser Industries, personal interview.

22. Jack Sheehan, United Steelworkers of America, personal interview.

23. A factor that in some cases compensates for cutbacks in the number of enforcement officers is that civil penalties under federal OSHA and some state regulations (such as Cal-OSHA) have increased. These more significant fines make some employers more attentive to the threat of enforcement, even though their chance of being inspected remains small.

24. If OSHA were reformed to include generic medical surveillance and environmental monitoring standards, for example, companies would be motivated to hire more doctors.

25. Occupational Safety and Health Act, 29 *Code of Federal Regulations,* section 1910.1043 (2002).

26. A lawyer who specializes in company health hazards said: "Industry's standard for labeling is stricter than OSHA's, because companies don't want to be sued."

27. In addition, corporate concern with litigation can cause employers and company physicians to avoid preventive health measures. When companies are in the mode of trying to defend themselves, company attorneys and managers fear that by adopting additional safeguards, they admit that they failed to do things properly in the past.

28. The media certainly have caused greater public recognition of workplace hazards and occupational medicine in the past twenty years, through articles and news reports on high-profile episodes such as Bhopal, asbestos, and lead in buildings and the water supply. Media coverage of toxic chemical hazards has publicized the need for corporate and government responsibility on environmental issues. For example, newspapers and television in the 1980s and 1990s covered hazards in U.S. Department of Energy facilities and in maquiladoras in Mexico; children born without brains in Brownsville, Texas; Superfund sites around the country; Chernobyl; and leukemia from groundwater contamination in Woburn, Massachusetts. These cases have intensified corporate responses to toxics and built occupational medicine generally. For discussions of media coverage of workplace and environmental hazards and community responses to them, see Brown and Middelsen (1990), Nelkin (1995), Couch and Kroll-Smith (1991), Haar (1995), Gamson and

Modigliani (1989), Stallings (1990), and Freudenburg and Pastor (1992).

29. The right-to-know campaign that swept the country and led to the implementation of the OSHA hazard communication standard and other community right-to-know laws in the 1970s and 1980s also boosted concern about chemical hazards. The greater awareness instigated by the media and educational efforts led people to demand better medical services. Increased information has fostered grassroots environmental organizations and facilitated labor educational efforts as well. States vary widely in their public opinion environment and rules. California, for example, is more pro-environment than most, Cal-OSHA is stronger than many other state programs, and corporations in the state are more concerned about pro-environment jury decisions. See Howard (1998) for a discussion of state occupational health regulation and its relationship to federal regulation.

30. According to Brady and his colleagues (1997), employers in 1994 paid over $1 trillion in health costs—including $418.7 billion in direct health-care costs ($3,510 per person), plus $837.5 billion in indirect costs (of lower productivity, profitability, and competitiveness, such as from absences and training costs). Workers' compensation medical costs have risen at a higher rate than medical costs outside workers' compensation. For example, workers' compensation medical costs increased 265 percent from 1980 to 1990, while medical costs outside workers' compensation increased 183 percent in the same decade (Boden 2000, 245). Employers' workers' compensation payments sometimes fell in the 1990s, partly owing to the efforts of employers and carriers to control medical costs as well as statutory changes in some states that reduced indemnity payments. Between 1992 and 1993, for example, workers' compensation employers' cash indemnity and medical benefits payments fell nationally (National Foundation for Unemployment Compensation and Workers' Compensation 1995). Employers' health expenditures overall grew in the 1990s; in 1998, for example, employers' total health-care spending increased 6.1 percent (Goetzel et al. 2000, 338; Business Insurance 1999).

31. Company medical programs may also raise productivity and morale and reduce use of the company medical plan. McCunney (2001) discusses studies that show that current occupational health services enhance productivity, primarily by reducing absenteeism through preventing short- and long-term disability. A study of Sherman, Texas, found that companies that offered occupational medi-

cine services had lower injury rates and fewer lost workdays than companies that did not (Ramphal 1999). Bunn and his colleagues (2001) found that a comprehensive corporate wellness program at International Truck and Engine Corporation significantly reduced direct health costs and improved productivity, measured as absenteeism.

32. Bruce Karrh, physician at E. I. du Pont de Nemours and Company at the time of personal interview.

33. Workers' compensation began in 1911 to pay for medical care and provide income to people who were hurt at work. Workers' compensation was not designed to cover disease. Despite recent modifications to widen its coverage, only about 1 percent of all compensation claims are for occupational disease, and only about 5 percent of occupational diseases are covered by workers' compensation programs (Boden 2000; Ashford 1998). Rosenman and his colleagues (2000) and Biddle and his colleagues (1998) have found that most workers diagnosed with an occupational disease do not apply for workers' compensation. In addition, many workers are not covered by workers' compensation, including self-employed and casual workers, domestic workers, state and local government workers, farm workers, and some small business workers. Railroads come under the Federal Employers' Liability Act (FELA) (45 *United States Code,* sections 51–60 [2000]), which differs from workers' comp: injured employees who claim that the company was negligent in any way may get an attorney and sue for their injuries. A successful claim for a work injury and surgery might wind up with a large settlement. The railroads have set up a wage continuation program, whereby a person who is legitimately injured and cannot return to work receives a continuing salary and is paid to be home. Employees who recover and go back to work are cut off from wage continuation but can get a lawyer to pursue further payments.

34. There were 26.5 million adults (16 percent of all adults) and 26.5 million children (13 percent of all children) who lacked health insurance in the United States in 1999. Rates of non-insurance did not change significantly between 1997 and 1999 for adults or children overall (Zuckerman et al. 2001, 170).

35. The lack of utilization review and limits on coverage helps explain escalating workers' compensation medical costs. Workers' compensation payments for medical expenses have been neither slashed like other medical costs nor regulated to the degree that other types of physician services have been. In addition, medical complaints and injuries treated under workers' compensation result in higher

costs and procedural intensity than under group health insurance (Harris et al. 2000, 353–56).

36.   However, doctors who know patients will be reimbursed for continuing treatment may continue to treat them until they reach a limit of visits beyond which the person must pay out of pocket.

37.   See Potter v. Firestone Tire and Rubber Co. 863 *P.2d* 795 (Cal., 1993); Ayers v. Township of Jackson, 525 *A.2d* 287, 312 (N.J., 1987); Sterling v. Velsicol Chemical Corp., 855 *F.2d* 1188 (Sixth Circuit, 1988); and Boston and Madden (1994, 165–212).

38.   The doctors and lawyers who support company claims typically earn whatever the company pays them, whereas in many states the doctors and lawyers who support workers' claims generally receive a percentage of the award.

39.   Anthony Mazzocchi, Oil, Chemical, and Atomic Workers International Union, personal interview.

40.   Companies need to account for future growth in employers' liability for future health-care benefits just as they need to account for pension-funding liabilities.

41.   Americans with Disabilities Act of 1990, 42 *United States Code,* sections 12101–12213 (2000); International Union, UAW, v. Johnson Controls, Inc., 499 U.S. 187 (1991); *California Insurance Code,* section 10143 (West, 2002 supplement); *New Jersey Statutes Annotated,* section 17B: 30–12 (West, 1996 and 2001 supplement).

42.   Title VII of the Civil Rights Act of 1964 (42 *United States Code,* section 2000e–2 [2000]) provides limited protection against discriminatory screening by making it illegal for employers to limit, segregate, or classify employees in any way that would tend to deprive them of employment opportunities or otherwise adversely affect their status as employees through screening programs that treat differently or disproportionately affect a class protected under Title VII (such as race, sex, or ethnicity), where employers cannot justify the practice with a recognized employer defense, such as the need for bona fide occupational qualifications that are reasonably necessary to the normal operation of the business but explicitly discriminate against protected classes. In addition, Title VI of the Civil Rights Act of 1964 (section 2000d) prohibits recipients of federal funds from discriminating based on race.

43.   The ADA (42 *United States Code,* sections 12101–12213 [2000]) protects from discrimination people who have, or who are perceived to have, physical or mental impairments that substantially limit one or more of their major life activities. Employers can require physical examinations of applicants after they make an offer of employment.

Employers can withdraw an offer if they can prove that applicants cannot perform the essential functions of the job even with reasonable accommodation or if they pose a "direct threat" to themselves or others on the job. The question of future risk is still open, as few cases have been decided under the ADA that deal with discrimination resulting from the belief that an individual who is diagnosed with an asymptomatic condition will become disabled in the future (Alper 1995). The ADA explicitly states that prohibited discrimination does not include conventional risk underwriting by insurance companies or self-insured employers (section 12201[c][1]). Instead, insurance regulation is left to the states. See the McCarran-Ferguson Act (15 *United States Code,* sections 1011–1015 [2000]), which declares that states will regulate insurance unless specific federal action seeks to regulate the industry.

44. 42 *United States Code,* sections 12111(8), 12111(3), and 12112(a) (2000).

45. The ADA (section 12210) excludes persons currently using illegal drugs from the term "individual with a disability" as long as the employer took its action against the person owing to the drug use.

46. The ADA does not offer clear-cut answers to many important questions, such as whether a certain impairment impedes an individual's ability to do his or her job, whether excluding a person is a business necessity, how much effort is reasonable to put forth on job placement, and what constitutes reasonable accommodation and work assignment for those with potential health problems. Moreover, the Equal Employment Opportunity Commission has yet to define what a medical examination is—which is important because the ADA prohibits pre-employment medical examinations. The EEOC has said that physical agility testing is not a medical examination, so police and fire departments can make candidates run obstacle courses. The EEOC has not ruled, however, on strength testing, hearing tests, or eye chart examinations; on the ADA, see Colledge, Johns, and Thomas (1999) and Frierson (1992). In addition to the ADA, other state and federal laws apply, such as the Fair Employment and Housing Act (FEHA) in California (*California Government Code,* sections 12900–12996 [1992 and 2002 West supplement]).

47. The ADA itself does not even mention genetics or genetic traits, and genetic susceptibility to disease and death was not a focus of the congressional debate on the ADA. The EEOC originally took the position that the ADA does not cover individuals until they are symptomatic and that the risk of future impairment is not a disability under the ADA. Then, in its March 1995 interpretation of the

ADA, the EEOC stated that disability under the ADA would include individuals who are predisposed to, or presymptomatic for, a disabling disease (EEOC 1995, section 902.8). This new section in the EEOC *Compliance Manual* concludes that individuals who are subjected to discrimination based on "genetic information relating to illness, disease, or other disorders" are being regarded as having disabling impairments. However, it is unclear whether courts will adopt the EEOC opinion. Furthermore, the EEOC's interpretation of the ADA does not limit an employer's ability to test or collect medical information after a conditional job offer, even if the information is not job-related, as long as the same information is requested of all applicants. That employer right is given by statute (see 42 *United States Code,* section 12112[d][2000]). For a discussion of the 1995 EEOC interpretation of the ADA regarding genetic disabilities, see Mehlman et al. (1996, 395) and Alper (1995, 167–68). For EEOC's former position on asymptomatic individuals under the ADA, see Philip B. Calkins, acting director of communications and legislative affairs, EEOC, letter to Patrick Johnson, Senate of the state of California, June 23, 1993; E. M. Thornton, deputy legal counsel, EEOC, letter to Paul Berg and Sheldon Wolff, co-chairpersons of NIH-DOE Joint Subcommittee on the Human Genome, August 2, 1991; and Ronnie Blumenthal, acting director of communications and legislative affairs, EEOC, letter to Representative Bob Wise, chair of the House Subcommittee on Government Information, Justice, and Agriculture, November 22, 1991. See also Alper (1995).

48.   In Bragdon v. Abbott, 524 U.S. 624 (1998), the U.S. Supreme Court decided that people with asymptomatic HIV infection can be covered by the ADA. The Court ruled that a woman with asymptomatic HIV infection who was refused care in a dentist's office met the ADA's definition of disability. The Court did not rule that the ADA automatically covers HIV infection, however, leaving it to the lower courts to determine whether HIV infection constitutes a direct threat in the dental-care context. Although the Court's analysis relied heavily on the history of HIV infection and its importance in the ADA congressional debates, its recognition that asymptomatic conditions can be covered by the ADA may extend to genetic predispositions. (Even before this decision, people with full-blown AIDS had been considered disabled under the ADA.) This was the Court's first substantive review of the ADA; see Greenhouse (1998). The Court narrowed the scope of the ADA in Toyota v. Williams (534 U.S. 184 [2002]), in which the Court decided that to be dis-

abled and protected under the ADA a person must have an impairment that prevents or severely restricts him or her from performing tasks that are of central importance to most people's daily lives—such as brushing teeth, bathing, and doing household chores—and not just work tasks. In addition, the Court held that the impact of the impairment must be permanent or long-term.

49. The Genetic Privacy Act is promising as a comprehensive effort to protect individuals from unauthorized analysis of their DNA. A version of the Genetic Privacy Act was introduced in the Maryland Senate in 1995, with important genetic privacy provisions. It would, among other things: bar unauthorized disclosure of information resulting from genetic analysis; require that authorization for collection or disclosure of an identifiable DNA sample "may not be coerced"; and require that a person to be tested be warned "that access to the results of genetic analysis by insurance companies, employers, or other third parties may occur" if the person "authorizes their disclosure," and the person must also be told that "the disclosure may lead to discrimination" against him or her; see Maryland's Genetic Privacy Act (S. 645, Md. 409 Leg. Sess. [1994]), sections 4–504(b), 4–505(a)(2), and 4–505(a)(8); see also Lin (1996), Annas, Glantz, and Roche (1995a, 1995b), and Holtzman (1995). The Health Insurance Portability and Accountability Act of 1996 (HIPAA) (29 *United States Code,* sections 1181–1182 [2000]) bars insurers from treating genetic mutations as "preexisting conditions" unless they are causing illness. It also guarantees coverage to anyone leaving one group plan for another, whatever their preexisting conditions. However, it covers only group plans and does not deal with disability insurance. Doctors and medical vendors increasingly will market genetic tests directly to patients. Although individuals may wish to be tested and keep information about their genetic makeup to themselves, employers and insurers generally could gain access to this information, under current laws.

50. Eric Frumin, Union of Needletrades, Industrial and Textile Employees, personal interview.

51. Lloyd Tepper, physician at Air Products and Chemicals Corporation, personal interview.

52. The Employee Retirement Income Security Act of 1974 (29 *United States Code,* section 1144[a] [2000]) exempts self-insured employers from state laws (such as those regarding minimum required benefits and antidiscrimination provisions) covering health and retirement plans and other benefits that employers provide. Self-insured employers may eliminate or modify their medical benefits for par-

ticular medical conditions; see Rosenblatt, Law, and Rosenbaum (1997, 159–292, 1001–37). The ERISA rules were originally designed to protect benefits and pension plans from mismanagement by companies. So Congress passed the McCarran-Ferguson Act, which sets regulations for managing certain company pension plans.

53. McGann v. H&H Music Co., 946 *F.2d* 401 (Fifth Circuit, 1991), *cert. denied sub. nom.*, Greenberg v. H&H Music Co., 506 U.S. 981 (1992). In McGann, the employee-plaintiff with AIDS filed suit under section 510 of ERISA, which provides, in part: "It shall be unlawful for any person to discharge, fine, suspend, expel, discipline, or discriminate against a participant or beneficiary for exercising any right to which he is entitled under the provisions of an employee benefit plan . . . or for the purpose of interfering with the attainment of any right to which such participant may become entitled under the plan." The McGann court held that ERISA (section 510) "does not prohibit an employer from electing not to cover or continue to cover AIDS, while covering or continuing to cover other catastrophic illnesses, even though the employer's decision in this respect may stem from some 'prejudice' against AIDS or its victims generally" (McGann, 946 *F.2d,* at 408). The McGann court held that a plaintiff is entitled to relief under section 510 only if he or she can demonstrate that the defendant intended either to retaliate for the plaintiff's filing of claims for AIDS-related treatment or to interfere with the plaintiff's attainment of any right to which he or she is entitled pursuant to an existing enforceable obligation the employer assumed. The plaintiff did not challenge the statute under the ADA because the conduct occurred before the ADA's effective date. However, it appears that McGann remains valid, if somewhat vulnerable. See Mansfield, Baer, and Hope (1998, 628–30) and Parker v. Metropolitan Life Insurance Company, 121 *F.3d* 1006 (Sixth Circuit, 1997), holding that provision of different benefits for mental versus physical disabilities under an ERISA plan does not violate ADA. But see Carparts Distribution Center v. Automotive Wholesalers Association of New England, Inc., 37 *F.3d* 12 (First Circuit, 1994), holding that caps on AIDS health benefits under ERISA plans may violate ADA. McGann undercuts the traditional function of insurance as spreading risks and enables companies to avoid high-risk individuals after they identify them. For discussion of insurance companies' efforts to avoid insuring individuals they consider high-risk, see Kass (1997) and Pear (1997a).

54. Although companies have a responsibility to seek profits for their shareholders, employers need not make a profit on their employees or on each person they employ.

55. On liability related to occupational health, see Snyder and Klees (1996) and General Dynamics v. Superior Court, 876 *P.2d* 487 (California, 1994), in which the court upheld a cause of action for wrongful discharge by an in-house corporate lawyer who claimed that the employer made illegitimate demands that conflicted with the mandatory ethical norms in the *California Rules of Professional Conduct*.

CHAPTER 9

1. See Marmot et al. (1997), Pelletier et al. (1999), and Karasek and Theorell (1990, 83–117) for discussions of control over work and its relationship to health and well-being. See also Punnett (2000) for a discussion of the relationship between job control and satisfaction and musculoskeletal disorders.

2. In *Moral Mazes*, Jackall (1988) analyzes what he calls the bureaucratic ethic of decisionmaking by corporate actors. What he calls a problem of bureaucracy, however, is really a problem caused by insufficient bureaucracy and quasi-feudal loyalty to employers. Corporate actors generally view their work not so much through a fixed bureaucratic lens of rules and procedures as through a changing web of allegiances within and outside the corporation, and these tend to place a higher value on loyalty to employers than on concern with social costs.

3. Several states have enacted legislation that either prohibits employers from requiring genetic testing as a condition of employment or prohibits the use of genetic health predictions in employment decisions. At least twenty-four states have statutes that protect against genetic discrimination in employment, and thirty-seven have statutes regarding genetic discrimination and health insurance (Jeffords and Daschle 2001). Most of them bar insurers from limiting coverage or establishing premiums based on "predictive" genetic information. Although state protections against discrimination by employers and insurers are beneficial, comprehensive federal genetic discrimination laws should be enacted. For discussions of proposed federal legislation, see Jeffords and Daschle (2001) and Annas, Glantz, and Roche (1995a, 1995b). Companies could offer individuals at risk an opportunity to move to an equal-status job in another area without any loss of pay, seniority, or benefits, as in the OSHA lead standard (29 *Code of Federal Regulations,* section 1910.1025[k][2][ii] [2002]), but companies that are small or downsizing would have difficulty doing this.

4. Mandated national health coverage would remedy problems within the workers' compensation system that now encourage people to seek compensation benefits simply to get medical coverage. It would also assist people who now decline health insurance coverage because of the high cost of premium co-payments that many companies require. With national health care, investigators could use national data systems to track suspected employee hazards and disease patterns by workplace or region, which would facilitate mortality and morbidity studies. Despite political obstacles to enacting a national single-payer health-care system, political leaders could overcome opposition to reform by educating the public about the expense, the gaps in coverage, and the inequities of the current health-care delivery system.

5. The exclusion of people perceived to be high-risk from private insurance is a major issue, although some insurance companies, such as Blue Cross, have voluntarily stopped excluding people with preexisting conditions from eligibility for insurance coverage. Most insurance is bought in groups, and people who obtain insurance virtually automatically with their employment are therefore not excluded for preexisting conditions. Insurance companies are resourceful, however, in coming up with ways to exclude people who they think will cost them money. Moreover, as in the McGann case discussed in chapter 8, self-insured companies are largely exempt from state regulation of health benefits and therefore can exclude people or conditions from their insurance plans. Congress should close this ERISA loophole for self-insured companies so that employers cannot effectively exclude from insurance coverage those employees who need it most. On health insurance coverage, including denial for preexisting conditions, see Capron (2000a, 2000b) and Rosenblatt, Law, and Rosenbaum (1997, 36–368, 466–647).

6. California, for example, has a specific retaliation clause with criminal penalties for retaliation against employees who pursue their rights after a workplace injury (*California Labor Code,* section 132a [West, 2002]).

7. *California Penal Code,* section 387 (West, 2000). Criminal penalties also apply under the Occupational Safety and Health Act (29 *United States Code,* section 666[e] [2000]). See Howard (1998).

8. Attorneys clearly have a duty to advise clients that they should terminate their continuing violation of the law. They may also have a duty to resign if their clients do not in fact terminate their illegal conduct. See the American Bar Association's *Model Rules of Professional Conduct,* particularly rule 1.16 and the comment ("Declining

or Terminating Representation"), in American Bar Association (2000, 49–52). Attorneys and bar associations argue that attorneys should not have the right to inform the authorities that the client rejected their advice. They maintain that in effect making attorneys police officers in relation to their corporate clients would destroy the traditional attorney-client privilege, discourage the free exchange of information, and unduly constrain corporate employers' willingness to seek legal advice about complex compliance issues. A lawyer must be able to obtain all the facts in order to counsel a client on proper conduct and give sound advice, and the client must feel free to communicate facts without fearing disclosure. However, although attorney-client confidentiality can be critical when the client has confessed past crimes, allowing clients to misuse their lawyers in order to commit future crimes is more difficult to justify. Moreover, since bar associations' ethical rules and case law allow lawyers to breach their client's confidences if necessary to collect their attorney fees and protect themselves, arguably lawyers should sometimes have the same right to protect the public from life-threatening harm. For example, see rule 1.6 and the comment ("Confidentiality of Information") in American Bar Association (2000, 20–24). See also Arnold and Kay (1995), Gallagher (1995), Schneyer (1992), and Wilkins (1992) on self-regulation, professional controls, and disciplinary sanctions of lawyers.

9. On professional socialization, see, for example, Becker et al. (1961), Brint (1980), Stover (1989), and Gordon and Simon (1992). See also Hughes (1962) for a classic article considering why employees with good opportunities and education and a background as law-abiding citizens violate rules and laws to further organizational goals.

10. In addition, companies could invest in people who would be available as ombudspersons within the work environment to help resolve employee problems and increase the affiliation people have with their work. Safeguards could be built in to protect against retribution for reporting problems.

11. The UAW and the auto companies have provided a good model for joint health activities. The UAW has been particularly successful in negotiations with major auto companies over joint training funds and other issues. As part of the comprehensive agreement between the UAW and GM, Ford, and Chrysler begun in 1994, the companies and the union jointly administer a fund for job-related health and safety training for employees (Silverstein and Mirer 2000, 723). After the UAW won the right to sit on GM's board, the board met

with scientists acting as adjudicators, information specialists, and facilitators to try to address workplace concerns jointly. OSHA could mandate joint labor-management health committees and occupational medical services for employees nationwide.

12. In 2000, 9.0 percent of private-sector U.S. workers were union members; 10.3 percent of private-sector U.S. workers were covered by unions. Union membership for public-sector workers is higher: in 2000, 37.5 percent were union members, and 42.0 percent were covered by unions. For wage and salary workers overall in 2000, 13.5 percent were union members and 14.9 percent were covered by unions (U.S. Department of Commerce, Bureau of the Census 2001, table 637 ["Labor Union Membership by Sector: 1983 to 2000"]).

13. See, for example, LaDou (1998, 1999), Jacoby (1995), Beck (1992), Gould, Schnaiberg, and Weinberg (1996), Couch and Kroll-Smith (1991), Capek (1993), and Dunlap and Mertig (1992). See Portes (1996) on transnational networks and communities, and Rodrick (1997) on the effects of globalization, including its undermining of domestic institutions, labor rules, and long-standing social contracts.

14. OSHA, "Access to Employee Exposure and Medical Records" (29 *Code of Federal Regulations*, section 1910.1020 [2002]).

15. As we have seen, the quality of the medical care is not necessarily better if the occupational medicine work is contracted out. However, employee participation in the selection of employee services, better-trained practitioners, and additional confidentiality protections would improve outside health services. If providing health services outside the corporation is purely a management decision, a third party with some independence and expertise in employee services could help define what those services should be.

16. Regional centers would give even small employers coverage. Companies could send new hires who require preplacement physicals to such centers, which would tell employers whether the individuals are healthy enough to do the required work. Screening thereby could become less of a coercive and punitive invasion of privacy.

APPENDIX

1. Seven of the sixty company physicians (approximately 12 percent) are women. Individuals used the male pronoun in referring to company physicians, employees, and others, even though the field of occupational medicine includes women, and I have preserved their language as a reflection of their own perceptions.

References

Abbott, Andrew. 1988. *The System of Professions: An Essay on the Division of Expert Labor.* Chicago: University of Chicago Press.

Abel, Richard L., ed. 1997. *Lawyers: A Critical Reader.* New York: New Press.

Abraham, Katherine G., and Susan K. Taylor. 1996. "Firms' Use of Outside Contractors: Theory and Evidence." *Journal of Labor Economics* 14(3): 394–434.

Aldana, Steven G., and Nicholaas Pronk. 2001. "Health Promotion Programs, Modifiable Health Risks, and Employee Absenteeism." *Journal of Occupational and Environmental Medicine* 43(1): 36–45.

Alper, Joseph S. 1995. "Does the ADA Provide Protection Against Discrimination on the Basis of Genotype?" *Journal of Law, Medicine, and Ethics* 23(2): 167–72.

Alvi, Shahid. 1994. "Union Perspectives on Workplace Drug Testing." In *Drug Testing in the Workplace,* edited by Scott Macdonald and Paul Roman. New York: Plenum Press.

American Bar Association, Center for Professional Responsibility. 2000. *Model Rules of Professional Conduct,* 2001 ed. Chicago: American Bar Association.

American College of Occupational and Environmental Medicine. 1994. "American College of Occupational and Environmental Medicine Code of Ethical Conduct." *Journal of Occupational Medicine* 36(1): 28–30.

———. 1995. "ACOEM Position on the Confidentiality of Medical Information in the Workplace." *Journal of Occupational and Environmental Medicine* 37(5): 594–96.

———. 1998. "Occupational and Environmental Medicine Competencies vol. 1.0—Committee Report by the American College of Occupational and Environmental Medicine Panel to Define the Competencies of Occupational and Environmental Medicine." *Journal of Occupational and Environmental Medicine* 40(5): 427–40.

———. 1999. "ACOEM Position Statement: Multiple Chemical Sensitivities: Idiopathic Environmental Intolerance." *Journal of Occupational and Environmental Medicine* 41(11): 940–42.

American College of Occupational Medicine, Council on Social Issues. 1991. "Drug Screening in the Workplace: Ethical Guidelines." *Journal of Occupational Medicine* 33(5): 651–52.

American Management Association. 1996. *1996 AMA Survey: Workplace Drug Testing and Drug Abuse Policies.* New York: American Management Association.

———. 2001. *2001 AMA Survey on Workplace Testing: Medical Testing.* New York: American Management Association.

American Medical Association, Council on Scientific Affairs. 1992. "Clinical Ecology." *Journal of the American Medical Association* 268(24): 3465–67.

American Medical Association. 2000a. *Graduate Medical Education Directory, 2000–2001.* Chicago: American Medical Association.

———. 2000b. *Physician Characteristics and Distribution in the U.S.* Chicago: AMA.

Andrews, Lori B., Jane E. Fullarton, Neil A. Holtzman, and Arno G. Motulsky, eds. 1994. *Assessing Genetic Risks: Implications for Health and Social Policy.* Washington, D.C.: National Academy Press.

Andrews, Lori B., Maxwell J. Mehlman, and Mark A. Rothstein. 2002. *Genetics: Ethics, Law, and Policy.* St. Paul, Minn.: West.

Annas, George J. 1993. "Privacy Rules for DNA Databanks: Protecting Coded 'Future Diaries.'" *Journal of the American Medical Association* 270(18): 2346–50.

Annas, George J., Leonard H. Glantz, and Patricia A. Roche. 1995a. "Drafting the Genetic Privacy Act: Science, Policy, and Practical Considerations." *Journal of Law, Medicine, and Ethics* 23(4): 360–66.

———. 1995b. *The Genetic Privacy Act and Commentary.* Boston: Boston University School of Public Health.

Anspach, Renee R. 1993. *Deciding Who Lives: Fateful Choices in the Intensive Care Nursery.* Berkeley: University of California Press.

Appelbaum, Paul S., Charles W. Lidz, and Alan Meisel. 1987. *Informed Consent: Legal Theory and Clinical Practice.* New York: Oxford University Press.

Arnold, Bruce L., and Fiona M. Kay. 1995. "Social Capital, Violations of Trust, and the Vulnerability of Isolates: The Social Organization of Law Practice and Professional Self-Regulation." *International Journal of the Sociology of Law* 23(4): 321–46.

Ashford, Nicholas A. 1976. *Crisis in the Workplace: Occupational Disease and Injury.* Cambridge, Mass.: MIT Press.

———. 1998. "Workers' Compensation." In *Environmental and Occupational Medicine,* 3d ed., edited by William N. Rom. Philadelphia: Lippincott-Raven.

———. 2000. "Government Regulation of Occupational Health and

Safety." In *Occupational Health: Recognizing and Preventing Work-Related Disease and Injury*, 4th ed., edited by Barry S. Levy and David H. Wegman. Philadelphia: Lippincott Williams & Wilkins.

Ashford, Nicholas A., and Robert F. Stone. 1998. "Economic Issues in Occupational Safety and Health." In *Environmental and Occupational Medicine*, 3d ed., edited by William N. Rom. Philadelphia: Lippincott-Raven.

Auerbach, Joseph. 1984. "Can Inside Counsel Wear Two Hats?" *Harvard Business Review* 84(5): 80–86.

Barker, Kathleen, and Kathleen Christensen, eds. 1998. *Contingent Work: American Employment Relations in Transition*. Ithaca, N.Y.: Cornell University Press/ILR Press.

Barnet, Richard J., and John Cavanagh. 1994. *Global Dreams: Imperial Corporations and the New World Order*. New York: Simon & Schuster.

Bayer, Ronald. 1982. "Women, Work, and Reproductive Hazards." *Hastings Center Report* 12(5): 14–19.

———, ed. 1988. *The Health and Safety of Workers*. New York: Oxford University Press.

———. 1993. "Coal, Lead, Asbestos, and HIV: The Politics of Regulating Risk." *Journal of Occupational Medicine* 35(9): 897–901.

Beamish, Thomas D. 2000. "Accumulating Trouble: Complex Organization, a Culture of Silence, and a Secret Spill." *Social Problems* 47(4): 473–98.

Beauchamp, Tom L., and James F. Childress. 1994. *Principles of Biomedical Ethics*, 4th ed. New York: Oxford University Press.

Beck, Ulrich. 1992. *Risk Society: Towards a New Modernity*. London: Sage Publications.

Becker, Howard S., Blanche Geer, Everett C. Hughes, and Anselm Strauss. 1961. *Boys in White: Student Culture in Medical School*. Chicago: University of Chicago Press.

Bell, Daniel. 1973. *The Coming of Post-Industrial Society*. New York: Basic Books.

Bellah, Robert N., Richard Madsen, William M. Sullivan, Ann Swidler, and Steven M. Tipton. 1985. *Habits of the Heart: Individualism and Commitment in American Life*. Berkeley: University of California Press.

Bellinger, David, Alan Leviton, Christine Waternaux, Herbert Needleman, and Michael Rabinowitz. 1987. "Longitudinal Analyses of Prenatal and Postnatal Lead Exposure and Early Cognitive Development." *New England Journal of Medicine* 316(17): 1037–43.

Bendix, Reinhard. 1956. *Work and Authority in Industry: Ideologies of Management in the Course of Industrialization*. Berkeley: University of California Press.

Berger, Peter L., and Thomas Luckmann. 1966. *The Social Construction of Reality: A Treatise in the Sociology of Knowledge.* Garden City, N.Y.: Doubleday.

Bergthold, Linda. 1990. *Purchasing Power in Health: Business, the State, and Health Care Politics.* New Brunswick, N.J.: Rutgers University Press.

Berman, Daniel M. 1978. *Death on the Job: Occupational Health and Safety Struggles in the United States.* New York: Monthly Review Press.

Beryllium Industry Scientific Advisory Committee. 1997. "Is Beryllium Carcinogenic in Humans?" *Journal of Occupational and Environmental Medicine* 39(3): 205–8.

Bianco, Elena. 1996. "Temporary Workers Gaining Market Share, Statistics Show." *Los Angeles Times,* December 31.

Biddle, Jeff, Karen Roberts, Kenneth D. Rosenman, and Edward M. Welch. 1998. "What Percentage of Workers with Work-Related Illnesses Receive Workers' Compensation Benefits?" *Journal of Occupational and Environmental Medicine* 40(4): 325–31.

Billings, Paul R., Mel A. Kohn, Margaret de Cuevas, Jonathan Beckwith, Joseph S. Alper, and Marvin R. Natowicz. 1992. "Discrimination as a Consequence of Genetic Testing." *American Journal of Human Genetics* 50(3): 476–82.

Bingham, Eula. 1980. Letter to the editor. *New York Times,* March 22.

Bird, Frederick Bruce. 1996. *The Muted Conscience: Moral Silence and the Practice of Ethics in Business.* Westport, Conn.: Quorum Books.

Bixby, Michael B. 1990. "Was It an Accident or Murder?: New Thrusts in Corporate Criminal Liability for Workplace Deaths." *Labor Law Journal* 41(7): 417–23.

Blackwell, Judith C. 1994. "Drug Testing, the War on Drugs, Workers, and the Workplace: Perspectives from Sociology." In *Drug Testing in the Workplace,* edited by Scott Macdonald and Paul Roman. New York: Plenum Press.

Blakeslee, Sandra. 1991. "Research on Birth Defects Turns to Flaws in Sperm." *New York Times,* January 1.

Bluestone, Barry, and Irving Bluestone. 1992. *Negotiating the Future: A Labor Perspective on American Business.* New York: Basic Books.

Bluestone, Barry, and Bennett Harrison. 1982. *The Deindustrialization of America: Plant Closings, Community Abandonment, and the Dismantling of Basic Industry.* New York: Basic Books.

Blum, Terry C. 1994. "The Interrelations of Drug Testing with Other Human Resource Management Practices and Organizational Characteristics." In *Drug Testing in the Workplace,* edited by Scott Macdonald and Paul Roman. New York: Plenum Press.

Boden, Leslie I. 2000. "Workers' Compensation." In *Occupational Health: Recognizing and Preventing Work-Related Disease and Injury,* 4th ed., edited by Barry S. Levy and David H. Wegman. Philadelphia: Lippincott Williams & Wilkins.

Bosk, Charles L. 1979. *Forgive and Remember: Managing Medical Failure.* Chicago: University of Chicago Press.

Boston, Gerald W., and M. Stuart Madden. 1994. *Law of Environmental and Toxic Torts.* St. Paul, Minn.: West.

Bowman, James E., and Robert F. Murray, Jr. 1990. *Genetic Variation and Disorders in Peoples of African Origin.* Baltimore: Johns Hopkins University Press.

Brady, William, Jean Bass, Royce Moser, Jr., George W. Anstadt, Ronald R. Loeppke, and Ronald Leopold. 1997. "Defining Total Corporate Health and Safety Costs—Significance and Impact." *Journal of Occupational and Environmental Medicine* 39(3): 224–31.

Brint, Steven G. 1980. *Stratification of Professional Schools and Stratification in the Profession: An Analysis of the Literature on Academics, Scientists, Lawyers, Corporate Managers, Engineers, and Doctors.* Cambridge, Mass.: Huron Institute.

———. 1994. *In an Age of Experts: The Changing Role of Professionals in Politics and Public Life.* Princeton, N.J.: Princeton University Press.

Brock, Dan W. 1992. "The Human Genome Project and Human Identity." *Houston Law Review* 29(1): 7–22.

Brodeur, Paul. 1985. *Outrageous Misconduct: The Asbestos Industry on Trial.* New York: Pantheon Books.

Brodkin, C. Andrew, Howard Frumkin, Katherine H. Kirkland, Peter Orris, Maryjean Schenk, Sandra Mohr, and the AOEC Board of Directors. 1998. "Choosing a Professional Code for Ethical Conduct in Occupational and Environmental Medicine." *Journal of Occupational and Environmental Medicine* 40(10): 840–42.

Brody, Howard. 1992. *The Healer's Power.* New Haven, Conn.: Yale University Press.

Brown, Michael S. 1992. "Setting Occupational Health Standards: The Vinyl Chloride Case." In *Controversy: Politics of Technical Decisions,* 3d ed., edited by Dorothy Nelkin. Newbury Park, Calif.: Sage Publications.

Brown, Phil, and Edwin J. Middelsen. 1990. *No Safe Place: Toxic Waste, Leukemia, and Community Action.* Berkeley: University of California Press.

Brown, R. Steven, and Karen Marshall, eds. 1993. *Advances in Genetic Information: A Guide for State Policy Makers,* 2d ed. Lexington, Ky.: Council of State Governments.

Bryant, Bunyan, and Paul Mohai, eds. 1992. *Race and the Incidence of Environmental Hazards: A Time for Discourse*. Boulder, Colo.: Westview.

Buchanan, Allen, Dan W. Brock, Norman Daniels, and Daniel Wikler. 2000. *From Chance to Choice: Genetics and Justice*. New York: Cambridge University Press.

Budrys, Grace. 1997. *When Doctors Join Unions*. Ithaca, N.Y.: ILR Press.

Bullard, Robert D. 2000. *Dumping in Dixie: Race, Class, and Environmental Quality*, 3d ed. Boulder, Colo.: Westview.

Bunn, William B., III, Dan B. Pikelny, Thomas J. Slavin, and Sadhna Paralkar. 2001. "Health, Safety, and Productivity in a Manufacturing Environment." *Journal of Occupational and Environmental Medicine* 43(1): 47–55.

Burrage, Michael, and Rolf Torstendahl, eds. 1990. *Professions in Theory and History: Rethinking the Study of the Professions*. London: Sage Publications.

Burstein, Jay M., and Barry S. Levy. 1994. "The Teaching of Occupational Health in U.S. Medical Schools: Little Improvement in Nine Years." *American Journal of Public Health* 84(5): 846–49.

Business Insurance. 1999. *1999 Mercer/Foster/Higgins Annual Employer Survey* (January 25): 1.

Calavita, Kitty. 1983. "The Demise of the Occupational Safety and Health Administration: A Case Study in Symbolic Action." *Social Problems* 30(4): 437–48.

Callaghan, Polly, and Heidi Hartmann. 1991. *Contingent Work*. Washington, D.C.: Economic Policy Institute.

Capek, Stella M. 1993. "The 'Environmental Justice' Frame: A Conceptual Discussion and an Application." *Social Problems* 40(1): 5–24.

Caplan, Arthur. 1995. *Moral Matters: Ethical Issues in Medicine and the Life Sciences*. New York: Wiley.

Capron, Alexander M. 2000a. "Genetic Discrimination in Insurance: Is It Ever Ethically Acceptable?" In *Biomedical Research Ethics: Updating International Guidelines*, edited by Robert J. Levine, Samuel Gorovitz, and James Gallagher. Geneva, Switzerland: Council for International Organizations of Medical Sciences.

———. 2000b. "Genetics and Insurance: Accessing and Using Private Information." *Social Philosophy and Policy* 17(21): 235–75.

Cassels, Jamie. 1993. *The Uncertain Promise of Law: Lessons from Bhopal*. Toronto: University of Toronto Press.

Castleman, Barry I. 1996. *Asbestos: Medical and Legal Aspects*, 4th ed. Englewood Cliffs, N.J.: Aspen Law and Business Publishers.

Castleman, Barry I., and Richard A. Lemen. 1998. "The Manipulation of International Scientific Organizations." *International Journal of Occupational and Environmental Health* 4(1): 53–55.

Castorina, Joseph S., and Linda Rosenstock. 1990. "Physician Shortage in Occupational and Environmental Medicine." *Annals of Internal Medicine* 113(12): 983–86.

Chambliss, Daniel F. 1996. *Beyond Caring: Hospitals, Nurses, and the Social Organization of Ethics.* Chicago: University of Chicago Press.

Chinoy, Ely. 1992 [1955]. *Automobile Workers and the American Dream,* 2d ed. Urbana: University of Illinois Press.

Clarke, Adele, and Joan Fujimura, eds. 1992. *The Right Tools for the Job: At Work in Twentieth-Century Life Sciences.* Princeton, N.J.: Princeton University Press.

Clarke, Lee. 1989. *Acceptable Risk?: Making Decisions in a Toxic Environment.* Berkeley: University of California Press.

——. 1999. *Mission Improbable: Using Fantasy Documents to Tame Disaster.* Chicago: University of Chicago Press.

Clauss, Carin Ann, Marsha Berzon, and Joan Bertin. 1993. "Litigating Reproductive and Developmental Health in the Aftermath of UAW Versus Johnson Controls." *Environmental Health Perspectives* 101(supp. 2): 205–20.

Colledge, Alan L., Richard E. Johns, Jr., and Madison H. Thomas. 1999. "Functional Ability Assessment: Guidelines for the Workplace." *Journal of Occupational and Environmental Medicine* 41(3): 172–80.

Collegium Ramazzini. 1999. "Call for an International Ban on Asbestos" (editorial). *Journal of Occupational and Environmental Medicine* 41(10): 830–32.

Conrad, Peter, and Joseph W. Schneider. 1992. *Deviance and Medicalization: From Badness to Sickness,* expanded ed. Philadelphia: Temple University Press.

Conrad, Peter, and Diana Chapman Walsh. 1992. "The New Corporate Health Ethic: Lifestyle and the Social Control of Work." *International Journal of Health Services* 22(1): 89–111.

Cook, Karen S., ed. 2001. *Trust in Society.* New York: Russell Sage Foundation.

Cook-Deegan, Robert. 1994. *The Gene Wars: Science, Politics, and the Human Genome.* New York: W. W. Norton.

Couch, Stephen Robert, and J. Stephen Kroll-Smith. 1991. *Communities at Risk: Collective Responses to Technological Hazards.* New York: Peter Lang.

Cowley, Geoffrey. 1996. "Flunk the Gene Test and Lose Your Insurance." *Newsweek* (December 23): 48–50.

Cozzens, Susan E., and Thomas F. Gieryn, eds. 1990. *Theories of Science in Society*. Bloomington: Indiana University Press.

Cronin, A. J. 1937. *The Citadel*. Boston: Little, Brown.

Cullen, Mark, and Kathleen Kreiss. 2000. "Indoor Air Quality and Associated Disorders." In *Occupational Health: Recognizing and Preventing Work-Related Disease and Injury*, 4th ed, edited by Barry S. Levy and David H. Wegman. Philadelphia: Lippincott Williams & Wilkins.

Cushman, John H., Jr. 1997. "U.S. Reshaping Cancer Strategy as Incidence in Children Rises." *New York Times*, September 29.

Cutter, Susan L. 1994. *Environmental Risks and Hazards*. Englewood Cliffs, N.J.: Prentice-Hall.

Daniels, Arlene K. 1969. "The Captive Professional: Bureaucratic Limitations in the Practice of Military Psychiatry." *Journal of Health and Social Behavior* 10(4): 255–65.

Davis, Dena S. 2001. *Genetic Dilemmas: Reproductive Technology, Parental Choices, and Children's Futures*. New York: Routledge.

Deitchman, Scott D. 2000. "Occupational Health Services." In *Occupational Health: Recognizing and Preventing Work-Related Disease and Injury*, 4th ed., edited by Barry S. Levy and David H. Wegman. Philadelphia: Lippincott Williams & Wilkins.

Dembe, Allard E. 1996. *Occupation and Disease: How Social Factors Affect the Conception of Work-Related Disorders*. New Haven, Conn.: Yale University Press.

Derber, Charles, William A. Schwartz, and Yale Magrass. 1990. *Power in the Highest Degree: Professionals and the Rise of a New Mandarin Order*. New York: Oxford University Press.

Devlin, Mary M. 1994. "Historical Overview: The Development of Lawyer Disciplinary Procedures in the United States." *Georgetown Journal of Legal Ethics* 7(4): 911–39.

Dietz, Thomas M., and Robert W. Rycroft. 1987. *The Risk Professionals*. New York: Russell Sage Foundation.

Dinman, Bertram D. 2000. "Education for the Practice of Occupational Medicine: Knowledge, Competence, and Professionalism." *Journal of Occupational and Environmental Medicine* 42(2): 115–20.

Domhoff, G. William. 1998. *Who Rules America?: Power and Politics in the Year 2000*. Mountain View, Calif.: Mayfield.

Donovan, Arthur L. 1988. "Health and Safety in Underground Coal Mining, 1900–1969: Professional Conduct in a Peripheral Industry." In *The Health and Safety of Workers: Case Studies in the Politics of Professional Responsibility*, edited by Ronald Bayer. New York: Oxford University Press.

Douglas, Mary. 1992. *Risk and Blame: Essays in Cultural Theory.* New York: Routledge.

Draper, Elaine. 1991. *Risky Business: Genetic Testing and Exclusionary Practices in the Hazardous Workplace.* New York: Cambridge University Press.

————. 1992. "Genetic Secrets: Social Issues of Medical Screening in a Genetic Age." *Hastings Center Report* 22(4): S15–18.

————. 1993a. "Fetal Exclusion Policies and Gendered Constructions of Suitable Work." *Social Problems* 40(1): 90–107.

————. 1993b. "Safety Claims and Corporate Organizational Control in Workplace Medical Screening." *Research in Social Problems and Public Policy* 5: 179–204.

————. 1999. "The Screening of America: The Social and Legal Framework of Employers' Use of Genetic Information." *Berkeley Journal of Employment and Labor Law* 20(2): 286–324.

Drury, David L., Vance Masci, Jerrold W. Jacobson, and Robert A. McNutt. 1999. "Urine Drug Screening: Can Counterfeit Urine Samples Pass Inspection?" *Journal of Occupational and Environmental Medicine* 41(8): 622–24.

Ducatman, Alan M. 1993. "Occupational Physicians and Environmental Medicine." *Journal of Occupational Medicine* 35(5): 251–59.

————. 1998. "Multiple Chemical Sensitivity." In *Environmental and Occupational Medicine,* 3d ed., edited by William N. Rom. Philadelphia: Lippincott-Raven.

Ducatman, Alan M., and Robert K. McLellan. 2000. "Epidemiologic Basis for an Occupational and Environmental Policy on Environmental Tobacco Smoke." *Journal of Occupational and Environmental Medicine* 42(12): 1137–41.

Dudley, Kathryn Marie. 1994. *The End of the Line: Lost Jobs, New Lives in Postindustrial America.* Chicago: University of Chicago Press.

Dunlap, Riley E., Michael E. Kraft, and Eugene Rosa, eds. 1993. *Public Reactions to Nuclear Waste: Citizens' Views of Repository Siting.* Durham, N.C.: Duke University Press.

Dunlap, Riley E., and Angela G. Mertig. 1992. "The Evolution of the U.S. Environmental Movement from 1970 to 1990: An Overview." In *American Environmentalism: The U.S. Environmental Movement, 1970–1990,* edited by Riley E. Dunlap and Angela G. Mertig. Philadelphia: Taylor and Francis.

Durbin, Nancy, and Tom Grant. 1996. *Fitness for Duty in the Nuclear Industry: Update of the Technical Issues 1996.* Seattle, Wash.: Battelle Human Affairs Research Centers.

Du Rivage, Virginia L., ed. 1992. *New Policies for the Part-Time and Contingent Work Force.* Armonk, N.Y.: M. E. Sharpe.

Duster, Troy. 1990. *Back Door to Eugenics.* New York: Routledge, Chapman, and Hall.

Dwyer, Tom. 1991. *Life and Death at Work: Industrial Accidents as a Case of Socially Produced Error.* New York: Plenum Press.

Edelstein, Michael R. 1988. *Contaminated Communities: The Social and Psychological Impacts of Residential Toxic Exposure.* Boulder, Colo.: Westview.

Emmons, Karen M., Laura A. Linnan, William G. Shadel, Bess Marcus, and David B. Abrams. 1999. "The Working Healthy Project: A Worksite Health-Promotion Trial Targeting Physical Activity, Diet, and Smoking." *Journal of Occupational and Environmental Medicine* 41(7): 545–55.

Engelhardt, Tristam H., and Arthur L. Caplan, eds. 1987. *Scientific Controversies: Case Studies in the Resolution and Closure of Disputes in Science and Technology.* New York: Cambridge University Press.

Epstein, Samuel S. 1979. *The Politics of Cancer.* New York: Anchor Books.

Epstein, Steven. 1996. *Impure Science: AIDS, Activism, and the Politics of Knowledge.* Berkeley: University of California Press.

Equal Employment Opportunity Commission. 1995. *Compliance Manual,* vol. 2, EEOC Order No. 915.0002. Washington: Bureau of National Affairs (March 14).

Erfurt, John C., Andrea Foote, and Max A. Heirich. 1991. "The Cost-Effectiveness of Work-Site Wellness Programs for Hypertension Control, Weight Loss, and Smoking Cessation." *Journal of Occupational Medicine* 33(9): 962–70.

Etzioni, Amitai. 1999. *The Limits of Privacy.* New York: Basic Books.

Ferrey, Steven. 1988. "Hard Time: Criminal Prosecution for Polluters." *Amicus Journal* 10(4): 11–14.

Field, Mark G. 1957. *Doctor and Patient in Soviet Russia.* Cambridge, Mass.: Harvard University Press.

———. 1966. "Structured Strain and the Soviet Physician." In *Medical Care: Readings in the Sociology of Medical Institutions,* edited by W. Richard Scott and Edmund H. Volkart. New York: Wiley.

Fischhoff, Baruch, Sarah Lichtenstein, Paul Slovic, Stephen L. Derby, and Ralph L. Keeney. 1981. *Acceptable Risk.* Cambridge: Cambridge University Press.

Flexner, Abraham. 1910. *Medical Education in the United States and Canada,* Bulletin No. 4. New York: Carnegie Foundation for the Advancement of Teaching.

Fox, Renée C. 1977. "The Medicalization and Demedicalization of American Society." *Daedalus* 106(1): 9–22.

Frazier, Linda M., Norbert J. Berberich, Royce Moser, Jr., John W. Cromer, Jr., Maurice A. Hitchcock, F. Marconi Monteiro, and Gary N. Greenberg. 1999. "Developing Occupational and Environmental Medicine Curricula for Primary Care Residents: Project EPOCH-Envi." *Journal of Occupational and Environmental Medicine* 41(8): 706–11.

Freidson, Eliot. 1970. *Professional Dominance: The Social Structure of Medical Care.* New York: Atherton Press.

———. 1973. *The Profession of Medicine: A Study of the Sociology of Applied Knowledge.* New York: Dodd, Mead.

———. 1984. "The Changing Nature of Professional Control." *Annual Review of Sociology* 10: 1–20.

———. 1986. *Professional Powers: A Study of the Institutionalization of Formal Knowledge.* Chicago: University of Chicago Press.

———. 1994. *Professionalism Reborn: Theory, Prophecy, and Policy.* Chicago: University of Chicago Press.

Freudenburg, William R. 1992. "Nothing Recedes Like Success?: Risk Analysis and the Organizational Amplification of Risks." *Risk* 3(1): 1–35.

———. 1993. "Risk and Recreancy: Weber, the Division of Labor, and the Rationality of Risk Perceptions." *Social Forces* 71(4): 900–32.

Freudenburg, William R., and Robert Gramling. 1994. *Oil in Troubled Waters: Perceptions, Politics, and the Battle over Offshore Drilling.* Albany: State University of New York Press.

Freudenburg, William R., and Susan K. Pastor. 1992. "Public Responses to Technological Risks: Toward a Sociological Perspective." *Sociological Quarterly* 33(3): 389–412.

Frierson, James G. 1992. "An Analysis of ADA Provisions on Denying Employment Because of a Risk of Future Injury." *Employee Relations Law Journal* 17(4): 603–22.

Frumkin, Howard. 1994. "Too Many Residencies?" *Journal of Occupational and Environmental Medicine* 36(6): 675–76.

Frumkin, Howard, and Michael Thun. 2000. "Carcinogens." In *Occupational Health: Recognizing and Preventing Work-Related Disease and Injury,* 4th ed., edited by Barry S. Levy and David H. Wegman. Philadelphia: Lippincott Williams & Wilkins.

Fuchs, Victor R. 1974. *Who Shall Live?: Health, Economics, and Social Change.* New York: Basic Books.

Fujimura, Joan. 1996. *Crafting Science: A Sociohistory of the Quest for the Genetics of Cancer.* Cambridge, Mass.: Harvard University Press.

Gabel, Jon, Larry Levitt, Jeremy Pickreign, Heidi Whitmore, Erin Holve,

Samantha Hawkins, and Nick Miller. 2000. "Job-Based Health Insurance in 2000: Premiums Rise Sharply While Coverage Grows." *Health Affairs* 19(5): 144–51.

Galanter, Marc. 1994. "The Transnational Traffic in Legal Remedies." In *Learning from Disaster: Risk Management After Bhopal,* edited by Sheila Jasanoff. Philadelphia: University of Pennsylvania Press.

Galbraith, John Kenneth. 1967. *The New Industrial State.* Boston: Houghton Mifflin.

Gallagher, William T. 1995. "Ideologies of Professionalism and the Politics of Self-Regulation in the California State Bar." *Pepperdine Law Review* 22(2): 485–628.

Galston, William A. 1996. "Won't You Be My Neighbor?" *The American Prospect* 26(May–June): 16–21, 94.

Gamson, William A., and Andre Modigliani. 1989. "Media Discourse and Public Opinion on Nuclear Power: A Constructionist Approach." *American Journal of Sociology* 95(1): 1–37.

Garrett, Laurie. 2000. *Betrayal of Trust: The Collapse of Global Public Health.* New York: Hyperion.

Garte, Seymour J. 1998. "Environmental Carcinogenesis." In *Environmental and Occupational Medicine,* 3d ed., edited by William N. Rom. Philadelphia: Lippincott-Raven.

Gatson, Sarah N. 1997. "Labor Policy and the Social Meaning of Parenthood." *Law and Social Inquiry* 22(spring): 277–310.

Geller, Lisa N., Joseph S. Alper, Paul R. Billings, Carol I. Barash, Jonathan Beckwith, and Marvin R. Natowicz. 1996. "Individual, Family, and Societal Dimensions of Genetic Discrimination: A Case Study Analysis." *Science and Engineering Ethics* 2(1): 71–88.

Gibson, Roy L. 1988. "Occupational Medicine in the Eighties: Decade of Change." *Occupational Medicine: State of the Art Reviews* 3(3): 391–408.

Gilbert, G. Nigel, and Michael Mulkay. 1984. *Opening Pandora's Box: A Sociological Analysis of Scientists' Discourse.* New York: Cambridge University Press.

Gilliam, John. 1994. *Surveillance, Privacy, and the Law: Employee Drug Testing and the Politics of Social Control.* Ann Arbor: University of Michigan Press.

Glaser, Barney G. 1964. *Organizational Scientists: Their Professional Careers.* Indianapolis: Bobbs-Merrill.

Glazer, Myron Peretz, and Penina Migdal Glazer. 1989. *The Whistle Blowers: Exposing Corruption in Government and Industry.* New York: Basic Books.

Goetzel, Ron Z., Ronald J. Ozminkowski, Laurie Meneades, Maureen

Stewart, and David C. Schutt. 2000. "Pharmaceuticals—Cost or Investment?" *Journal of Occupational and Environmental Medicine* 42(4): 338–51.

Goffman, Erving. 1963. *Stigma: Notes on the Management of Spoiled Identity*. Englewood Cliffs, N.J.: Prentice-Hall.

Gordon, Robert W., and William H. Simon. 1992. "The Redemption of Professionalism?" In *Lawyers' Ideals/Lawyers' Practices: Transformations in the American Legal System*, edited by Robert L. Nelson, David M. Trubek, and Rayman L. Solomon. Ithaca, N.Y.: Cornell University Press.

Gostin, Lawrence O. 1995. "Genetic Privacy." *Journal of Law, Medicine, and Ethics* 23(4): 320–30.

Gould, Kenneth A., Allen Schnaiberg, and Adam S. Weinberg. 1996. *Local Environmental Struggles: Citizen Activism in the Treadmill of Production*. New York: Cambridge University Press.

Gould, Stephen Jay. 1981. *The Mismeasure of Man*. New York: W. W. Norton.

Granfield, Robert, and Thomas Koenig. 1992. "The Fate of Elite Idealism: Accommodation and Ideological Work at Harvard Law School." *Social Problems* 39(4): 315–31.

Greenhouse, Linda. 1998. "Ruling on Bias Law: Infected People Can Be Covered Even with No Symptoms Present." *New York Times*, June 26.

Greider, William. 1997. *One World, Ready or Not: The Manic Logic of Capitalism*. New York: Simon & Schuster.

Gusterson, Hugh. 1996. *Nuclear Rites: A Weapons Laboratory at the End of the Cold War*. Berkeley: University of California Press.

Haar, Jonathan. 1995. *A Civil Action*. New York: Random House.

Hadler, Nortin M. 2000. "Comments on 'Ergonomics Program Standard' Proposed by the Occupational Safety and Health Administration." *Journal of Occupational and Environmental Medicine* 42(10): 951–65.

Hafferty, Frederic W., and John B. McKinlay. 1993. *The Changing Medical Profession: An International Perspective*. New York: Oxford University Press.

Halpern, Sydney A. 1992. "Dynamics of Professional Control: Internal Coalitions and Cross-Professional Boundaries." *American Journal of Sociology* 97(4): 994–1021.

Hamilton, Alice. 1943. *Exploring the Dangerous Trades*. Boston: Little, Brown.

Hanson, F. Allan. 1993. *Testing Testing: Social Consequences of the Examined Life*. Berkeley: University of California Press.

Harris, Jeffrey S., Lee S. Glass, Charlene Ossler, and Peter Low. 2000.

"Evidence-Based Design: The ACOEM Practice Guidelines Dissemination Project." *Journal of Occupational and Environmental Medicine* 42(4): 352–61.

Hawkins, Dana. 1997. "A Bloody Mess at One Federal Lab." *U.S. News & World Report,* June 23.

Healy, Bernadine. 1992. "Testimony on the Possible Uses and Misuses of Genetic Information." *Human Gene Therapy* 3(1): 51–56.

Heckscher, Charles. 1995. *White-Collar Blues: Management Loyalties in an Age of Corporate Restructuring.* New York: Basic Books.

Heinz, John P., and Edward O. Laumann. 1994. *Chicago Lawyers: The Social Structure of the Bar,* rev. ed. Evanston, Ill.: Northwestern University Press.

Heinz, John P., Robert L. Nelson, Edward O. Laumann, and Ethan Michelson. 1998. "The Changing Character of Lawyers' Work: Chicago in 1975 and 1995." *Law and Society Review* 32(4): 751–76.

Holmes-Farley, S. Rebecca. 1997. "CRG Files Amicus Brief in Workplace Privacy and Discrimination Case." *GeneWatch* 10(4–5): 1, 4.

Holtzman, Neil A. 1995. "Panel Comment: Attempt to Pass the Genetic Privacy Act in Maryland." *Journal of Law, Medicine, and Ethics* 23(4): 367–70.

Holtzman, Neil A., and Mark A. Rothstein. 1992. "Eugenics and Genetic Discrimination: Invited Editorial." *American Journal of Human Genetics* 50(3): 457–59.

Howard, John. 1998. "OSHA and the Regulatory Agencies." In *Environmental and Occupational Medicine,* 3d ed., edited by William N. Rom. Philadelphia: Lippincott-Raven.

Howe, Edmund G. 1986. "Ethical Issues Regarding Mixed Agency of Military Physicians." *Social Science and Medicine* 23(8): 803–15.

Huber, Peter W. 1990. *Liability: The Legal Revolution and Its Consequences.* New York: Basic Books.

Hudson, Kathy L., Karen H. Rothenberg, Lori B. Andrews, Mary Jo Ellis Kahn, and Francis S. Collins. 1995. "Genetic Discrimination and Health Insurance: An Urgent Need for Reform." *Science* 270(5235): 391–93.

Hughes, Everett C. 1958. *Men and Their Work.* Glencoe, Ill.: Free Press.

———. 1962. "Good People and Dirty Work." *Social Problems* 10(1): 3–11.

Ibsen, Henrik. 1997 [1882]. *An Enemy of the People.* London: Faber and Faber.

Illich, Ivan, John McKnight, Irving K. Zola, Jonathan Caplan, and Harley Shaiken. 1987. *Disabling Professions.* London: Marion Boyars.

Institute of Medicine, National Academy of Sciences. 1988. *Role of the*

Primary Care Physician in Occupational and Environmental Medicine. Washington, D.C.: National Academy Press.

———. 1991. *Addressing the Physician Shortage in Occupational and Environmental Medicine.* Washington, D.C.: National Academy Press.

International Agency for Research on Cancer. 1993. *IARC Monographs on the Evaluation of Carcinogenic Risks to Humans,* vol. 58, *Beryllium, Cadmium, Mercury, and Exposures in the Glass Manufacturing Industry.* Lyon, France: International Agency for Research on Cancer.

Jackall, Robert. 1988. *Moral Mazes: The World of Corporate Managers.* New York: Oxford University Press.

Jacobs, Deborah L. 1995. "Can a Visit to the Company Doc Help a Cold but Hurt a Career?: In Work-Site Care, Issues of Loyalty and Privacy." *New York Times,* May 21.

Jacoby, Sanford M., ed. 1995. *The Workers of Nations: Industrial Relations in a Global Economy.* New York: Oxford University Press.

Jasanoff, Sheila. 1995. *Science at the Bar: Law, Science, and Technology in America.* Cambridge, Mass.: Harvard University Press.

Jeffords, James M., and Tom Daschle. 2001. "Political Issues in the Genome Era." *Science* 291(5507): 1249–51.

Judkins, Bennett M. 1986. *We Offer Ourselves as Evidence.* New York: Greenwood Press.

Kagan, Robert A., and Robert Eli Rosen. 1985. "On the Social Significance of Large Law Firm Practice." *Stanford Law Review* 37(January): 399–443.

Kahn, Jeffrey P., Anna C. Mastroianni, and Jeremy Sugarman. 1998. *Beyond Consent: Seeking Justice in Research.* New York: Oxford University Press.

Kamieniecki, Sheldon, and Janie Steckenrider. 1997. "Two Faces of Equity in Superfund Implementation." In *Flashpoints in Environmental Policymaking: Controversies in Achieving Sustainability,* edited by Sheldon Kamieniecki, George A. Gonzalez, and Robert O. Vos. Albany: State University of New York Press.

Kaplan, John, Robert Weisberg, and Guyora Binder. 1996. *Criminal Law,* 3d ed. Boston: Little, Brown.

Karasek, Robert, and Tores Theorell. 1990. *Healthy Work: Stress, Productivity, and the Reconstruction of Working Life.* New York: Basic Books.

Kass, Nancy E. 1997. "The Implications of Genetic Testing for Health and Life Insurance." In *Genetic Secrets: Protecting Privacy and Confidentiality in the Genetic Era,* edited by Mark A. Rothstein. New Haven, Conn.: Yale University Press.

Katz, Pearl. 1999. *The Scalpel's Edge: The Culture of Surgeons.* Boston: Allyn and Bacon.

Kevles, Daniel J. 1985. *In the Name of Eugenics: Genetics and the Uses of Human Heredity.* New York: Knopf.

Kevles, Daniel J., and Leroy Hood, eds. 1992. *The Code of Codes.* Cambridge, Mass.: Harvard University Press.

Kilborn, Peter T. 1990. "Who Decides Who Works at Jobs Imperiling Fetuses?" *New York Times,* September 2.

———. 1991. "Employers Left with Many Decisions." *New York Times,* March 21.

Kirp, David L. 1992. "Fetal Hazards, Gender Justice, and the Justices: The Limits of Equality." *William and Mary Law Review* 34(1): 101–38.

Knorr-Cetina, Karin D., and Michael Mulkay, eds. 1983. *Science Observed: Perspectives on the Social Study of Science.* Beverly Hills, Calif.: Sage Publications.

Korn, David. 2000. "Conflicts of Interest in Biomedical Research." *Journal of the American Medical Association* 284(17): 2234–37.

Kornhauser, William. 1962. *Scientists in Industry: Conflict and Accommodation.* Berkeley: University of California Press.

Krajcinovic, Ivana. 1997. *From Company Doctors to Managed Care: The United Mine Workers' Noble Experiment.* Ithaca, N.Y.: ILR Press.

Kraut, Alan. 1994. *Silent Travelers.* New York: Basic Books.

Kreiss, Kathleen. 1994. "Beryllium." In *Textbook of Clinical Occupational and Environmental Medicine,* edited by Linda Rosenstock and Mark R. Cullen. Philadelphia: W. B. Saunders.

Kroll-Smith, Steven, and Stephen R. Couch. 1990. *The Real Disaster Is Above Ground.* Lexington: University of Kentucky Press.

Kuhn, Thomas. 1964. *The Structure of Scientific Revolutions.* Chicago: University of Chicago Press.

Kunda, Gideon. 1992. *Engineering Culture: Control and Commitment in a High-Tech Corporation.* Philadelphia: Temple University Press.

Kurzman, Dan. 1987. *A Killing Wind: Inside Union Carbide and the Bhopal Catastrophe.* New York: McGraw-Hill.

LaDou, Joseph. 1998. "International Occupational and Environmental Health." In *Environmental and Occupational Medicine,* 3d ed., edited by William N. Rom. Philadelphia: Lippincott-Raven.

———. 1999. "The Role of Occupational Medicine in the New Industrial Era." *European Journal of Oncology* 4(2): 101–10.

Landrigan, Philip. 1994. "Lead." In *Textbook of Clinical Occupational and Environmental Medicine,* edited by Linda Rosenstock and Mark R. Cullen. Philadelphia: W. B. Saunders.

Larson, Arthur. 1999. *Workmen's Compensation Law,* vol. 1A. New York: Matthew Bender.

Larson, Magali Sarfatti. 1977. *The Rise of Professionalism: A Sociological Analysis*. Berkeley: University of California Press.

———. 1980. "Proletarianization and Educated Labor." *Theory and Society* 9(January): 131–75.

Lasch, Christopher. 1979. *The Culture of Narcissism: American Life in an Age of Diminishing Expectations*. New York: W. W. Norton.

———. 1994. "The Revolt of the Elites: Have They Canceled Their Allegiance to America?" *Harper's* (November): 39–49.

Latour, Bruno, and Steve Woolgar. 1979. *Laboratory Life: The Social Construction of Scientific Facts*. Beverly Hills, Calif.: Sage Publications.

Lemasters, Grace Kawas. 1998. "Occupational Exposures and Effects on Male and Female Reproduction." In *Environmental and Occupational Medicine*, 3d ed., edited by William N. Rom. Philadelphia: Lippincott-Raven.

Lester, Gillian. 1998. "Careers and Contingency." *Stanford Law Review* 51(1): 73–145.

Levine, Adeline Gordon. 1982. *Love Canal: Science, Politics, and People*. Lexington, Mass.: Lexington Books.

Levy, Barry S., and David H. Wegman, eds. 2000. *Occupational Health: Recognizing and Preventing Work-Related Disease and Injury*, 4th ed. Philadelphia: Lippincott Williams & Wilkins.

Lieberwitz, Risa L. 1994. "Constitutional and Statutory Treatment of Drug Testing in the United States." In *Drug Testing in the Workplace*, edited by Scott Macdonald and Paul Roman. New York: Plenum Press.

Lifton, Robert Jay. 1986. *The Nazi Doctors: Medical Killing and the Psychology of Genocide*. New York: Basic Books.

Lin, Michael M. J. 1996. "Conferring a Federal Property Right in Genetic Material: Stepping into the Future with the Genetic Privacy Act." *American Journal of Law and Medicine* 22(1): 109–34.

Lo, Bernard, Leslie E. Wolf, and Abiona Berkeley. 2000. "Conflict-of-Interest Policies for Investigators in Clinical Trials." *New England Journal of Medicine* 343(22): 1616–20.

Lodwick, Dora G. 1993. "Rocky Flats and the Evolution of Mistrust." *Research in Social Problems and Public Policy* 5: 149–70.

Lofland, John, and Lyn H. Lofland. 1995. *Analyzing Social Settings*, 3d ed. Belmont, Calif.: Wadsworth.

Lynn, Frances M. 1986. "The Interplay of Science and Values in Assessing and Regulating Environmental Risks." *Science, Technology, and Human Values* 11(2): 40–50.

Lyon, David, and Elia Zureik, eds. 1996. *Computers, Surveillance, and Privacy*. Minneapolis: University of Minnesota.

Macdonald, Scott, and Paul Roman, eds. 1994. *Drug Testing in the Workplace*. New York: Plenum Press.

Macdonald, Scott, and Samantha Wells. 1994. "The Impact and Effectiveness of Drug Testing Programs in the Workplace." In *Drug Testing in the Workplace,* edited by Scott Macdonald and Paul Roman. New York: Plenum Press.

Madrick, Jeffrey. 1995. *The End of Affluence: The Causes and Consequences of America's Economic Dilemma.* New York: Random House.

Maier, Lisa A., and Lee S. Newman. 1998. "Beryllium Disease." In *Environmental and Occupational Medicine,* 3d ed., edited by William N. Rom. Philadelphia: Lippincott-Raven.

Mannheim, Karl. 1952. *Essays on the Sociology of Knowledge.* London: Routledge and Kegan Paul.

Mansfield, Nancy R., Elizabeth T. Baer, and Leonard J. Hope. 1998. "Insurance Caps on AIDS-Related Health-Care Costs: Will the ADA Fill the Gap Created by ERISA?" *Georgia State University Law Review* 14(3): 601–32.

Marcson, Simon. 1960. *The Scientist in American Industry.* New York: Harper.

Marks, Jonathan. 1995. *Human Biodiversity.* New York: Aldine de Gruyter.

Marmot, M. G., H. Bosma, H. Hemingway, E. Brunner, and S. Stansfeld. 1997. "Contribution of Job Control and Other Risk Factors to Social Variations in Coronary Heart Disease Incidence." *Lancet* 350(9073): 235–39.

Marshall, Karen. 1993. "The Impact of Advances in Genetics on Workplace Policy." In *Advances in Genetic Information: A Guide for State Policy Makers,* edited by R. Steven Brown and Karen Marshall. Lexington, Ky.: Council of State Governments.

Marshman, Joan A. 1994. "Evaluation Approaches for Cost-Effectiveness and Effectiveness of Drug Testing Programs." In *Drug Testing in the Workplace,* edited by Scott Macdonald and Paul Roman. New York: Plenum Press.

Martin, Jack K., Joan M. Kraft, and Paul M. Roman. 1994. "Extent and Impact of Alcohol and Drug Use Problems in the Workplace: A Review of the Empirical Evidence." In *Drug Testing in the Workplace,* edited by Scott Macdonald and Paul Roman. New York: Plenum Press.

Mattison, Donald, and Mark R. Cullen. 1994. "Disorders of Reproduction and Development." In *Textbook of Clinical Occupational and Environmental Medicine,* edited by Linda Rosenstock and Mark R. Cullen. Philadelphia: W. B. Saunders.

McCaffrey, David P. 1982. *OSHA and the Politics of Health Regulation.* New York: Plenum Press.

McConnell, Rob. 1994. "Pesticides and Related Compounds." In *Textbook of Clinical Occupational and Environmental Medicine,* edited by Linda Rosenstock and Mark R. Cullen. Philadelphia: W. B. Saunders.

McCunney, Robert J. 2001. "Health and Productivity: A Role for Occupational Health Professionals." *Journal of Occupational and Environmental Medicine* 43(1): 30–35.

McEwen, Jean E. 1997. "DNA Databanks." In *Genetic Secrets: Protecting Privacy and Confidentiality in the Genetic Era,* edited by Mark A. Rothstein. New Haven, Conn.: Yale University Press.

McEwen, Jean E., and Philip R. Reilly. 1992. "State Legislative Efforts to Regulate Use and Potential Misuse of Genetic Information." *American Journal of Human Genetics* 51(3): 637–47.

Mechanic, David. 1976 *The Growth of Bureaucratic Medicine: An Inquiry Into the Dynamics of Patient Behavior and the Organization of Medical Care.* New York: Wiley-Interscience.

———. 2000. "Managed Care and the Imperative for a New Professional Ethic." *Health Affairs* 19(5): 100–11.

Mechanic, David, and Mark Schlesinger. 1996. "The Impact of Managed Care on Patients' Trust in Medical Care and Their Physicians." *Journal of the American Medical Association* 275(21): 1693–97.

Medical Information Bureau. 1998. *A Consumer's Guide to the Medical Information Bureau.* Westwood, Mass.: Medical Information Bureau.

Mehlman, Maxwell J., and Jeffrey R. Botkin. 1998. *Access to the Genome: The Challenge to Equality.* Washington, D.C.: Georgetown University Press.

Mehlman, Maxwell J., Eric D. Kodish, Peter Whitehouse, Arthur B. Zinn, Sharmon Sollitto, Joshua Berger, Emmeline J. Chiao, Melissa S. Dosick, and Suzanne B. Cassidy. 1996. "The Need for Anonymous Genetic Counseling and Testing." *American Journal of Human Genetics* 58(2): 393–97.

Meier, Barry. 2000. "Bringing Lawsuits to Do What Congress Won't." *New York Times,* March 26.

Meiksins, Peter F. 1982. "Science in the Labor Process: Engineers as Workers." In *Professionals as Workers: Mental Labor in Advanced Capitalism,* edited by Charles Derber. Boston: G. K. Hall.

Meiksins, Peter, and Chris Smith, eds. 1996. *Engineered Labor: Technical Workers in Comparative Perspective.* New York: Verso.

Melius, James J. 1998. "The Bhopal Disaster." In *Environmental and Occupational Medicine,* 3d ed., edited by William N. Rom. Philadelphia: Lippincott-Raven.

Merton, Robert K. 1940. "Bureaucratic Structure and Personality." *Social Forces* 18(4): 560–68.

————. 1973. *The Sociology of Science: Theoretical and Empirical Investigations*. Chicago: University of Chicago Press.

Miethe, Terance D., and Joyce Rothschild. 1994. "Whistleblowing and the Control of Organizational Misconduct." *Sociological Inquiry* 64(3): 322–47.

Miller, George A. 1967. "Professionals in Bureaucracy: Alienation Among Industrial Scientists and Engineers." *American Sociological Review* 32(October): 755–68.

Millman, Marcia. 1977. *The Unkindest Cut*. New York: Morrow.

————. 1981. "Medical Mortality Review: A Cordial Affair." In *The Sociology of Health and Illness: Critical Perspectives,* edited by Peter Conrad and Rochelle Kern. New York: St. Martin's Press.

Mills, C. Wright. 1956. *White Collar: The American Middle Classes*. New York: Oxford University Press.

Mintz, Beth, and Donald Palmer. 2000. "Business and Health Care Policy Reform in the 1980s: The Fifty States." *Social Problems* 47(3): 327–59.

Mishler, Elliot G. 1991. *Research Interviewing: Context and Narrative*. Cambridge, Mass.: Harvard University Press.

Molotch, Harvey. 1970. "Oil in Santa Barbara and Power in America." *Sociological Inquiry* 40(1): 131–44.

Murray, Thomas H., Mark A. Rothstein, and Robert F. Murray, Jr., eds. 1996. *The Human Genome Project and the Future of Health Care*. Bloomington: Indiana University Press.

Murray, Yxta Maya. 1993. "Note: Employer Liability After Johnson Controls: A No-Fault Solution." *Stanford Law Review* 45(2): 453–83.

National Academy of Sciences. 1997. *For the Record: Protecting Electronic Health Information*. Washington, D.C.: National Academy Press.

National Foundation for Unemployment Compensation and Workers' Compensation. 1995. "Fiscal Data for State Workers' Compensation System, 1993–1994." *Research Bulletin* (Washington) (June 16).

National Institutes of Health/Department of Energy Working Group on Ethical, Legal, and Social Implications of Human Genome Research. 1993. *Genetic Information and Health Insurance*. NIH Publication No. 93–3686. Bethesda, Md.: National Institutes of Health.

Nelkin, Dorothy, ed. 1992. *Controversy: Politics of Technical Decisions,* 3d ed. Newbury Park, Calif.: Sage Publications.

————. 1995. *Selling Science: How the Press Covers Science and Technology,* rev. ed. New York: W. H. Freeman.

Nelkin, Dorothy, and Michael S. Brown. 1984. *Workers at Risk: Voices from the Workplace*. Chicago: University of Chicago Press.

Nelkin, Dorothy, and M. Susan Lindee. 1995. *The DNA Mystique: The Gene as a Cultural Icon*. New York: W. H. Freeman.

Nelkin, Dorothy, and Laurence Tancredi. 1989. *Dangerous Diagnostics: The Social Power of Biological Information*. New York: Basic Books.

Nelson, Robert L., and Laura Beth Nielsen. 2000. "Cops, Counsel, and Entrepreneurs: Constructing the Role of Inside Counsel in Large Corporations." *Law and Society Review* 34(2): 457–93.

Nelson, Robert L., and David M. Trubek. 1992. "Arenas of Professionalism: The Professional Ideologies of Lawyers in Context." In *Lawyers' Ideals/Lawyers' Practices: Transformations in the American Legal System*, edited by Robert L. Nelson, David M. Trubek, and Rayman L. Solomon. Ithaca, N.Y.: Cornell University Press.

Newman, Katharine S. 1988. *Falling from Grace: The Experience of Downward Mobility in the American Middle Class*. New York: Free Press.

Noble, David F. 1977. *America by Design: Science, Technology, and the Rise of Corporate Capitalism*. New York: Knopf.

Normand, Jacques, Richard O. Lempert, and Charles P. O'Brien, eds. 1994. *Under the Influence?: Drugs and the American Work Force*. Washington, D.C.: National Academy Press.

Oil, Chemical, and Atomic Workers International Union (OCAW). 1991. *Controlled Substances Policy*. Denver, Col.: OCAW.

Oppenheimer, Martin. 1970. "White Collar Revisited: The Making of a New Working Class." *Social Policy* 1(2): 27–32.

———. 1973. "The Proletarianization of the Professional." *Sociological Review Monographs* 20: 213–27.

Orentlicher, David. 1997. "Genetic Privacy in the Patient-Physician Relationship." In *Genetic Secrets: Protecting Privacy and Confidentiality in the Genetic Era*, edited by Mark A. Rothstein. New Haven, Conn.: Yale University Press.

Osterman, Paul, ed. 1996. *Broken Ladders: Managerial Careers in the New Economy*. New York: Oxford University Press.

Ostrer, Harry, William Allen, Lee A. Crandall, Ray E. Moseley, Marvin A. Dewar, David Nye, and S. Van McCrary. 1993. "Insurance and Genetic Testing: Where Are We Now?" *American Journal of Human Genetics* 52(3): 565–77.

Otten, Alan L. 1985. "Women's Rights Versus Fetal Rights Looms as Thorny and Divisive Issue." *Wall Street Journal*, April 12.

———. 1986. "Probing the Cell: Genetic Examination of Workers Is an Issue of Growing Urgency." *Wall Street Journal*, February 24.

Parliman, Gregory C., and Erica L. Edwards. 1992. "Employee Assistance Programs: An Employer's Guide to Emerging Liability Issues." *Employee Relations Law Journal* 17(4): 593–602.

Parsons, Talcott. 1939. "The Professions and Social Structure." *Social Forces* 17(4): 457–67.

Paul, Maureen, and Linda Frazier. 2000. "Reproductive Hazards." In *Occupational Health: Recognizing and Preventing Work-Related Disease and Injury,* 4th ed., edited by Barry S. Levy and David H. Wegman. Philadelphia: Lippincott Williams & Wilkins.

Pear, Robert. 1997a. "Health Insurers Skirting New Law, Officials Report." *New York Times,* October 5.

———. 1997b. "States Pass Laws to Regulate Use of Genetic Testing." *New York Times,* October 18.

———. 2000. "Clinton Bans Use of Genetic Makeup in Federal Employment." *New York Times,* February 9.

Pedersen, David H., Herbert L. Venable, and William Karl Sieber, Jr. 1990. "An Examination of Occupational Medicine Practices." *Journal of Occupational Medicine* 32(10): 1037–41.

Pelletier, Kenneth R. 1996. "A Review and Analysis of the Health and Cost-Effective Outcome Studies of Comprehensive Health Promotion and Disease Prevention Programs at the Work Site: 1993–1995 Update." *American Journal of Health Promotion* 10(5): 380–88.

Pelletier, Kenneth R., Annette Rodenburg, Amy Vinther, Yosuke Chikamoto, Abby C. King, and John W. Farquhar. 1999. "Managing Job Strain: A Randomized, Controlled Trial of an Intervention Conducted by Mail and Telephone." *Journal of Occupational and Environmental Medicine* 41(4): 216–23.

Pennisi, Elizabeth. 2001. "The Human Genome." *Science* 291(5507): 1177–80.

Perrow, Charles. 1984. *Normal Accidents: Living with High-Risk Technologies.* New York: Basic Books.

Peterson, Michael, and Tim Dunnagan. 1998. "Analysis of a Work-Site Health Promotion Program's Impact on Job Satisfaction." *Journal of Occupational and Environmental Medicine* 40(11): 973–79.

Plater, Zygmunt J. B., Robert H. Abrams, William Goldfarb, and Robert L. Graham. 1998. *Environmental Law and Policy: Nature, Law, and Society,* 2d ed. St. Paul, Minn.: West.

Plovika, Anne E. 1996. "A Profile of Contingent Workers." *Monthly Labor Review* 119(10): 10–20.

Portes, Alejandro. 1996. "Global Villagers: The Rise of Transnational Communities." *The American Prospect* 25(March–April): 74–77.

Post, Jerrold M., and Robert S. Robins. 1993. *When Illness Strikes the Leader.* New Haven, Conn.: Yale University Press.

Pransky, Glenn. 1990. "Occupational Medicine Specialists in the United States: A Survey." *Journal of Occupational Medicine* 32(10): 985–88.

Preston, Jennifer. 1996. "Bill in New Jersey Would Limit Use of Genetic Tests by Insurers." *New York Times,* June 18.

Punnett, Laura. 2000. "Commentary on the Scientific Basis of the Proposed Occupational Safety and Health Administration Ergonomics Program Standard." *Journal of Occupational and Environmental Medicine* 42(10): 970–81.

Ramphal, Lilly. 1999. "The Impact of Occupational Medicine Specialty Practice on the Injury Rate and Lost-Worktime Incidence in Industry of a Community" (letter to the editor). *Journal of Occupational and Environmental Medicine* 41(1): 1–2.

Randall, Donna M., and James F. Short. 1983. "Women in Toxic Work Environments: A Case Study of Social Problem Development." *Social Problems* 30(4): 411–24.

Reich, Robert. 1991. *The Work of Nations.* New York: Knopf.

Reilly, Philip. 1992a. "ASHG Statement on Genetics and Privacy: Testimony to United States Congress." *American Journal of Human Genetics* 50(3): 640–42.

———. 1992b. "DNA Banking." *American Journal of Human Genetics* 51(6): 1169–70.

Reinhardt, Charles. 1978. "Chemical Hypersusceptibility." *Journal of Occupational Medicine* 20(5): 319–22.

Reiser, Stanley Joel. 1978. "The Emergence of the Concept of Screening for Disease." *Milbank Memorial Fund Quarterly/Health and Society* 56(4): 403–25.

Reissman, Dori B., Peter Orris, Roy Lacey, and David E. Hartman. 1999. "Downsizing, Role Demands, and Job Stress." *Journal of Occupational and Environmental Medicine* 41(4): 289–93.

Reskin, Barbara F., and Patricia A. Roos. 1990. *Job Queues, Gender Queues: Explaining Women's Inroads into Male Occupations.* Philadelphia: Temple University Press.

Richter, Elihu, Colin L. Soskolne, and Joseph LaDou. 2001. "Efforts to Stop Repression Bias by Protecting Whistleblowers." *International Journal of Occupational and Environmental Health* 7(1): 68–71.

Rischitelli, D. Gary. 1995. "The Confidentiality of Medical Information in the Workplace." *Journal of Occupational and Environmental Medicine* 37(5): 583–93.

Ritti, Richard R. 1971. *The Engineer in the Industrial Corporation.* New York: Columbia University Press.

Roberts, J. Timmons. 1993. "Psychosocial Effects of Workplace Hazardous Exposures: Theoretical Synthesis and Preliminary Findings." *Social Problems* 40(1): 74–89.

Robinson, James C. 1999. *The Corporate Practice of Medicine: Competition and Innovation in Health Care.* Berkeley: University of California Press.

Rodrick, Dani. 1997. "Sense and Nonsense in the Globalization Debate." *Foreign Policy* 107(summer): 19–36.

Rom, William N. 1998a. "Asbestos-Related Disease." In *Environmental and Occupational Medicine,* 3d ed., edited by William N. Rom. Philadelphia: Lippincott-Raven.

———. 1998b. "The Discipline of Environmental and Occupational Medicine." In *Environmental and Occupational Medicine,* 3d ed., edited by William N. Rom. Philadelphia: Lippincott-Raven.

Rosenblatt, Rand E., Sylvia A. Law, and Sara Rosenbaum. 1997. *Law and the American Health Care System.* Westbury, N.Y.: Foundation Press.

Rosenman, K. D., J. C. Gardiner, J. Wang, J. Biddle, A. Hogan, M. J. Reilly, K. Roberts, and E. Welch. 2000. "Why Most Workers with Occupational Repetitive Trauma Do Not File for Workers' Compensation." *Journal of Occupational and Environmental Medicine* 42(1): 25–39.

Rosenstock, Linda, Kathleen Rest, John Benson, Joseph Cannella, Jordan Cohen, Mark Cullen, Frank Davidoff, Philip J. Landrigan, Richard C. Reynolds, Linda Hawes Clever, Gary B. Ellis, and Bernard D. Goldstein. 1991. "Occupational and Environmental Medicine: Meeting the Growing Need for Clinical Services." *New England Journal of Medicine* 325(September 26): 924–27.

Rothenberg, Karen H. 1995. "Genetic Information and Health Insurance: State Legislative Approaches." *Journal of Law, Medicine, and Ethics* 23(4): 312–19.

Rothschild, Joyce, and Terance D. Miethe. 1999. "Whistleblower Disclosures and Management Retaliation: The Battle to Control Information About Organizational Corruption." *Work and Occupations* 1(1): 107–28.

Rothstein, Mark A. 1992. "Genetic Discrimination in Employment and the Americans with Disabilities Act." *Houston Law Review* 29(1): 23–84.

———. 1994. "The Americans with Disabilities Act, Workers' Compensation, and Related Issues of Occupational Medicine Practice." In *Textbook of Clinical Occupational and Environmental Medicine,* edited by Linda Rosenstock and Mark R. Cullen. Philadelphia: W. B. Saunders.

———, ed. 1997a. *Genetic Secrets: Protecting Privacy and Confidentiality in the Genetic Era.* New Haven, Conn.: Yale University Press.

———. 1997b. "A Proposed Revision of the ACOEM Code of Ethics." *Journal of Occupational and Environmental Medicine* 39(7): 616–22.

Rubin, Susan B., and Laurie Zoloth, eds. 2000. *Margin of Error: The Ethics of Mistakes in the Practice of Medicine.* Hagerstown, Md.: University Publishing Group.

Rudolph, Linda. 1996. "A Call for Quality." *Journal of Occupational and Environmental Medicine* 38(4): 343–44.

Ryan, William. 1971. *Blaming the Victim*. New York: Random House.

Saks, Michael. 1992. "The Behavior of the Tort Litigation System." *University of Pennsylvania Law Review* 140(4): 1147–1292.

Salter, Liora. 1988. *Mandated Science: Science and Scientists in the Making of Standards*. Boston: Klewer Academic Publishers.

Samuels, Sheldon W. 1999. "Genetic Testing in the Workplace: A Caste System for Workers?" *Working USA* (May–June): 83–92.

Samuels, Suzanne Uttaro. 1995. *Fetal Rights, Women's Rights: Gender Equality in the Workplace*. Madison: University of Wisconsin Press.

———. 1997. "The Lasting Legacy of *International Union, UAW v. Johnson Controls*." *Wisconsin Women's Law Journal* 12(1): 1–19.

Sassower, Raphael. 1993. *Knowledge Without Expertise: On the Status of Scientists*. Albany: State University of New York Press.

Schaeffer, Robert K. 1997. *Understanding Globalization: The Social Consequences of Political, Economic, and Environmental Change*. Lanham, Md.: Rowman and Littlefield.

Schafer, Sarah. 2001. "EEOC Sues to Halt Worker Gene Tests." *Washington Post*, February 10.

Schiller, Zachary, Walecia Konrad, and Stephanie Anderson. 1991. "If You Light up on Sunday, Don't Come in on Monday." *Business Week* (August 26): 68–72.

Schneyer, Theodore. 1992. "Professionalism as Politics: The Making of a Modern Legal Ethics Code." In *Lawyers' Ideals/Lawyers' Practices: Transformations in the American Legal System,* edited by Robert L. Nelson, David M. Trubek, and Rayman L. Solomon. Ithaca, N.Y.: Cornell University Press.

Schuck, Peter H. 1986. *Agent Orange on Trial: Mass Toxic Disasters in the Courts*. Cambridge, Mass.: Harvard University Press.

Schulte, Paul A., Geoffrey P. Lomax, Elizabeth M. Ward, and Michael J. Colligan. 1999. "Ethical Issues in the Use of Genetic Markers in Occupational Epidemiologic Research." *Journal of Occupational and Environmental Medicine* 41(8): 639–46.

Schwartz, Brian S., Glenn Pransky, and Delores Lashley. 1995. "Recruiting the Occupational and Environmental Medicine Physicians of the Future: Results of a Survey of Current Residents." *Journal of Occupational and Environmental Medicine* 37(6): 739–43.

Schwartz, Gary T. 1993. "Waste, Fraud, and Abuse in Workers' Compensation: The Recent California Experience." *Maryland Law Review* 52(4): 983–1015.

Scott, W. Richard. 1966. "Professionals in Bureaucracies: Areas of Conflict." In *Professionalization,* edited by Howard M. Vollmer and Donald L. Mills. Englewood Cliffs, N.J.: Prentice-Hall.

Scott, W. Richard, Martin Ruef, Peter J. Mendel, and Carol A. Caronna. 2000. *Institutional Change and Health-Care Organizations: From Professional Dominance to Managed Care.* Chicago: University of Chicago Press.

Seltzer, Curtis. 1988. "Moral Dimensions of Occupational Health: The Case of the 1969 Coal Mine Health and Safety Act." In *The Health and Safety of Workers: Case Studies in the Politics of Professional Responsibility,* edited by Ronald Bayer. New York: Oxford University Press.

Severo, Richard. 1980. "The Genetic Barrier: Job Benefit or Job Bias?" *New York Times,* February 3–6.

Shain, Martin. 1994. "Alternatives to Drug Testing: Employee Assistance and Health Promotion Programs." In *Drug Testing in the Workplace,* edited by Scott Macdonald and Paul Roman. New York: Plenum Press.

Sharpe, Virginia A., and Alan I. Faden. 1998. *Medical Harm: Historical, Conceptual, and Ethical Dimensions of Iatrogenic Illness.* Cambridge: Cambridge University Press.

Sheehan, Helen E., and Richard P. Wedeen, eds. 1993. *Toxic Circles: Environmental Hazards from the Workplace into the Community.* New Brunswick, N.J.: Rutgers University Press.

Sheridan, Peter J. 1983. "Reproductive Hazards: Probing the Ethical Issues." *Occupational Hazards* (May): 72–75.

Short, James F. 1994. "Trace Substances, Science, and Law: Perspectives from the Social Sciences." *Risk: Health, Safety, and Environment* 5(4): 319–35.

Short, James F., Jr., and Lee Clarke, eds. 1992. *Organizations, Uncertainties, and Risk.* Boulder, Colo.: Westview.

Shrader-Frechette, Kristin S. 1991. *Environmental Ethics,* 2d ed. Pacific Grove, Calif.: Boxwood Press.

———. 1995. "Evaluating the Expertise of Experts." *Risk: Health, Safety, and Environment* 6(2): 115–26.

Silverstein, Michael, and Franklin E. Mirer. 2000. "Labor Unions and Occupational Health." In *Occupational Health: Recognizing and Preventing Work-Related Disease and Injury,* 4th ed., edited by Barry S. Levy and David H. Wegman. Philadelphia: Lippincott Williams & Wilkins.

Simpson, Ida Harper, and Richard Simpson, eds. 1999. *Deviance in the Workplace.* Stamford, Conn.: JAI Press.

Slovic, Paul, James H. Flynn, and Mark Layman. 1991. "Perceived Risk, Trust, and the Politics of Nuclear Waste." *Science* 254(December 13): 1603–7.

Smigel, Erwin O. 1964. *The Wall Street Lawyer: Professional Organization Man?* New York: Free Press.

Smith, H. Jeff. 1994. *Managing Privacy: Information Technology and Corporate America*. Chapel Hill: University of North Carolina Press.

Snyder, Jack, and Julia Klees. 1996. "Law and the Workplace." In *Occupational Medicine: State of the Art Reviews*. Philadelphia: Hanley and Belfus.

Spangler, Eve. 1986. *Lawyers for Hire: Salaried Professionals at Work*. New Haven, Conn.: Yale University Press.

Sparks, Patricia J., William Daniell, Donald W. Black, Howard M. Kipen, Leonard C. Altman, Gregory E. Simon, and Abba I. Terr. 1994. "Multiple Chemical Sensitivity Syndrome: A Clinical Perspective." *Journal of Occupational Medicine* 36(7): 718–37.

Speece, Roy G., Jr., David S. Shimm, and Allen E. Buchanan, eds. 1996. *Conflicts of Interest in Clinical Practice and Research*. New York: Oxford University Press.

Spieler, Emily A. 1994. "Perpetuating Risk?: Workers' Compensation and the Persistence of Occupational Injuries." *Houston Law Review* 31(1): 119–264.

Stallings, Robert A. 1990. "Media Discourse and the Social Construction of Risk." *Social Problems* 37(1): 80–95.

———. 1995. *Promoting Risk: Constructing the Earthquake Threat*. New York: Aldine de Gruyter.

Stanley, Jay, and John D. Blair, eds. 1993. *Challenges in Military Health Care: Perspectives on Health Status and the Provision of Care*. New Brunswick, N.J.: Transaction.

Starr, Paul. 1982. *The Social Transformation of American Medicine: The Rise of a Sovereign Profession and the Making of a Vast Industry*. New York: Basic Books.

Steinfels, Peter. 1979. *The Neo-Conservatives*. New York: Simon & Schuster.

Stellman, Jeanne M., and Mary Sue Henefin. 1982. "No Fertile Women Need Apply: Employment Discrimination and Reproductive Hazards in the Workplace." In *Biological Woman—The Convenient Myth*, edited by Ruth Hubbard, Mary Sue Henefin, and Barbara Fried. Cambridge, Mass.: Schenkman.

Stern, Carole, and Cathleen M. Gillen Tierney. 1993. "Inheriting Workplace Risks: The Effect of Workers' Compensation 'Exclusive Remedy' Clauses on the Preconception Tort After *Johnson Controls*." *Tort and Insurance Law Journal* 28(4): 800–22.

Stone, Deborah A. 1986. "The Resistible Rise of Preventive Medicine." *Journal of Health Politics, Policy, and Law* 11(4): 671–97.

———. 1997. "The Implications of the Human Genome Project for Access to Health Insurance." In *The Human Genome Project and the*

Future of Health Care, edited by Thomas H. Murray, Mark A. Rothstein, and Robert F. Murray Jr. Bloomington: Indiana University Press.

Stover, Robert V. 1989. *Making It and Breaking It: The Fate of Public Interest Commitment During Law School.* Urbana: University of Illinois Press.

Strauss, Anselm L., and Juliet M. Corbin. 1998. *Basics of Qualitative Research: Techniques and Procedures for Developing Grounded Theory,* 2d ed. Thousand Oaks, Calif.: Sage Publications.

Stretesky, Paul, and Michael J. Hogan. 1998. "Environmental Justice: An Analysis of Superfund Sites in Florida." *Social Problems* 45(2): 268–87.

Suchman, Mark C. 1998. "Working Without a Net: The Sociology of Legal Ethics in Corporate Litigation." *Fordham Law Review* 67(2): 837–74.

Sullivan, William M. 1995. *Work and Integrity: The Crisis and Promise of Professionalism in America.* New York: HarperCollins.

Supreme Court of the United States. 1990. *International Union, United Automobile, Aerospace, and Agricultural Implement Workers of America, UAW v. Johnson Controls, Inc., Case No. 89–1215, Proceedings* (official transcript). Washington: U.S. Government Printing Office (October 10).

Swotinsky, Robert B., and Kenneth H. Chase. 1990. "The Medical Review Officer." *Journal of Occupational Medicine* 32(10): 1003–8.

Szasz, Andrew. 1986. "The Reversal of Federal Policy Toward Worker Safety and Health." *Science and Society* 50(1): 25–51.

Taub, Nadine. 1996. "At the Intersection of Reproductive Freedom and Gender Equality: Problems in Addressing Reproductive Hazards in the Workplace." *UCLA Women's Law Journal* 6(2): 443–56.

Tebo, Margaret Graham. 2000. "Guilty by Reason of Title." *American Bar Association Journal* (May): 44–48.

Tesh, Sylvia Noble. 1988. *Hidden Arguments: Political Ideology and Disease Prevention Policy.* New Brunswick, N.J.: Rutgers University Press.

Thomas, Robert J. 1994. *What Machines Can't Do: Politics and Technology in the Industrial Enterprise.* Berkeley: University of California Press.

Thompson, Jeffrey N., Carl A. Brodkin, Kelly Kyes, William Neighbor, and Bradley Evanoff. 2000. "Use of a Questionnaire to Improve Occupational and Environmental History Taking in Primary Care Physicians." *Journal of Occupational and Environmental Medicine* 42(12): 1188–94.

Thurow, Lester C. 1996. *The Future of Capitalism: How Today's Economic Forces Shape Tomorrow's World.* New York: Penguin Books.

Tilly, Chris. 1996. *Half a Job: Bad and Good Part-Time Jobs in a Changing Labor Market.* Philadelphia: Temple University Press.

United Steelworkers of America. 1991. *Substance Abuse Policy*. Pittsburgh: United Steelworkers of America.

U.S. Congress, Office of Technology Assessment. 1985. *Reproductive Health Hazards in the Workplace*. Washington: U.S. Government Printing Office.

———. 1990a. *Genetic Monitoring and Screening in the Workplace*. OTA-BA-455. Washington: U.S. Government Printing Office.

———. 1990b. *The Use of Integrity Tests for Pre-Employment Screening*. OTA-SET-442. Washington: U.S. Government Printing Office.

U.S. Department of Commerce, Bureau of the Census. 2001. *Statistical Abstract of the United States: 2001*, 121st ed. Washington: U.S. Government Printing Office.

U.S. Department of Labor, Bureau of Labor Statistics. 1997. "Occupational Injuries and Illnesses in the U.S. by Industry, 1995." *U.S. Department of Labor Bulletin*. Washington: U.S. Department of Labor (December).

Vainio, Harri, and Jerry M. Rice. 1997. "Beryllium Revisited" (editorial). *Journal of Occupational and Environmental Medicine* 39(3): 203–4.

Vaughan, Diane. 1996. *The Challenger Launch Decision: Risky Technology, Culture, and Deviance at NASA*. Chicago: University of Chicago Press.

Viscusi, W. Kip. 1983. *Risk by Choice: Regulating Health and Safety in the Workplace*. Cambridge, Mass.: Harvard University Press.

Viscusi, W. Kip, and Michael J. Moore. 1990. *Compensation Mechanisms for Job Risks*. Princeton, N.J.: Princeton University Press.

Vogel, Lise. 1993. *Mothers on the Job: Maternity Policy in the U.S. Workplace*. New Brunswick, N.J.: Rutgers University Press.

Vollmer, Howard M., and Donald L. Mills, eds. 1966. *Professionalization*. Englewood Cliffs, N.J.: Prentice-Hall.

Wahl, Ana-Maria, and Steven E. Gunkel. 1999. "Due Process, Resource Mobilization, and the Occupational Safety and Health Administration, 1971–1996: The Politics of Social Regulation in Historical Perspective." *Social Problems* 46(4): 591–616.

Walsh, Diana Chapman. 1987. *Corporate Physicians: Between Medicine and Management*. New Haven, Conn.: Yale University Press.

Walters, LeRoy, and Julie Gage Palmer. 1997. *The Ethics of Human Gene Therapy*. New York: Oxford University Press.

Walters, Vivienne. 1984. "Company Doctors: Standards of Care and Legitimacy: A Case Study from Canada." *Social Science and Medicine* 19(8): 811–21.

Watterson, Andrew. 1993. "Chemical Hazards and Public Confidence." *Lancet* 342(8864): 131–32.

Weinstein, Jack B. 1995. *Individual Justice in Mass Tort Litigation: The Effect of Class Actions, Consolidations, and Other Multiparty Devices.* Evanston, Ill.: Northwestern University Press.

Whalley, Peter. 1986. *The Social Production of Technical Work.* Albany: State University of New York.

White, Mary Terrell. 2000. "Genetic Susceptibility Research in Occupational Disease: Should Subjects Have Access to Interim Findings?" *Journal of Occupational and Environmental Medicine* 42(3): 246–50.

Whorton, M. Donald. 1998. "Health Effects of Dibromochloropropane." In *Environmental and Occupational Medicine,* 3d ed., edited by William N. Rom. Philadelphia: Lippincott-Raven.

Whyte, William H., Jr. 1957. *The Organization Man.* Garden City, N.Y.: Doubleday.

Wilfond, Benjamin S., Karen H. Rothenberg, Elizabeth J. Thomson, and Caryn Lerman, for the Cancer Genetic Studies Consortium, National Institutes of Health. 1997. "Cancer Genetic Susceptibility Testing: Ethical and Policy Implications for Future Research and Clinical Practice." *Journal of Law, Medicine, and Ethics* 25(4): 243–51.

Wilkins, David B. 1992. "Who Should Regulate Lawyers?" *Harvard Law Review* 105(4): 799–887.

Willborn, Steven L., Stewart J. Schwab, and John F. Burton, Jr. 1993. *Employment Law: Cases and Materials.* Charlottesville, Va.: Michie.

Wilson, William Julius. 1996. *When Work Disappears: The World of the New Urban Poor.* New York: Knopf.

Wolkinson, Benjamin W., and Richard N. Block. 1996. *Employment Law: The Workplace Rights of Employees and Employers.* Cambridge, Mass.: Blackwell.

Zola, Irving Kenneth. 1983. *Socio-Medical Inquiries: Recollections, Reflections, and Reconsiderations.* Philadelphia: Temple University Press.

Zuckerman, Stephen, Genevieve M. Kennedy, Lisa Dubay, Jennifer Haley, and John Holahan. 2001. "Shifting Health Insurance Coverage, 1997–1999." *Health Affairs* 20(1): 169–77.

Zussman, Robert. 1985. *Mechanics of the Middle Class: Work and Politics Among American Engineers.* Berkeley: University of California Press.

———. 1992. *Intensive Care: Medical Ethics and the Medical Profession.* Chicago: University of Chicago Press.

Index

—— About the Author ——

Elaine Draper is a professor of sociology at California State University, Los Angeles.